After *the* Diagnosis

After *the* Diagnosis

How Patients React and How to Help Them Cope

Gary McClain, PhD

with Michelle Buchman, MA, BSN, RN

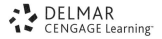

DELMAR
CENGAGE Learning™

Australia • Brazil • Japan • Korea • Mexico • Singapore • Spain • United Kingdom • United States

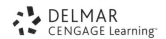
DELMAR
CENGAGE Learning™

After the Diagnosis: How Patients React and How to Help Them Cope

Gary McClain, PhD

Vice President, Career and Professional Editorial: Dave Garza

Director of Learning Solutions: Matt Kane

Acquisitions Editor: Matt Seeley

Managing Editor: Marah Bellegarde

Product Manager: Samantha Zullo

Vice President, Career and Professional Marketing: Jennifer Baker

Marketing Director: Wendy Mapstone

Senior Marketing Manager: Kristin McNary

Marketing Coordinator: Erica Ropitsky

Production Director: Carolyn Miller

Senior Content Project Manager: Ken McGrath

Senior Art Director: Jack Pendleton

For product information and technology assistance, contact us at
Cengage Learning Customer & Sales Support, 1-800-354-9706

For permission to use material from this text or product, submit all requests online at **www.cengage.com/permissions**. Further permissions questions can be e-mailed to **permissionrequest@cengage.com**

Library of Congress Control Number: 2010939812

ISBN-13: 978-1-4354-9569-2

ISBN-10: 1-4354-9569-1

Delmar
5 Maxwell Drive
Clifton Park, NY 12065-2919
USA

Cengage Learning is a leading provider of customized learning solutions with office locations around the globe, including Singapore, the United Kingdom, Australia, Mexico, Brazil, and Japan. Locate your local office at: **international.cengage.com/region**

Cengage Learning products are represented in Canada by Nelson Education, Ltd.

To learn more about Delmar, visit **www.cengage.com/delmar**

Purchase any of our products at your local college store or at our preferred online store **www.CengageBrain.com**

Notice to the Reader

Publisher does not warrant or guarantee any of the products described herein or perform any independent analysis in connection with any of the product information contained herein. Publisher does not assume, and expressly disclaims, any obligation to obtain and include information other than that provided to it by the manufacturer. The reader is expressly warned to consider and adopt all safety precautions that might be indicated by the activities described herein and to avoid all potential hazards. By following the instructions contained herein, the reader willingly assumes all risks in connection with such instructions. The publisher makes no representations or warranties of any kind, including but not limited to, the warranties of fitness for particular purpose or merchantability, nor are any such representations implied with respect to the material set forth herein, and the publisher takes no responsibility with respect to such material. The publisher shall not be liable for any special, consequential, or exemplary damages resulting, in whole or part, from the readers' use of, or reliance upon, this material.

Printed in the United States of America
1 2 3 4 5 6 7 12 11 10

CONTENTS

CHAPTER 3

Acknowledging Emotional Reactions   45

CHAPTER 4

Acknowledging and Confronting the Fear Factor   67

CHAPTER 5

Emotions and Health-Care Decision Making   95

CHAPTER 6

Helping Newly Diagnosed Patients Communicate with Health-Care Professionals

CHAPTER 7

Encouraging Patients to Gather Information

CHAPTER 8

Developing a Support Plan with Patients   183

CHAPTER 9

Coping with Effects on Self-Image   211

CHAPTER 10

Connecting with a Sense of Meaning   233

CHAPTER 11

Communicating with Family Members and Caregivers   259

CHAPTER 12

Creating a Vision for the Future   289

CHAPTER 13

When Diagnoses Involve the End of Life   309

CHAPTER 14

Recognizing Personal Emotions as Health-Care Professionals   329

Every day, millions of patients receive medical diagnoses they either feared or did not expect. Left with conflicting, and often crippling, emotions, these patients must make life-changing health-care decisions, many times lacking the proper information to make those decisions and under immense time pressure. Lacking the proper support, newly diagnosed patients are at risk in terms of treatment outcomes, ongoing compliance, and quality of life. Everyone in the patients' life is affected, from the family members who care about them to the health-care professionals who care for them.

After the Diagnosis was created with a two-pronged goal: (1) help health-care professionals—nurses, physician's assistants, nursing assistants, those from other allied professions—understand how newly diagnosed patients react to their diagnoses, and (2) help those professionals help patients harness their emotional and rational strengths as they communicate with their health-care professionals, gather information, evaluate treatment options, make informed treatment decisions, and manage their conditions.

How to Use This Book

CHAPTER OBJECTIVES

In addition to helping readers familiarize themselves with chapter topics, the objectives that are clearly outlined at the beginning of each chapter serve as valuable chapter-review tools.

KEYWORDS

To help keep readers focused on crucial topics, key terms are listed at the beginning of each chapter, highlighted when they first appear in the text, and defined fully in the glossary.

OPENING CASE STUDY

Each chapter opens with a real-world case study that, in the form of a patient conversation, illustrates a challenge facing newly diagnosed patients and their health-care professionals.

KEEP IN MIND

The Keep in Mind feature is designed to encourage readers to think critically about key topics, both from newly diagnosed patients' perspectives and from health-care professionals' viewpoints.

RX: CONDUCTING A PATIENT DISCUSSION

Each chapter's opening case study resumes again as the chapter ends. This element provides readers both examples and guidelines for conducting conversations with newly diagnosed patients themselves.

REAL-WORLD EXAMPLES

Much of the power of *After the Diagnosis* comes from its real-world examples, examples health-care professionals can both relate to and learn from. Body language highlights alert readers to the facial expressions and body positions that help relay how newly diagnosed patients are feeling. Examples of the negative and positive self-talk that are common among newly diagnosed patients serve as guidance as health-care professionals strive to cultivate beneficial patient outlooks. Throughout, the book identifies "educational moments," opportunities in which health-care professionals can help newly diagnosed patients recognize self-defeating attitudes and consider more productive alternatives.

CHAPTER REVIEW SECTION

The workbook section at the end of each chapter includes exercises designed to help readers assess what they have learned in each chapter and apply that knowledge in practical situations.

- *Multiple-Choice Questions* Structured multiple-choice questions test comprehension of key points.

- *Fill-in-the-Blank Questions* Fill-in-the-blank question focus primarily on key terms.

- *Short-Answer Questions* Short-answer questions provide opportunities to apply chapter information to real-life situations.

- *Critical-Thinking Questions* The goal of critical-thinking questions is to challenge learners to evaluate what they have learned from the textbook by considering their own experiences in and opinions of real-life situations.

- *Internet Exercise* The Internet exercise in each chapter encourages learners to explore relevant Internet resources.

- *Worksheets* Worksheets can be used with patients, for example, to assist in listing support resources.

Instructor Supplements

INSTRUCTOR'S GUIDE

The *After the Diagnosis Instructor's Guide* provides all the answers to the exercises in each chapter. It also includes exercises that can be used in a classroom setting to help learners practice using the concepts and techniques in each chapter. Exercises are both self-directed as well as role plays.

POWERPOINT PRESENTATIONS

PowerPoint presentations cover the key content from each chapter.

TEST BANK

The Test Bank is a comprehensive repository of questions to use in student evaluation.

ACKNOWLEDGMENTS

I owe a special debt of gratitude to Matt Seeley of Delmar Cengage Learning for choosing *After the Diagnosis* to be among the distinguished company of Delmar books for health-care professionals. Thanks also to Samantha Zullo of Delmar Cengage Learning for her invaluable help in moving the book through the editorial process.

I would also like to acknowledge Colleen Corrice, who did a wonderful job editing and making sure the concepts of the book were clear and concise. A special thank you goes to Michelle Buchman, MA, BSN, RN, for diligently reading and rereading my chapters for technical accuracy and offering suggestions and encouragement.

The author and the publisher would also like to thank the following reviewers for their input and feedback:

Christina Egeland RMA, NCMA, MBA
Program Director
Heald College
Portland, OR

Mary Nichols, RMA (AMT)
Director of Healthcare Programs
Heald College
Roseville, CA

Dr. Carol Qare-Carcar DPM, CPT, RMA
Program Director
Heald College
San Francisco, CA

Heidi Weber BS, CMA (AAMA)
Medical Assisting Program Chair
Globe University
Sioux Falls, SD

ABOUT THE AUTHORS

Gary McClain, who completed graduate work in clinical psychology and education and holds a PhD from the University of Michigan, is a therapist, consultant, and educator specializing in helping clients deal with the emotional impact of chronic and life-threatening illnesses. Also a New York State–licensed counselor, Dr. McClain works with patients to help them understand and cope with their emotions, learn about their lifestyle and treatment options, maintain compliance with medical regimens, communicate effectively with the medical establishment, and listen to their inner voices as they make decisions about their futures.

Dr. McClain consults with community organizations on the needs of newly diagnosed patients and for local and national organizations has spoken on such topics as dealing with medical diagnoses, being one's own patient advocate, and communication between patients and family caregivers. He conducts training for community agency volunteers and health-care professionals on patient advocacy and communications. He has written for publications that include *Body Positive Magazine, Caring for Cancer, Arthritis Self-Management*, and *Hep C Connection*; writes a regular column on mental health issues for *HIV Plus* Magazine; and is involved in patient social networking through the Internet. His Web site, www.JustGotDiagnosed.com, which provides information for patients and caregivers facing chronic and catastrophic illness as well as their health-care professionals, was awarded the Standard of Excellence Award in the health-care category in 2008. He welcomes questions and comments and can be reached through his e-mail address at gary@justgotdiagnosed.com.

Michelle A. Buchman, MA, BSN, RN, is the medical assisting program coordinator and an assistant professor at Cox College. Mrs. Buchman has been employed as a nursing director and nurse manager for behavioral health inpatient units. She earned her diploma in nursing from Burge School of Nursing and she obtained her bachelor's of science degree in nursing from Southwest Missouri State University. She was awarded a master's degree in management and leadership from Webster University.

I wrote *After the Diagnosis* as my mother, Elaine, faced her own health challenges at the end of her life. While she made her final transition before my book was published, I hope I was able to channel her loving and caring spirit onto each page. *After the Diagnosis* is dedicated to her. Thanks, Mom.

My book is also dedicated to Kevin and Leigh Ganton and the wonderful staff of Arbor North Center for Living, health-care professionals who truly embody skill, dedication, and compassion. I could not have completed this book without the assurance that they were partners in watching lovingly over my mom 24/7. Thank you, and thank you again.

CHAPTER 1

Starting the Conversation about a Medical Diagnosis

OVERVIEW

After reading this chapter, you should be able to:

- Define and use the keywords of conversations about medical diagnoses.

- Understand the optimal, stepwise approach to presenting and discussing a medical diagnosis with a newly diagnosed patient.

- Be aware of a patient's initial, anticipatory anxiety upon hearing a diagnosis, as well as the key, underlying questions.

- Understand the factors affecting a patient's readiness to hear a diagnosis and how those factors may impact the patient's reaction.

- Know how to prepare to deliver a medical diagnosis.

KEYWORDS

Anticipatory anxiety	Hope	Prebargaining
Denial	Listen	Referral
Diagnosis	Normalize	Superstitious thinking
Emotion	Overwhelmed	Ventilation
Hear		

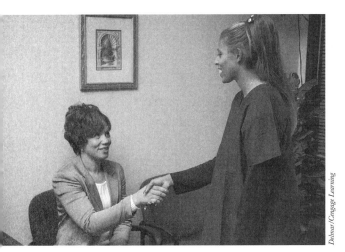

Delmar/Cengage Learning

Case Study

"Right out of the blue" is how Gina described her diagnosis after her physician, Dr. Maura Bennett, informed her she was being diagnosed with Type II diabetes. While her mother had had the same condition, Gina had hoped that somehow she might be spared, but as her physician had explained to her, "Type II diabetes isn't uncommon for someone who is overweight and getting no exercise."

"But I'm only 42," Gina had argued. "This isn't fair."

"Type II diabetes can strike anyone who isn't taking care of their health, at any age," Dr. Bennett had answered. The physician then informed Gina that she would need to begin using an anti-insulin agent daily and that the health-care team would be talking to her about the diet and exercise routines she recommended. After that, she described Gina's medication regimen and told Gina she wanted her to talk to one of the clinic's nurses, Shelly, before she left.

> **KEEP IN MIND**
>
> Gina's first reaction to her diagnosis was that, at age 42, a chronic condition seemed unfair. As a health-care professional, you may be expected to address this concern when you sit down with patients to discuss their treatment plans. How would you prepare for this type of discussion?

When Shelly entered the examination room, she realized immediately that Gina was confused and upset. Still sitting on the examination table as she had been when Dr. Bennett had delivered her diagnosis, Gina had a fearful expression on her face and was slumped forward. Shelly could hear her sighs.

"How are you doing, Gina?" Shelly asked.

"Not so good," Gina responded. "Honestly, I'm feeling kind of lost. I just received a diagnosis I didn't expect. I'm not even sick, and now I'm supposed to be on medications for who knows how long."

2

Shelly gently touched Gina's arm. "Looks to me like we need to go over the discussion you had with Dr. Bennett," she started. Then, gesturing toward a nearby chair, she said, "You don't look so comfortable sitting on this table. Why don't you have a seat over here first, okay?"

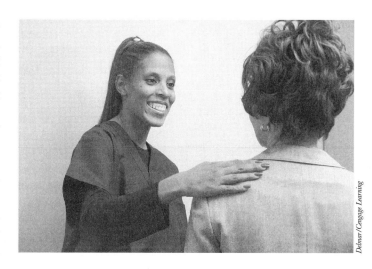

Gina nodded and moved to the chair. Shelly pulled up another chair and sat across from her.

"So you just got diagnosed with Type II diabetes," Shelly said. "Why don't you start by telling me what the doctor told you."

Gina took a deep breath and briefly told Shelly what the physician had told her about her diagnosis, how it would be treated, and what kinds of lifestyle changes she would need to make. As she talked, Gina choked back tears. "I can't believe this is happening to me!" she exclaimed. "Who knows what might happen when I get older. I could end up blind!"

Shelly handed Gina some tissues. As Gina wiped the tears from her eyes and blew her nose, Shelly continued.

"You're really upset about this, Gina," she said.

Gina nodded.

"And right now," Shelly continued, "this all seems really overwhelming and scary to you."

"Yes," Gina answered. "It does."

"A new diagnosis always brings up a lot of emotions," Shelly said gently. "It's scary to have someone give you a medical label, especially when it's unexpected."

Gina nodded in agreement.

"So let's talk about what's scaring you," Shelly said. "And then I'm going to give you some information about Type II diabetes and go over your treatment plan with you. Does that sound like a good idea?"

"Yeah," Gina answered, sighing softly. "That sounds like a good idea."

Introduction

"We need to talk about your test results."

That sentence can strike fear in the heart of a newly diagnosed patient, because it brings to mind all kinds of scary possibilities, both real and imagined. How the **diagnosis** is initially presented to the patient, and how the health-care team communicates with the patient during the days and weeks that follow, can make a tremendous difference in how the patient reacts and subsequently copes.

Hearing the news of a medical diagnosis, whether expected or unexpected, is in many ways a life-changing experience for the patient. For the health-care professional, this conversation, or any conducted immediately after the diagnosis, is only the first of many difficult but important exchanges between the patient and health-care professionals who may include providers, nurses, physical therapists, medical assistants, or dieticians. For the health-care professional, however, such exchanges are rather routine.

> **KEEP IN MIND**
>
> As a health-care professional, you are expected to provide patient support at all points in the diagnosis cycle. What do you think Gina needs at this point? How comfortable would you be with a patient who is feeling this way immediately after a diagnosis? What would you do next?

Delmar/Cengage Learning

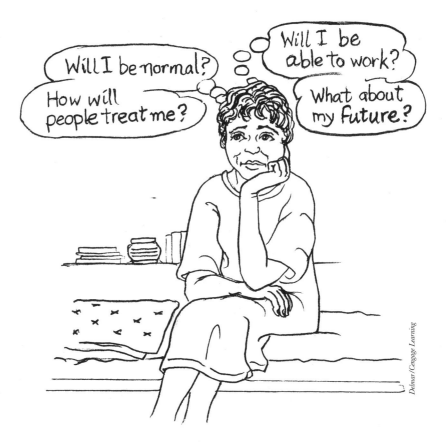

Delmar/Cengage Learning

Health-care professionals will have both initial and ongoing involvement with patients who have been newly diagnosed with medical conditions. Depending on the duration and severity of those conditions—minor, acute, chronic, or life-threatening—patients will, at the time of diagnosis, experience a wide range of **emotions** that include fear, anger, and sadness. They may be **overwhelmed** by the critical treatment decisions they must make and feel they have neither the information, nor the mental capacity, they need. Newly diagnosed patients may need to **listen** to, and evaluate, medical information that is both confusing and frightening. When conditions are serious, patients may have questions about their futures and spiritual crises. At some point, patients will likely need support for practical and emotional issues, and the roles of family and friends will become important.

> **KEEP IN MIND**
>
> Have you ever received a medical diagnosis yourself or gone through the experience with a loved one? Each patient is an individual, so the experience of another person's medical diagnosis may be very different than yours. Keep an open mind, and make no assumptions about how a patient may react.

From the moment the diagnosis is given, health-care professionals can positively impact patients and enhance the therapeutic relationship. Such a relationship has many opportunities for educational moments.

Understanding the Patient's Mindset

Patients approach news about a medical diagnosis with what mental health professionals call **anticipatory anxiety**. They worry about what they might **hear**, what it might mean for their daily lives and the lives of their loved ones. They worry about the future, if it will be altered in some way or if they will have none at all.

Anticipatory anxiety is often experienced through questions that go through patients' minds. Often, these questions are based not on information or reality but on scenarios the patients create to try to prepare themselves for the reality of their situations. Following are some common examples.

WHAT WILL MY DAILY LIFE BE LIKE? WILL I BE NORMAL?

As a child, John watched an aunt cope with chronic pain. He remembers how uncomfortable she always seemed to be at family gatherings and how she would have difficulty smiling or participating in conversations. He also remembers how his uncle had had to help her with simple things during dinner, like putting food on her plate and cutting her meat. Often, the couple would excuse themselves and leave early because the pain John's aunt had been experiencing had increased.

Being "normal" is being able to do the little things in life, including self-care, participating in work and leisure, and caring for others. It includes going to the grocery store, keeping our homes clean, going to work, participating in family and work activities, enjoying hobbies—lots of little things that, when added together, make up our unique lives. Basically, we all want to be "normal" in whatever way we define the word.

For most of us, being "abnormal" means standing out from the crowd in ways we don't want to—looking different, acting different, needing special assistance, or having special requirements, like needing foods that differ from everybody else's. In short, a medical diagnosis can raise all sorts of questions regarding potential normalcy going forward. It can also cause us to question what it means for the people we care about.

WHAT WILL CHANGE IN MY RELATIONSHIPS?
WILL PEOPLE TREAT ME THE SAME?

Theresa once read a story about a woman with breast cancer who had to ask a relative to take in her two small children because she was temporarily unable to care for them herself. Theresa, who has a child of her own, remembers crying after reading this story, and even dreaming about it.

Sigmund Freud said that the goal of a human being is "to work and to love." Human beings are social beings, and newly diagnosed patients worry that their illnesses will interfere with their personal relationships, the ones with their family and friends.

Adult patients in general tend to worry that they will be unable to maintain their household responsibilities, but parents wonder if they will be able to care for their children adequately or if their conditions will shame or embarrass their children. For parents, this may be the greatest tragedy they can imagine. Patients with partners worry that their partners will be less attracted to them or that they will require more support than their partners are willing or able to give.

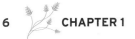

In terms of nonfamily relationships, newly diagnosed patients may fear that their friendships may suffer, that their friends may now be uncomfortable with them and unable to talk to them about their conditions. Patients may worry that they will lose their friends altogether as a result of their diagnoses. No one wants to feel avoided or like an outsider, but the fear of being unable to be "normal" may translate to being "less than" other people, which means driving people away by needing different treatment and, at the worst extreme, being a burden. Newly diagnosed patients may even fear that their friends and family will try to care for them like children.

WHAT WILL HAPPEN AT MY JOB?
WILL I STILL BE EMPLOYABLE?

Annika has a high-pressure job in an advertising agency. She has always worked long hours but also tried to eat healthy. Lately, she has been experiencing some pain that has worried her. She watched her mother's condition gradually deteriorate after being diagnosed with arthritis, to the point where she had to rely on others to handle daily tasks like housekeeping. This is the memory Anna holds in her mind as she waits in her doctor's examination room.

To Sigmund Freud, being able to work, whether inside or outside the house, was integral to achieving a sense of being a valuable part of the world. Indeed, we gain much of our identity through what we do, and we evaluate others based on what they do, as well. In today's world, many work too hard and derive too much of their identities from their professions. Annika may be one of these individuals.

It is important to keep in mind that we work to support ourselves, to provide the basics, but also to live certain lifestyles and pursue our interests. Those with families to support have even higher stakes in maintaining the ability to work: Others depend on them.

Consequently, it is common for newly diagnosed patients to approach their diagnoses with fear—the fear of work loss, for example—and to be filled with images of others who have lost their professions.

WHAT CAN I EXPECT IN THE FUTURE?
DO I EVEN *HAVE* A FUTURE?

Jerry is all about the future, as he is the first to admit. At 32, he is filled with dreams of what he is going to do with his life, and he already owns a successful small business that he maintains while working full time. Jerry had already been planning to take the next big step in the next year—leave his job to make his small business his life's work—when he discovered a lump that did not seem to be going away. Though he had finally decided to call his doctor, he hadn't met with the doctor yet. Right now, he's asking himself, "Am I going to finally get what I've been working for, or is it all going to go up in smoke?"

No one knows what the future will bring, but human beings assume they will have one. They also assume that they have some kind of control over what it brings. Living a good life, working hard, being close to friends and family . . . these actions are all supposed to create the basis for getting what we want in life. Furthermore, having plans for the future adds meaning to whatever discomfort or disappointment arises from jobs, living situations, or relationships going poorly. After all, there is always tomorrow, and doing the right thing is supposed to bring a better tomorrow.

Hearing a medical diagnosis that might interfere with future plans can be daunting. A patient contemplating a medical diagnosis most likely equates the diagnosis with lack of control, being unable to do the things necessary to have a future. Without a vision for the future, what's left?

Accompanying questions like these, the ones that run through patients' minds, are images of what life might be like with a diagnosis. Like patients' questions, these images are often based on incomplete or false information. To complicate matters, images like these accumulate throughout patients' lifetimes. When patients face their own medical diagnoses, these images can reemerge—and prove overwhelming. For example, patients who had parents or relatives face illnesses—chronic conditions like diabetes or more life-threatening illnesses like cancer—may have specific, vivid memories of the experiences, ones that come to the fore when the patients are newly diagnosed with medical conditions of their own.

Sometimes, the images patients harbor flood the patients before diagnoses even occur. Often, newly diagnosed patients are programmed to expect the worst, but the reality is that while newly diagnosed patients use their experiences with others' illnesses to create assumptions—and fears—about their own conditions, others' experiences with illness are poor road maps.

The assumptions and images patients bring to their diagnoses create a two-pronged challenge for the health-care team. First, the newly diagnosed patient has no experience with the condition and therefore no basis for experience. The team must educate an inexperienced, uninitiated patient. Second, this same patient has a pre-conceived notion of the future, one that is based on frightening images and assumptions. The health-care team must identify and address the patient's concerns while providing the proper information. While health-care professionals speak with the first patient—the one in need of information—it is the second patient who has prepared to hear the diagnosis.

Identifying Other Factors Affecting Readiness to Hear a Diagnosis

In addition to images and assumptions, other factors may affect a patient's readiness to hear a diagnosis. These factors, introduced briefly here, are elaborated on in upcoming chapters.

DIAGNOSING DENIAL

Denial is a common response to a medical diagnosis, one that can occur even before the diagnosis. Patients may prepare themselves to hear diagnoses by promising themselves that "it won't happen to me," or they may tell themselves that if a diagnosis is confirmed, or unexpected, they won't believe it or it will be less damaging than it was for someone else.

DEFINING SUPERSTITIOUS THINKING

Human beings have varied superstitions, including a number involving illness. One of the more common examples of **superstitious thinking** is the belief that people

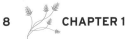

who are kind enough to other people will experience nothing bad. As a result of this superstition, patients facing medical diagnoses commonly report having done extra kindnesses or made large donations. Assuming the worst is another example of superstitious thinking. For example, a patient awaiting a medical diagnosis may self-diagnose with the most catastrophic condition possible, hoping that this conceived diagnosis will make any other option relatively minor in comparison.

WORKING THROUGH PREBARGAINING

Patients facing medical diagnoses may indulge in a process of **prebargaining**. Patients with children may, for example, promise to be exemplary parents, if only they are promised health. Other patients may promise to follow through on plans to further their education or to get more involved in community affairs. Essentially, the goal of prebargaining is to make a promise—to one's self, to one's loved ones, to a spiritual being—to do something that would make a poor medical diagnosis a negative event for the world. Another form of superstitious thinking, prebargaining can cause denial or devastation.

> **KEEP IN MIND**
>
> As they anticipate their diagnoses, patients' thought processes and expectations directly impact their abilities to accurately understand and process medical information.

Giving a Diagnosis

Depending on the type and severity of medical diagnosis, the standard procedures of the hospital, clinic, or private practice where the diagnosis is delivered may determine how the diagnosis is given and by whom. This section provides some additional guidelines for giving a diagnosis, the goal being to help the patient listen and respond in ways that will facilitate further discussion.

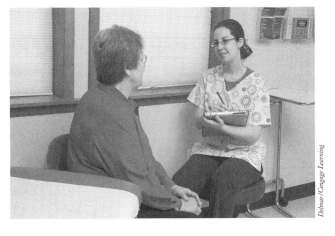

As alluded to at the beginning of this chapter, a routine diagnosis for the health-care professional is anything but routine for the patient. Even the most common diagnosis can devastate a patient, especially given the patient's state of mind when the diagnosis is given. Health-care professionals may feel a condition is readily treatable and, as such, should not overly frighten the patient. Compounding the problem, health-care professionals may be unprepared or unwilling to provide the patient more than the basic facts, limited by time or the feeling that it is best for the patient to pursue additional information and emotional support. Finally, physicians often feel that other staff, especially nurses or medical assistants, are better equipped, and have the time, to elaborate on diagnoses and help patients cope.

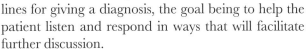
Delmar/Cengage Learning

CULTIVATING EMOTIONAL OPENNESS

When giving a medical diagnosis, it is important to stay open to patients' emotions. Patients may or may not be expecting to hear diagnoses. If they do have expectations, they may be experiencing emotions like fear on one hand or denial on the other. Nursing staff can begin the conversation by understanding how patients may be feeling. This signals to patients that the health-care professionals are concerned about their well-being and comfortable talking about emotions.

REVIEWING REASON FOR REFERRAL

It helps patients when health-care professionals briefly review with them why they have been referred. Patients may have referred themselves for routine physicals or complaints about symptoms, or they may have been referred by other sources, like physicians or clinics. Reviewing the reason for **referral** helps to remind patients what brought them to the point in the process of being diagnosed. Always gain agreement with the patient on the reason for referral, especially when some time has passed between the initial contact and when the diagnosis was determined.

GAINING A BASIC UNDERSTANDING OF DIAGNOSTIC PROCEDURES

Upon reviewing the reason for referral, health-care professionals should give patients basic understandings of their diagnostic procedures. While the science or technology underlying the procedures is likely unnecessary—too much technical information can overwhelm, and frighten, patients—it helps patients to understand, in basic terms, why certain procedures were chosen, how widely those procedures are used, how reliable they are, and what preparation is involved before and after. Health-care professionals should relate procedures to reasons for referral, any relevant aspects of patients' medical histories, and the procedures' reliability.

> **KEEP IN MIND**
>
> Readiness is an important factor in a patient's ability to hear—and listen to—information. Much like the patient awaiting diagnosis who resists any discussion that precedes it, a patient may have difficulty processing any information that follows.

DISCUSSING THE DIAGNOSIS

With the reason for referral and the diagnostic procedures briefly reviewed with the patient, it is time to provide the diagnosis. Because medical diagnoses vary widely in terms of symptoms, treatment, and degree of risk, it is important to present the diagnosis, as much as possible, in language the patient will understand. It is also important for health-care professionals to be sensitive to the nonroutine nature of the diagnosis for the patient and to speak slowly enough for the patient to comprehend.

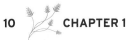

After providing the diagnosis, immediately give the patient an opportunity to react to it. Some patients may have emotional reactions, others may seem to have no reaction, and still others will want to ask questions about things like prognosis, treatment, and recovery. As with the diagnosis, answer patient questions in understandable terms and, before presenting the treatment plan, ensure the patient fully comprehends the diagnosis.

Presenting the Treatment Plan

Newly diagnosed patients want to have **hope**, and they seek that hope from the health-care professional's discussion of the treatment plan. Health-care professionals should discuss the treatment plan, or treatment options, in straightforward terms,

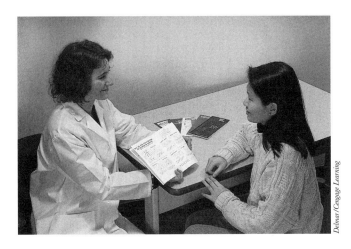
Delmar/Cengage Learning

highlighting the treatment process itself, what to expect in terms of side effects and impact on daily life management, and the likelihood of success. Some patients may be unprepared to evaluate the pros and cons of various treatment options, for reasons that include being too emotionally distraught to talk about their treatment or because, on the other hand, they want to do their own information-gathering to help prepare themselves to consider the alternatives and make a decision. Some patients at this point will decline to have the discussion at all.

As a result, discussion of the treatment plan may be ongoing. As patients cope with their initial reactions to their diagnoses (detailed further in Chapter 2) and do more of their own research, they will have more questions. When physicians provide the initial diagnoses, other members of the health-care team may be called on to answer patient questions about treatment, especially those related to side effects and recovery. The team members answering treatment questions may be involved with, if not primarily responsible for, ongoing treatment administration and supportive care, so it benefits patients when physicians begin discussing treatment plans with the nurses or medical assistants as soon as possible, to get all of the health-care team members involved in a dialogue with the patient.

Discussing Emotional Reactions to a Diagnosis

The missing aspect when discussing a medical diagnosis is the patient's emotional reaction. Emotional reactions are complex and discussed at length in upcoming chapters. At this point, it is important to emphasize that medical diagnoses are emotional experiences for patients. Too often, out of time constraints, lack of training, or personal discomfort, health-care professionals avoid discussing emotional issues with patients. They fear the discussions will get "out of hand" and that they will be required to deliver mental health services they are not qualified to deliver. Alternatively, they may feel that patients should be focused on information and treatment decisions, not enmeshed in emotional reactions.

EMBRACING EMPATHY AND OPPORTUNITY

To support their patients, health-care professionals can make it clear that they understand medical diagnoses can be emotional experiences. A simple question like, "How are you doing with this?" can give the patient the opportunity to express some initial reactions, at least enough to feel a sense of release during this potentially traumatizing experience.

As you will see going forward, simply having the opportunity to express feelings and be heard is the beginning of the journey in coping with a diagnosis.

TAKING NEXT STEPS

Patients must leave the discussion of the medical diagnosis with a sense of what they can and should do next. This includes next steps regarding:

- Patient education information
- Where to go/who to call for additional information, including Web sites
- When treatment begins and what to expect
- Guidance on any lifestyle modifications
- Referral source for mental health counseling, if needed
- Specialists or tests to be scheduled
- Medication information

KEEP IN MIND

Patients are first and foremost unique human beings. This means that each patient goes through an individual process in terms of acknowledging and accepting the diagnosis, coping with it emotionally, getting educated, and moving forward with treatment and lifestyle modification decisions. As a health-care professional, let your patients know you understand this and are standing by as questions arise.

Discussing a Recent Diagnosis

The health-care team is often in the position of meeting with a patient after the physician has delivered the initial diagnosis. As we saw at the beginning of the chapter when Gina received her Type II diabetes diagnosis, patients often require discussion of their diagnoses beyond initial delivery. There are a number of reasons for this need. Patients often experience some initial shock at their diagnoses and are consequently unprepared to hear more or do anything beyond sit with their emotional reactions. Physicians may lack time at those moments to remain with patients and answer further questions and may instead rely on the health-care team to handle those conversations. As the primary interface between patient and physician, the health-care team is uniquely able to have these discussions.

A meeting with a patient who has recently received a medical diagnosis can be conducted much like the discussion in which the diagnosis was originally delivered. In fact, patients may have to have the complete discussion over again, from diagnosis, to treatment, to next steps. They may have been so distraught that they were unable to listen to their diagnosis the first time, or they may have been in a state of denial or disbelief. Patients may have been so caught up in their anticipatory anxiety and all of their perceptions and misperceptions that they hardly heard what the physician said beyond their diagnosis. Or, they may simply need to repeat the discussions again to process them properly.

Preparing to Deliver a Patient Diagnosis

As you prepare to deliver a diagnosis to a patient, ask the following questions:

- "Do I understand the condition?"
- "Am I prepared to discuss the treatment and the treatment options?"
- "Am I armed with patient education material?"
- "What are the patient's potential concerns, including side effects of treatment, duration of treatment, expected outcomes of treatment, required lifestyle modifications, and potential of recurrence?"
- "Do I know where I can send the patient for more information?"
- "How might the patient react emotionally? Am I prepared to discuss the patient's emotional reactions?"
- "Do I have a referral source that can help the patient cope with emotional reactions?"
- "What next steps must I go through with the patient?"

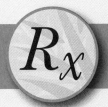

Discussing the News of a Diagnosis with a Patient

Early in this chapter, we left Gina with Dr. Bennett's nurse, Shelly. After Gina moved to a comfortable chair and Shelly sat across from her, here is how the conversation progressed.

SHELLY: So, Gina. Where would you like to start?

GINA: With how I got to this point.

SHELLY: Would it help if I started from the beginning?

GINA: Yes, I think it would.

SHELLY: Well, you came in for your annual physical, and I was going through the standard health questions with you. You said you had been more thirsty than usual lately, and that you felt tired a lot. Do you remember that?

GINA: Yes, I do.

SHELLY: And you checked the box on the questionnaire that indicated your mom had suffered from Type II diabetes. Right?

GINA: Yeah, she did. From about her early fifties onward. She was on medication until she died last year.

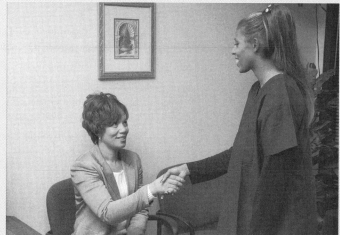

SHELLY: That was a red flag. Dr. Bennett scheduled you for some additional tests to check your blood glucose levels. She received the results, and you were diagnosed with Type II diabetes.

GINA: I just can't believe this is happening to me. I mean, I knew it was possible, but somehow I thought I might escape it.

SHELLY: I know this is upsetting for you. What are your biggest concerns?

GINA: I'm worried about what my life will be like. If I'm going to have to change the way I live, not eat the food I enjoy. And I'm worried about what this might mean as I get older. I mean, my mother had a lot of stuff happen to her as she got older.

SHELLY: Type II diabetes can be controlled. The medication will help. And I can recommend diet and exercise that will work with your lifestyle. What else is on your mind?

GINA: I'm just scared. And angry at myself for letting this happen.

SHELLY: You don't have to beat yourself up over this, Gina. I know it's disappointing.

GINA: You don't know how disappointing. I feel like I have this cloud that's going to keep following me around, and I have to keep paying attention to it. But no matter what I do, it's not going to go away.

SHELLY: It's always disappointing and scary to hear about a medical diagnosis. Nobody likes that, especially a chronic condition like diabetes. Yes, it's going to be around. But we can work together to make sure you take the best care of yourself you possibly can.

GINA: Okay.

SHELLY: And if you'd like to talk to a counselor, I have a couple of names I can give you. It might be really helpful to you to have someone to talk to about this. You can think about that if you want.

GINA: Okay, I will.

SHELLY: Now. Do you want to know more about the medication?

GINA: I know what I need to take, and the doctor gave me a pamphlet to read. I think I have dealt with enough for today.

SHELLY: Okay. You know how to call me as questions come up. But the doctor wants you to start the medication as soon as possible, and we need to go over some diet and exercise recommendations. Are you ready to go over that with me for a few minutes?

GINA: Sure.

Guidelines for Discussing a Diagnosis with a Patient

Following are guidelines for discussing a recent diagnosis with a patient.

1. ***Review the facts.***   Newly diagnosed patients often cannot take in much of what their physicians tell them about their diagnoses during their initial conversations. Often, they hear little beyond their medical conditions. Therefore, it can be helpful to review facts with patients. Notice that, in the preceding example, Shelly started with what prompted Gina to make an appointment—an annual physical—then proceeded to a discussion of the symptoms Gina was experiencing and her family history of diabetes.

2. ***Listen to the patient's initial fears.***   Patients often have initial concerns regarding their diagnoses, and these concerns are top-of-mind for them. These concerns can be so pronounced that patients are unable to focus on anything else the health-care professionals tell them until they have had opportunities to at least express their concerns. Health-care professionals may be unable to offer resolution at this point, but doing so is unnecessary. What is necessary at this point, and what can provide some sense of relief, is providing patients the chance to voice what they are thinking and feeling and reassuring them that these concerns will be addressed. Notice that Shelly listened to Gina's fears and then reassured her that they would work together to help Gina stay healthy.

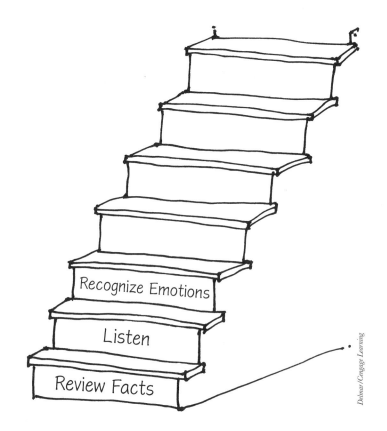

Delmar/Cengage Learning

3. *Recognize—and acknowledge—when a patient is overwhelmed.* Newly diagnosed patients may be so overwhelmed by the news of their conditions that they cannot focus on further discussion until they have had opportunities to process what they have heard. They may indicate that they are overloaded by not responding to questions or comments or by doing things like crying. Shelly was watching for signs that Gina might be overwhelmed, because at one point in the conversation she offered to refer Gina to a counselor. If a patient becomes so overwhelmed that the conversation cannot continue, it may be necessary to reschedule it.

Picking Up the Pieces after the Straight Talk

As a member of the health-care team, you may find yourself stepping in after a health-care provider or another health-care professional has delivered a diagnosis in a direct, "just the facts" manner. If the patient was emotionally unprepared for the news, or the deliverer was unable or unwilling to acknowledge the patient's emotional reaction, you may feel like you must undo the damage of the exchange. When this happens, start the conversation by having the patient describe the experience—what was heard, understood, felt. This may feel like a **ventilation** session, and essentially it will be, but patients must be heard if they are to put experiences like these in perspective, process them, and move forward.

At this point, review the process of diagnosis delivery from the beginning to ensure that the patient has all needed information, as well as the opportunity to react in the most productive, safe way.

> ### KEEP IN MIND
>
> It can help patients when health-care professionals **normalize** their conditions by reassuring them that they are reacting to their diagnoses much like other patients, the same patients who have coped successfully with this process.

SUMMARY

The process of helping a patient cope with a medical diagnosis begins the moment the medical diagnosis is delivered. As they approach conversations like these, patients experience anticipatory anxiety, much of it based on past encounters with others' illnesses, as well on a lack of information. Health-care professionals can help patients receive their diagnoses by being understanding of this lack of information, allowing patients to hear and process information as they are ready to cope, and remaining sensitive to the emotions patients may be experiencing. Health-care team members do things like these whether they are delivering diagnoses or following up on physicians' deliveries.

Multiple-Choice Questions

1. The newly diagnosed patient who expresses the expectation that an upcoming treatment will have uncomfortable side effects is an example of which of the following?
   a. Anticipation causation
   b. Depression
   c. Anticipatory anxiety
   d. Denial

2. The diagnosis of a medical condition can be a life-changing event when the:
   a. Diagnosis is terminal
   b. News requires a change in employment
   c. Patient must begin a treatment regimen
   d. All of the above

3. Patient feelings like fear, anger, and sadness upon initial diagnosis are considered a(n):
   a. Emotional reaction
   b. Breakdown
   c. Issue avoidance
   d. Overreaction

4. Patients who refuse to believe they have received medical diagnoses demonstrate which of the following?
   a. Rehearsal
   b. Reversal
   c. Denial
   d. Depression

5. The patient who donates to a nonprofit organization before hearing the results of a medical test, believing that doing so will bring personal good fortune, demonstrates _____ thinking.
   a. Superstitious
   b. Unconscious
   c. Supernatural
   d. Unnatural

Fill-in-the-Blank Questions

1. Using the numbers 1 through 6, order the following steps to presenting a medical diagnosis to a patient properly.

   ___ Present the diagnosis

   ___ Review reason for referral

   ___ Provide next steps

   ___ Review the diagnostic procedure

   ___ Present the treatment plan

   ___ Discuss emotional reactions to the diagnosis

2. _____ occurs when newly diagnosed patients refuse to accept the seriousness of their diagnoses.

3. Reminding a patient that other patients in the same situation have felt the same way is a way to _____ the patient's reaction.

4. _____ anxiety results when patients fear their test results.

5. The patient who promises to be a better human being if test results come back negative demonstrates the principle of _____.

6. Patients who become upset and refuse to listen to health-care professionals indicate that they are feeling _____.

Short-Answer Questions

1. A newly diagnosed patient who witnessed a friend being treated for a similar diagnosis may present additional challenges to the health-care professional upon initial diagnosis. Why?

_____

_____

_____

2. What three concerns do newly diagnosed patients have regarding how their personal relationships will be affected by their diagnosis and treatment?

_____

_____

_____

3. Explain how health-care professionals can best prepare themselves to deliver the news of a medical diagnosis.

_____

_____

_____

Critical-Thinking Questions

1. Health-care professionals sometimes talk about holding back the details of conditions when providing patients with diagnoses or downplaying the seriousness of those conditions until the patients have had time to process. Similarly, family members may ask that health-care professionals withhold facts from patients. What are the advantages and disadvantages of avoiding the facts? Are there situations in which this might be recommended?

_____

_____

_____

_____

2. Newly diagnosed patients may ask health-care professionals to explain their diagnoses and answer additional questions. What is the best way to ensure that patients receive no contradictory or unwanted information?

_____

_____

_____

_____

Internet Exercise

Find three Web sites for one condition (e.g., breast cancer, Type II diabetes), and review how each describes the condition. Contrast the descriptions based on:

- Level of detail
- Language
- Tone

Think about how a newly diagnosed patient might react to each description you found. How could each description help the patient better understand the condition? How could each description confuse or upset the patient?

_____

_____

_____

_____

_____

_____

_____

_____

CHAPTER 2

Recognizing Initial Coping Styles

OVERVIEW

After reading this chapter, you should be able to:

- Define and use the keywords of initial coping styles.

- Understand how patients react to medical diagnoses, beginning with initial shock and followed by a flight, freeze, or fight reaction.

- Recognize the behavioral and emotional cues to patient reactions.

- Understand how diagnosis reactions can impact treatment decisions and patient coping.

- Know how to best communicate with patients who react in varied ways.

KEYWORDS

Body language	Freeze	Panic
Consciously suppressing	Helplessness	Paraphrasing
Empowered	Hopelessness	Process
Fight	Intellectualize	Shock
Flight	Numbness	

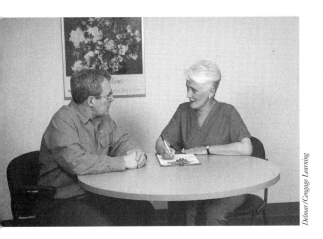

Delmar/Cengage Learning

Case Study

When John's ophthalmologist, Dr. Aldrich, told him he had glaucoma, he had no immediate response other than to look down at the floor and slowly shake his head.

Dr. Aldrich had given this diagnosis many times before and was comfortable talking with patients about their emotions, so she waited a few moments. She knew John would need some time to let the news sink in.

After a few moments of silence, Dr. Aldrich continued. "I know this is unexpected," she said. "It must be a shock to you."

In response, John simply nodded.

"Do you have any questions?" Dr. Aldrich asked.

"Not now," John answered. "I think this is probably all I need to know at this point."

"Well, I'd like to get you started on a medication," Dr. Aldrich continued. "You'll need to take it every day to keep the pressure down. Other patients have responded well to this treatment, and I don't see any reason why you won't, too."

"Okay," John replied. "Whatever you say."

Although Dr. Aldrich wanted to talk with John further about his condition and his treatment, she could see he would be unable to make any more progress at this point. John was clearly too closed down emotionally to talk further. Instead of pressing for

---

KEEP IN MIND

Silence is a normal and necessary part of patient exchanges, particularly when diagnoses are unexpected. Are you comfortable with silence? Could you sit with a patient in silence for a few moments like Dr. Aldrich, or would you feel the need to intervene? If you felt the need to intervene, would you be able to identify why? Would it be something about the silence? The patient? You?

John's understanding, the physician handed her patient a prescription and briefly explained what a diagnosis of glaucoma might mean, especially if left untreated. Finally, she explained to John the treatment plan.

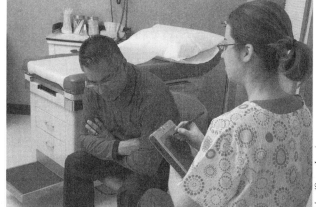

John mumbled a few words about following up and then hurried out of Dr. Aldrich's office.

Michele, an optometric technician working outside the consultation room, noticed John's state of mind as he exited and decided to catch up with him before he left the building. Michele was somewhat prepared for John's reaction, because she had talked with Dr. Aldrich before the appointment and had been told by Dr. Aldrich that she had planned to deliver the diagnosis during John's appointment. Dr. Aldrich had suggested to Michele that she might check in with John to see how he was feeling emotionally, and to see if he had any additional questions that he would need to have answered, before John left the office.

"John," Michele called down the office hall as the patient strode away. "Is there anything I can help you with?"

"No," John mumbled over his shoulder. "Not right now."

Michele's experience as an optometric technician working with newly diagnosed patients had taught her that John would need time to both move past the initial shock of his diagnosis and to **process** his emotional reaction. Michele also knew that, while John was doing those two things, he would be unable to articulate his thoughts or feelings beyond a sense of **numbness**.

Michele also knew something else: From a medical standpoint, it was important for John to acknowledge his diagnosis, understand his condition, and start a treatment regimen to prevent any further damage to his eyes. Michele knew that Dr. Aldrich would have made all of this clear to John, including the possibility that, without treating his condition, he could lose his sight. From John's demeanor now, however, Michele knew the patient had been unprepared to hear all the information the physician wanted to share.

Like Dr. Aldrich, Michele was concerned that, if John was unable face the emotions around his diagnosis and did not become proactive about his health, he might take no responsibility for his treatment. Once the initial shock wore off, Michele knew John would react in the ways human beings do with traumatic events: flight, freeze, or fight. She also knew that John's reaction would have implications for what kind of a patient he would be and the kinds of help he would need going forward with his treatment.

"John," Michele asked, "Do you mind if I give you a call in a couple of days?"

Introduction

"Suddenly, it was like time stood still."

Receiving a medical diagnosis is stressful. Regardless of the diagnosis, or how the patient perceives it, the patient usually—and immediately—feels uncertainty: Life may never be quite the same.

Our minds and bodies are hardwired to react to stressful events. As the initial shock fades, it gives way to one of three stress-response reactions: flight, freeze, or fight. The **flight** response is primarily emotional. Patients may be so caught up in their emotions that they may be unable to make objective decisions about their conditions and treatments. The **freeze** response, in contrast, is largely unemotional. Those reacting this way may be unable to acknowledge their feelings at all, or they may have fatalistic views. Either option may cause patient inaction. **Fight** is the ideal response in that patients responding this way can harness both their emotions and their resources as tools for facing their conditions. Nearly all patients can be taught to be fighters. Those who cannot may continuously erect barriers to treatment compliance and life management.

In addition to impacting the kinds of emotions and challenges newly diagnosed patients experience, the basic reactions of flight, freeze, and fight affect how patients cope with their emotions and confront their diagnoses. Patients' coping strategies during those first few days and weeks after diagnosis have implications throughout the treatment process—from treatment decision making and information-gathering to recovery and life management.

For health-care professionals, understanding and recognizing how patients react to diagnoses can benefit patient and health-care professional alike. For patients, the flight, freeze, and fight reactions are signposts to their readiness to receive information. For health-care professionals, the stress-response reactions are guides to presenting information in ways that are most receptive to patients. For example, patients in flight reaction may need additional emotional support, while those in freeze reaction may need help optimistically interpreting what they read and hear. Fighter patients, for their part, may ask a lot of questions for which the health-care team must be prepared.

> **KEEP IN MIND**
>
> We have all been momentarily thrown off guard upon reading or experiencing something highly unpleasant. For the patient, this unpleasant event might be receiving a medical diagnosis. When you experienced an unpleasant event, how did you react? How does your reaction relate to that of a theoretical patient receiving a shocking medical diagnosis?

Identifying the First Reaction: No or Numb Reaction

When newly diagnosed with any health conditions, whether catastrophic or relatively mild, patients almost invariably describe their reactions with single words: shock, numbness, disbelief, emptiness. Patients' shock is often accompanied by a sense that they must keep their emotions at bay lest those emotions overwhelm them.

The initial shock of a diagnosis may last moments, hours, or days, or it may persist long term as the patient struggles to balance emotions with rational thought. Those who have been diagnosed may recall their first reactions—or nonreactions—to the unexpected information, or they may have felt helpless as they watched a friend or family member experience the struggle.

Carole described her reaction upon first being diagnosed with cancer:

"It was like the world suddenly stood still. I mean, all I could hear was my own breathing and the thumping of my heart. At first, I was completely numb, and I wasn't thinking anything. Then, I started saying the word cancer *over and over. Still, no feelings emerged. But deep inside, I realized that, no matter what, my life was never going to be the same."*

In a way, delivery of a medical diagnosis, while not usually a death sentence, is like news of a death. As Carole described, news of her diagnosis ended life as she knew it. Newly diagnosed patients like Carole learn that bad things can happen, that they are not invincible. They also learn that the reality of a diagnosis is inevitable. At some point, the diagnosis will require the patient's acknowledgement and full attention. This looming eventuality, much like their emotions, can initially overwhelm patients.

Sometimes, the nature of a diagnosis can make it less overwhelming. When a condition is recurring, for example, or when ongoing symptoms render a diagnosis inevitable, patients may feel initially that "the other shoe has finally dropped" or that they are on a road they have been on before. In these cases, patients are less surprised by news of their conditions, but they are still susceptible to some level of shock. After all, it is human nature to cling to the belief that "it won't happen to me." When it does happen, there can ultimately be no denial.

During the time of initial shock, regardless of its magnitude, patients often need time and patience. As discussed in Chapter 1, health-care professionals should give patients time to sit with, and absorb, their diagnoses. Health-care professionals who push patients too hard or too fast to discuss treatment plans or make treatment decisions risk patients who become defensive and potentially even more resistant to communication. Human beings cannot be forced to take in more information than they can process, and newly diagnosed patients are often initially closed off to information and its implications.

Of course, health-care professionals must balance sensitivity to patients with the medical level of urgency. Providers may need to start patients on medication or treatment regimens immediately. To ensure patients receive the proper level of care and information at the appropriate times, it may be useful to schedule follow-up appointments.

Recovering from the Initial Shock

Accepting that life is going to change is the first step toward coping with the emotional impact of a medical diagnosis. It is also the first step toward making decisions.

Most newly diagnosed patients take this step, albeit at different times and in different ways. Some, unfortunately, never take it at all. All patients, however, must confront their diagnoses on some level and move forward. Once the initial **shock** starts to abate, the common next steps are the three stress-response reactions discussed previously: flight, freeze, or fight (Table 2.1).

TABLE 2.1   Initial Shock at Diagnosis

Flight	Freeze	Fight
Positive but unrealistic thinking	Isolation	Empowerment
Rigidity	Helplessness	Emotional coping sills
		Rational thinking

Delmar/Cengage Learning

RESPONDING WITH FLIGHT: CHARGING FORWARD BLINDLY

The best way to introduce the flight response is through the case example of a newly diagnosed patient named Dante. An active man with no history of health problems, Dante was totally surprised by his diagnosis of a heart condition. His physician presented him with what she thought was the best recommendation, a triple bypass, and then suggested that Dante go home and do some thinking before making a decision about treatment.

Dante later reported that his sense of shock continued for a few days. He could not believe that he was in anything but top condition. His disbelief led him to tell his wife that he was fine and that his physician was merely monitoring his heart. Dante's wife was skeptical, but she knew better than to push Dante when he was not ready to talk. Dante described the next few days as follows:

> *"Once the numbness started to wear off, I kind of went into panic mode. It was like I had this thing around my heart, and I wanted it cut out as soon as possible. I was afraid to think, because I was afraid I might talk myself into doing nothing, or that I might put too much strain on my heart. I imagined my doctor as my savior. I wanted to put all my faith and trust in her and have her direct my path. I was in such a rush, I asked her to call the cardiologist she had recommended to try and influence him to schedule me for surgery as soon as possible."*

Dante's response reflects the flight reaction in a couple of ways. First, he placed all his trust in the first physician he encountered. Second, he immediately gravitated to the treatment he felt most expedient. Because he was focused on immediacy, he did not consider the treatment's implications—its side effects, recovery time, and ongoing lifestyle management. As a result, he may later discover that he was unprepared for the treatment, a possibility that has implications for ongoing compliance as well as satisfaction with his health-care provider.

The flight reaction has other implications as well. Patients who react this way may, out of a sense of **panic**, run toward unproven, alternative treatments with potentially alarming consequences. They may also be susceptible to the recommendations of health-care providers with whom they feel comfortable emotionally but who may offer suboptimal treatment options. Enamored by the value they are believed to deliver, patients in flight reaction may profess to "love" their practitioners. Like falling head-over-heels in love, the flight reaction leaves no room for second opinions, other treatment options, or research into physicians' credentials and track records. The flight reaction can inspire such strong emotional responses—excessive crying, anger expressions, fearfulness episodes—that patients sometimes cannot access their logical sides. They can focus only on running from their diagnoses.

FREEZING: FAILING TO REACT

Not all patients take flight toward the first available treatment. Some take no flight at all. They freeze instead. They sit and stare into space, literally and figuratively, waiting for the nightmare to pass, or for someone, often a family member, to step in and take charge. Between the shock of the diagnosis, the perception that they are unprepared to make the decisions suddenly thrust upon them, and a sense of hopelessness, patients who react this way are essentially immobilized.

When in freeze mode, the emotions appear to stop working, not because they are broken but because they are being tightly held in place. While this might be an opportunity for a patient's rational side to take charge, logic without emotion is not necessarily going to inspire rational thinking, as evidenced by Joaquin, who recounts his diagnosis reaction as follows:

> *"I just sat there when the doctor told me, and I guess I'm still just sitting still. I can hardly get out of the chair, to tell you the truth. I kind of decided to be philosophical about it. I don't know much about this, but I do know that, statistically, the numbers are against me. I mean, what can I do when fate isn't on my side?"*

Joaquin is typical of patients in freeze reaction: He refused to react emotionally or to become actively involved in learning about his condition and its treatment. Unfortunately, **consciously suppressing** the emotions this way also means giving up.

Essentially, the freeze reaction is an extension of the original feeling of shock. Shock is the mind's way of shutting down the emotions and allowing the brain to process the information before reacting. Patients in freeze reaction give in to rational thinking based on their view of the facts.

Allowing the logical mind to operate without the emotions this way is risky, however. Because patients in freeze reaction operate without their emotional sides, they may be at risk for an attitude of **hopelessness** and **helplessness**. They do not allow themselves to work through emotions like anger and fear, which patients generally experience upon initial diagnosis. They simply miss that experience. Often, patients in freeze reaction discuss their conditions with health-care professionals only as absolutely necessary, and they may avoid telling family members for as long as possible. Whereas patients in flight reaction give in to their emotions completely, at the expense of rational thinking, patients in freeze reaction fail to acknowledge their emotions at all, which leaves them stuck in avoidance and isolation.

One common characteristic of patients in freeze mode is an unwillingness to make decisions about their treatment. They rely on their physicians, and possibly their family members, to do so. In short, patients like this decide not to decide.

FIGHTING BACK: BALANCING EMOTION AND LOGIC

Being open to emotions can create a sense of hope and optimism. When optimism is balanced with rational thinking—when patients adopt the fight reaction—they are best positioned to make treatment decisions, address treatment and lifestyle changes effectively, and otherwise cope with changes and challenges

The term *fight* does not necessarily imply fighting in the literal sense, in the sense of taking up arms, which sometimes has a negative connotation. Being a fighter means being **empowered**: understanding the diagnosis, identifying options for treatment, and recognizing what lifestyle adjustments must be made. Being empowered means mobilizing emotional coping skills as well as rational-thinking ones.

Fighters acknowledge, and continue to honor, the emotions that arose upon hearing the diagnosis. Fear may never fade away. Anger and disappointment may flare up. When acknowledged and experienced, emotions like fear and anger may give way to hope, optimism, and a renewed passion for life.

Marie explained it the following way:

> *"I sat and cried and asked 'Why me?' for quite a while, maybe a few days. Then I stood up and said, 'I'm going to fight this beast. I'm not going to let it beat me down.' The next day, I made a list of people I needed to talk to, places I needed to go for information, and things I needed to start planning for. This doesn't mean I don't feel overwhelmed sometimes, because I still do. But I'm now in active mode."*

Instead of suppressing her emotions, Marie faced her disappointment and fear. She sat alone with her emotions and had a good cry. She also discussed her emotional reactions with a member of her health-care team, someone who was comfortable being a "listening ear." Had she not taken the time to experience how she was feeling, Marie would have been forced to sit with a large block of emotion, and it would have drained all her mental energy. Instead, she was able to start asking questions and making decisions. She was able to start being productive.

Patients in fight reaction are more prepared than other patients to confront their conditions. With the self-confidence that comes from being aware of, and open to, emotions, fighters search for, and accurately process, information. They are more likely to ask questions and evaluate alternatives, because they can access their rational minds. Fighters' balance of emotion and logic cultivates an attitude of empowerment toward health care and the professionals who deliver it. Fighters are not in perfect balance every day, but they have the tools, and the partners, to continue trying.

For some patients, the fight attitude comes naturally; it is simply how they react to their diagnoses once they move beyond their initial shock. However, these patients sometimes challenge their health-care teams, because they believe they are ultimately responsible for decisions regarding things like information sources, treatment alternatives, and lifestyle adjustments. Upcoming chapters describe both why fighters are most likely to have successful outcomes and how health-care professionals can cultivate the fight instinct in their patients.

KEEP IN MIND

Before they start facing the reality of their diagnoses and develop strategies for moving forward, fighters must often have good cries and talk to friends and family about their feelings. How have you faced unexpected news in your life? Have you ever felt that you could not face a challenge, that if you just ignored the hurdle, it would go away? Or did you find yourself seeking a quick solution to try to put the challenge behind you as soon as possible?

Recognizing Patient Reactions

The health-care team can greatly benefit from recognizing the reactions of patients to their diagnoses. As discussed previously, patients in flight, freeze, and fight reactions have widely differing orientations to their conditions, perceptions of control, and willingness to be involved in their medical destinies. Health-care professionals who are sensitive to these differences can leverage patients' strengths and weaknesses as they approach diagnosis and treatment. Specifically, understanding patient reactions can help health-care professionals:

- Present information on conditions and treatments
- Coach patients through treatment
- Recommend lifestyle-management actions
- Encourage support in daily living activities
- Monitor ongoing compliance

Working with Patients in Flight Reaction

Essentially, the flight reaction is recognizable based on the presence of pronounced emotionality. While it is important for patients to express their emotions in ways that are consistent with their personal styles and comfort levels, patients in flight basically become "stuck" in their emotions, unable to entertain information or options.

As a result, patients with the flight reaction provide a range of challenges for the health-care team. Flight patients who become singularly focused on their courses of treatment can initially be easy to work, because they are motivated and compliant. However, this single-mindedness can cause rigidity, such that the patients reject any information interpreted as counter to their chosen courses of action, and they may be less open to changing direction or exploring other options. In fact, patients in flight may become so profoundly disappointed as to become discouraged and, given their emotional state, irrational (Table 2.2).

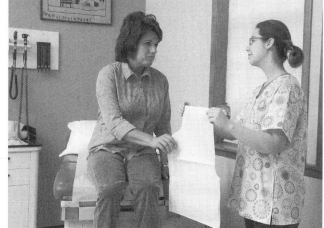

Patients in flight who are simply overcome by their emotions and unable to cope with the reality of their conditions pose a different set of challenges for health-care professionals. These patients may become so overwrought that they are, at least temporarily, unreachable. Information about the diagnosis or suggestions for treatment tend to fall on deaf ears.

Fortunately, the emotional energy of flight patients can be channeled into an enthusiastic attitude toward treatment. The key is to gently encourage a sense of reality, both so that expectations remain realistic and to avoid the extreme disappointment that can result when patients in flight reaction fail to experience what they expected from their treatment.

KEYS TO COMMUNICATING WITH PATIENTS IN FLIGHT REACTION

Paraphrase. **Paraphrasing** patients' statements strengthens your connections with those patients and deepens your understanding of them. The process of paraphrasing is really two steps. First, listen carefully to what the patient is saying. Second, briefly tell the patient what you think you just heard them say. Make it clear that your paraphrases are attempts at comprehension only, not attempts to tell the patients how to think or feel. Connect your paraphrases to feeling words.

Examples:

"It sounds like you've talked with your doctor about your potential treatment options, and it all sounds depressing."

"So your understanding is that you will see results quickly, and you won't experience any side effects. Is that right?"

"This is all feeling so bleak to you that you don't even want to talk about it, do you?"

TABLE 2.2 A Patient in Flight Reaction

Overarching Theme: Caught up in emotions

1. Running Toward	Positive thinking, but blind to reality
	"This is my only hope."
Consequences	Avoidance of information perceived as threatening to the chosen path
	Overexpectation of the treatment experience and its benefits, which can cause extreme disappointment, or denial, when treatment fails to meet expectations
Behaviors	Elation bordering on mania regarding "miracle" course of action
	Refusal to listen to alternatives
	Anger when others are perceived as being negative
2. Running Away	Descent into emotions bordering on irrationality
	"Please leave me alone. I can't face this."
Consequences	Refusal to accept the diagnosis and embark on a beneficial treatment path
	Emotional distress may contribute to physical symptoms
Behaviors	Extreme sadness, crying, heaviness similar to inconsolable grief
	Avoidance of others, which may lead to isolation

Delmar/Cengage Learning

Acknowledge emotions.   Patients in flight reaction are receptive to acknowledgement of their emotions. "Feeling" words like *frustrated*, *angry*, *excited*, and *positive* signal that you are attuned to your patients' feelings and are open to knowing more. Reflect back to patients the feelings that you heard them describe, as any feelings that you detect in their voice or their facial expressions.

Examples:

"So you're really upset about this."

"You're pretty excited about getting started."

"You aren't sure where to turn right now."

Explore expectations.   Patients in flight are highly sensitive to any suggestion that they are heading in the wrong direction in terms of treatment, outcome, or ongoing lifestyle management. Therefore, they are likely to view any questions or comments that are contrary to their positions as negative or argumentative, which increases their defensiveness. To counteract this effect, ask open, nonjudgmental questions.

Examples:

"What's ahead for you at this point?"

"How do you see this treatment working?"

"What's your doctor telling you?"

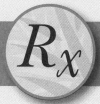 ## Working with Patients in Flight Reaction

While in the medical office, Dante, the patient described previously as having a flight reaction, spoke with Tom, a member of his health-care team. Fortunately, Tom recognized Dante's flight reaction and spoke with him in a way that eased any defensiveness and promoted information exchange.

TOM: How are you doing, Dante?

DANTE: How am I doing? How do you *think* I'm doing? I've just been told I'm going to die if I don't get some help right away. How would you be if you were me?

TOM: Sounds like you're feeling pretty scared about your diagnosis, Dante. I can understand why.

DANTE: Of course I'm scared. I've got to get this thing fixed before it kills me.

TOM: Okay, Dante. You have a lot of highly skilled professionals here who are watching over you closely.

DANTE: Don't I know that! I really love Dr. Costa. She's taken good care of me for the last 10 years. She's sending me to a Dr. Jacobs, a cardiologist who's one of the best in the country. I know this is soon going to be behind me.

TOM: Wow, one of the best cardiologists in the country?

DANTE: I can't imagine that Dr. Costa would send me to someone who wasn't the absolute best in his field.

TOM: So it sounds like you have a lot confidence in Dr. Jacobs. What's the next step?

DANTE: I meet with Dr. Jacobs next week. I know he'll want to operate right away, and that's what I want, too. I expect to be fully back to my life in a month or so.

TOM: What's Dr. Costa told you about that?

DANTE: I told you already. Dr. Jacobs is an excellent cardiologist. I know she'll give him a call and have him push up my surgery. I wouldn't be surprised if I ended up going in for it later next week. No time like the present, I've always said. And if I don't have faith in the people who are helping me, then I may as well give up.

TOM: So Dr. Costa is referring you to someone she trusts, Dr. Jacobs, and you're anxious to get going. Is that right?

DANTE: Exactly. I can't afford to think negative.

TOM: You've really got a positive attitude here, Dante. I'm certainly not going to argue that with you. And like I mentioned before, you've got some very good people on your case. But I was wondering if it might be useful to sit down and talk about the process that people with your diagnosis generally go through. You know, like how cardiologists generally work with their patients and the recovery process after surgery. Would that be useful?

DANTE: I'm not expecting anything less than a miracle! That's the only way I can get through this. That's why I'm so excited about getting started.

TOM: I'm not suggesting you won't have a good outcome, Dante. I just wanted to suggest that we go over a few things so that you'll have a better idea how this process usually works.

DANTE: Well . . . I guess we could talk a little bit. But I'm only allowing positive people to come through my door today.

TOM: You can count on me as a member of the positive team!

Offer consistent and gentle references to reality.   Patients in flight reaction can benefit from gentle references to realistic treatment expectations and outcomes, but because they are highly attached to their emotional reactions, they become resistant when they perceive that health-care professionals are not acknowledging or respecting their feelings. Therefore, present references to reality as suggestions, rather than statements. In addition, ask patients if they are interested in hearing how other patients have experienced their condition and its treatment.

Examples:

"I've worked with a lot of other patients who have felt like you about their condition. Would you be interested in hearing about some of their experiences?"

"I know you're feeling totally alone here. But I can tell you about some of the options you have."

"It's certainly understandable that you would be hopeful. That attitude is really going to help you to get through your treatment. To help you further, I have a couple of ideas you might want to consider."

Working with Patients in Freeze Reaction

Patients who seem to have no emotional responses to their diagnoses may be having freeze reactions. Such patients can express emotions, but the shock of their diagnoses prompts them to suppress their reactions out of fear they will become overwhelmed by their feelings and lose control.

Patients in freeze reaction are difficult for health-care professionals to reach for two key reasons. First, they are not open to discussing their conditions, which can frustrate the team members responsible for treatment planning and compliance. Second, patients like these have such low levels of optimism for their treatment plans that they

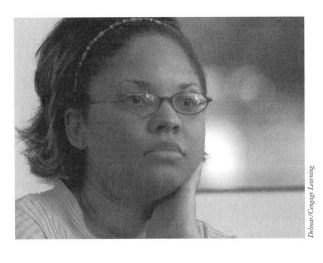

Delmar/Cengage Learning

most likely see no need to participate in them. If they do, they do so minimally and without motivation.

Patients in freeze reaction may **intellectualize** their conditions. While they might be willing to discuss the facts, unfortunately they are often willing only to consider their own viewpoints, which are usually based less on information and more on information avoidance. Consequently, patients in freeze reaction tend to have limited, bleak outlooks or no desire to be involved in their treatments. The result in an uphill journey for the health-care team. As mentioned earlier, the first step to a successful medical outcome is accepting the diagnosis and working with health-care professionals to identify and implement an optimal treatment strategy.

Like freeze patients who intellectualize, patients in freeze reaction who retreat are hard to reach. Rather than intellectualize, they may act like victims. They refuse to take any responsibility for decision making or treatment, shut down emotionally, and wait for someone else to take charge. A sense of helplessness may drive patients like these to resist the assistance of family members, however. In response, families may ask their health-care teams to act as mediators, which is an uncomfortable position and likely unproductive (Table 2.3).

TABLE 2.3   A Patient in Freeze Reaction

Overarching Theme: Emotionally shut down, fatalistic

1. Intellectualizing	Avoidance of discussing the condition with anyone, perhaps limited discussions with the physician
	"I'm not going to sit around and wring my hands about this."
Consequences	Lack of information-seeking behaviors
	Holding in emotions, which hampers the ability to accept the diagnosis
	Lack of emotional support
Behaviors	Refusal to discuss the diagnosis
	Citing statistics and/or limited medical facts, usually in support of the futility of treatment and a negative outcome
	Using "I think" to the exclusion of "I feel"
2. Hopelessness	Immobilized by the prospect of having the condition
	"I can't deal with this."
Consequences	Avoidance of discussion about the condition
	Passively allows the physician or family members to step in and make decisions
	May be noncompliant with treatment due to lack of optimism or motivation
Behaviors	Emotionally disconnected or flat
	Refuses to participate in discussion about the diagnosis
	May cease other activities and essentially shut down

Delmar/Cengage Learning

KEYS TO COMMUNICATING WITH PATIENTS IN FREEZE REACTION

Use "thinking" words.   Because patients in freeze reaction are emotionally shut down, they resist references to feelings and use of the word *feel*. For greater compliance, use the word *think* when discussing the patient's condition.

Examples:

"What do you think are your options?"

"What are you thinking as I talk about this approach to your treatment?"

"Can you give me some of your thoughts?"

Paraphrase.   For a patient in freeze reaction, a paraphrase demonstrates you are listening, you acknowledge the struggle for self-expression, and you are open to the patient's thoughts. Respecting patients' perceptions and opinions subtly encourages those patients to open up. Over time, paraphrasing may help patients see how they are avoiding their feelings and restricting their options for treating their conditions.

Examples:

"At this point, you don't see any reason to think you can be treated effectively?"

"So you're telling me you don't want to be involved in making decisions about how you might modify your lifestyle?"

"You remember reading about your condition a few years ago, and what you read about the treatment wasn't so encouraging."

Model the use of feeling words.   Patients in freeze reaction suppress their feelings, often out of a fear of losing control, but feeling words in other contexts may reach them. For example, health-care professionals can express how they might feel in similar situations. Stories about how other patients have reacted emotionally, and how they coped, can subtly communicate that patients can have emotional reactions to their diagnoses and cope effectively. It is important, however, to be sensitive to patient resistance and to avoid pushing too hard.

Examples:

"I know this must all feel really overwhelming. At least, that's how I would be feeling at this point."

"I have another patient who had the same diagnosis at your age. He was really freaked out—scared and angry—but he reached out and got a lot of support. Now, he's doing well with his treatment."

"Sometimes people just want to sit and feel sad for awhile. That's normal."

Offer gentle invitations to talk about feelings.   Patients in freeze reaction may need to give themselves permission to feel. If they perceive their health-care professionals are comfortable with emotions, they may decide they can open up safely. Let these patients know you can refer them for additional mental health assistance if, and when, they feel overwhelmed.

Examples:

"Do you want to talk to me about how this is affecting you emotionally?"

"I want to reassure you it is normal to have a lot of feelings when someone is going through a situation like this. If you want to talk about how you feel, I'm ready to listen."

"If at any time you feel overwhelmed by your feelings, I can put you in touch with someone who is trained to help you."

KEEP IN MIND

Tread gently, and stay open. Patients who are having trouble getting in touch with their emotions, or thinking rationally, tend to respond poorly when told how they should react, regardless of intention. Use your instincts, and the skills you learned in this chapter, when you approach patients who are in crisis over medical diagnoses. Make suggestions, but be ready to retreat when patients resist. Avoid approaching patients with expectations regarding how they might, or should, be reacting to their diagnoses. Assume nothing. When you learn from patients, you will be able to better reach them.

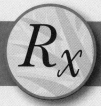 # Working with Patients in Freeze Reaction

Joaquin, the patient quoted in the freeze reaction section earlier in this chapter, was so overwhelmed at the news of his condition that he had basically given up on his treatment before he even got started. Upon recognizing this, Michael, a member of Joaquin's health-care team, sat down to talk with Joaquin about his diagnosis.

MICHAEL: Hey, Joaquin. I hear the doctor gave you some news this morning. How are you doing?

JOAQUIN: How am I doing, or what am I doing? The answer is about the same for both questions. I'm a complete zero.

MICHAEL: What does that mean?

JOAQUIN: It means what it sounds like. The stats are against me.

MICHAEL: What did the doctor say about next steps?

JOAQUIN: I don't really remember if we talked about that. But the key point here is that I have a condition that is life-threatening any way you want to look at it. I'm not stupid, and I'm not going to sit and wring my hands over it. I know the deal here.

MICHAEL: Sounds like you've done some research on your own. Have you?

JOAQUIN: I don't need to do a bunch of research. Anybody knows what my diagnosis means. It means death.

MICHAEL: So you're kind of familiar with your condition and have an idea of what your diagnosis means.

JOAQUIN: That's right. So let's not sit here and complain about it.

MICHAEL: How are you feeling about all this?

JOAQUIN: It's like I told you. I'm not going to weep and wail about reality.

MICHAEL: Okay, Joaquin. I understand your thinking here. Do you want to talk about next steps?

JOAQUIN: I don't think there's a lot to discuss, like I've been trying to explain to you. The doctor is going to recommend what he's going to recommend.

MICHAEL: So you're thinking you don't have a lot of options here.

JOAQUIN: Really, I don't want to deal with this by doing a lot of talking. What's going to happen is going to happen. It's not about what I want.

MICHAEL: Well, like I said, you have a right to your opinions. But I can tell you that there are some options here, as the doctor outlined for you. With your permission, I'd like to go over them with you. I know you don't want to think about this a lot, but it might help give you a clearer picture of what's available to you in terms of treatment.

JOAQUIN: My doctor will tell me what to do.

MICHAEL: I'm sure he can recommend the best course of action. But maybe I can help you get ready for that discussion.

JOAQUIN: I don't know. . . .

MICHAEL: You don't have to talk about this with me if you don't want to, Joaquin. But I wanted to let you know I'm around.

JOAQUIN: Okay. I'll think about it.

Working with Patients in Fight Reaction

Health-care professionals describe patients in fight reaction as joys and inspirations. They are informed, motivated, and willing to take responsibility for their treatment.

From this perspective, the fight reaction is a mentally healthy response to a medical diagnosis. Patients have access to their emotions and are willing and able to talk about them. To provide these types of patients the proper support, health-care professionals must feel comfortable discussing emotions, and they must be prepared with information. Fighters often have many questions about their treatment, and they may have suggestions for alternate medications and remedies. They may also have ideas, based on research, about the best ways to change their day-to-day lifestyles. As questions and suggestions arise, health-care professionals must not only provide answers, they must provide rationales. To avoid the defensiveness that can arise from working with highly educated, opinionated patients, health-care providers must be comfortable with assertive patients, as well as fully informed.

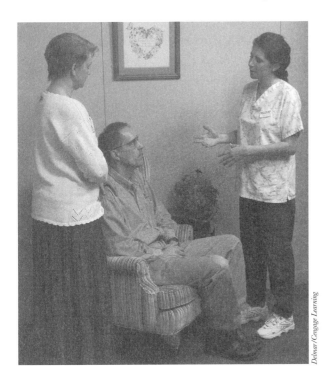

Delmar/Cengage Learning

If there is a negative side to the fight reaction, it is that fighters can at times be overconfident. They may assume they know so much about their conditions and their treatments that they need no support from medical experts. When they feel they need information, they may demand evidence that is not readily available. In addition to frustrating their health-care providers, behaviors like these can cause unnecessary delays when patients continue to insist on doing further research, evaluating treatment options, and demanding further discussion when it is critical that treatment be initiated as soon as possible. Fighters may develop a "go it alone" mentality that can isolate them from the support they need to easily complete day-to-day tasks. Without adequate support, fighters can take too much on and, consequently, have too little energy to heal (Table 2.4).

KEYS TO COMMUNICATING WITH PATIENTS IN FIGHT REACTION

Acknowledge that the patients are in control. Fighters pride themselves on taking responsibility for their health care, and they expect their health-care providers to respect their role. While this attitude can sometimes frustrate and anger providers, providers should not challenge this position directly. After all, the benefits of working with empowered patients greatly outweigh the occasional control issues that may arise.

Examples:

"You're in charge here."

"The decision is ultimately up to you."

TABLE 2.4   A Patient in Fight Reaction

Overarching Theme: Empowerment through an emotion/logic balance

Ongoing Coping	Good days and bad days, but staying focused on the future
	"I'm going to do what I have to do to get through this."
Consequences	In touch with emotions and able to express them
	Active information-gatherer
	Self-perception as the final decision-maker and responsible party for ongoing lifestyle management
	Attitude of independence may at times be unproductive; may not ask for needed support and may insist on a treatment path that may conflict with the recommendations of the primary physician
Behaviors	Emotionally expressive
	Brings questions and Web hard copy to appointments
	Insists that health-care providers support their recommendations

Delmar/Cengage Learning

Don't think you always have to have the answers.   Fighters may be all over the Web, on the sites of support groups offering discussion boards on the latest, often experimental, treatments. Because they research their conditions and their treatments so heavily, these patients may encounter information that is new to their health-care providers. As patients have questions on emerging information, do not hesitate to say you have no answers. Offer to investigate the information and/or to use your own sources to find the answers. As another option, direct patients to resources that can offer the information the patients want and need.

Examples:

"I haven't been asked that question before, and I don't want to answer it until I have given it some thought. I will follow up with you."

"Where did you see that information? Why don't you give me the resource, and I'll read through it and give you my thoughts."

"I don't have that answer, but I can recommend a good resource that I have used and also recommend to patients with these kinds of questions."

Offer suggestions.   Given that fighters want to feel that they are in control, they may resist the directives of the health-care team. Remember that the directive approach is appropriate for patients in freeze reaction. For fighters, offer suggestions and let them make their own choices. Even if you have only one option to offer, make it clear that that there is more than one possible outcome, depending on whether the patient accepts the suggestion or not.

Examples:

"I can't tell you what to do here, but I'd like to give you some ideas for you to consider."

"I can tell you about some of the experiences of other patients in your situation."

"You have the ultimate decision here, but I'd like to suggest what might occur if you decide to say no."

Don't be afraid to identify your concerns.   While they are assertive when communicating with health-care professionals, fighters generally accept assertive behavior as well. If you sense fighter patients are going down the wrong path, do not hesitate to tell them so. Be ready to support your assertions with information and, when possible, evidence. These patients will appreciate that only some aspects of their treatment and ongoing care are negotiable.

Examples:

"I have to be honest with you. I don't think this is the best decision, and I'll tell you why."

"The alternative you're talking about just doesn't make any sense to me based on my experiences with other patients."

"Can we talk about this? I want to share some concerns with you."

Encourage fighters to ask for help when they need it.   Fighters can sometimes become independent to an extreme, to the point that they fail to ask for practical or emotional support when they need it. For example, fighters may attempt to perform daily tasks like housework while recovering from treatment, thinking they will be energized by the activity or an example of what it means to be in charge. Members of the health-care team can be instrumental both in gently suggesting the value of adequate support during treatment and recovery, and in offering to brainstorm support options.

Examples:

"You're really taking a lot on when your body needs time for rest and recovery. Don't you think you could use some temporary help here?"

"I know you're managing all of this really well. But I also think it would be helpful to sit down and talk to someone on a regular basis, just to help you let off some steam."

"I know you aren't an invalid. But maybe we could come up with some ideas to get the yardwork handled by someone else while your body mends."

KEEP IN MIND

For some patients, the fight reaction comes naturally. For others, fighter skills can be taught. Teaching patients to fight is the overarching goal of this book. Do you believe patients are born fighters—or must they be taught? Guidelines and suggestions for bringing out the fighter in patients—and using fighter skills to enhance the relationship between patients and health-care professionals—appear in the chapters that follow.

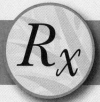 Working with Patients in Fight Reaction

Marie, the patient quoted in the fight reaction section earlier in this chapter, returned to her physician's office a few days after her diagnosis to begin discussing her treatment. While there, she met with Jonelle, a member of the health-care team, to discuss how they would work together once her treatment began.

JONELLE: Marie! How are you doing?

MARIE: Today? Not so bad. Over the weekend? Not so good.

JONELLE: I was concerned about you when you left the office last week. I knew your diagnosis had hit you like a ton of bricks and you weren't sure what to feel or think. What happened over the weekend?

MARIE: I called in sick on Friday and cancelled all my weekend plans with the lame excuse that I had to bring home work from the office. In actuality, I sat and stared into space for a couple of days. I didn't even turn the TV on. On Saturday afternoon, I had a good long cry and beat on a pillow for a while. I just felt so sad that this was happening to me, and then I was mad about how unfair it was.

JONELLE: So you really let yourself have your feelings. Was that helpful?

MARIE: You bet it was. Afterward, I felt like I could take a deep breath again. I said to myself, "I'm going to stomp this beast. I'm gonna fight back." I called my brother and told him the news. I listened to him cry for a few minutes, and then I said the same thing to him. And he said, "How can I help you?"

JONELLE: Fantastic! You powered yourself up. And you reached out for support. Those are all good things!

MARIE: Well, I'm not telling you I've turned into superwoman or anything. I woke up on Sunday morning with this dull ache in my stomach and the thought that I have a whole lot to deal with. And I'm not sure how I'm going to do it. I lay in bed and stared at the ceiling for a while and felt sorry for myself. Then, I answered that question, too. I'm going to do it one day at a time. I got out of bed and sat in front of the computer and got busy.

JONELLE: It's normal to have some dips in your feelings. As you experienced, you can have your feelings and then pick yourself up and move forward. So you did some research.

MARIE: Yes, I did. I had a whole list of questions for the doctor, and now I have a whole list for you. I am going to take some notes while we talk and then do some more research and talk to some other experts. I have a lot of work ahead of me.

JONELLE: Sounds good to me. Let the fact-finding begin!

Introducing Body Language

Humans experience emotions in various ways. They may try to hold them inside, out of a desire to prevent others from knowing how they feel or because they are uncomfortable. In contrast, they may discuss their feelings openly. Humans demonstrate their feelings in part through **body language**: the facial expressions, gestures, and postures that reflect emotions. For example, people who are sad may cry, hold their hands to their faces, and hang their heads. Angry people will have angry expressions, stand stances, and hands on the hips. Going forward in this book, each chapter discusses body language.

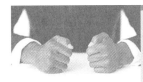

Body Language

Patients in flight, freeze, and fight reactions to their diagnoses all show their emotions through body language, as follows:

Flight Reaction
- Crying, rubbing eyes
- Holding hands to the face or limply at the sides
- Agitated, nervous gestures
- Rubbing hands

Freeze Reaction
- Sitting with legs and arms crossed
- Shoulders hunched
- Head resting in hands, looking downward
- Rigid posture
- No facial expression

Fight Reaction
- Straight, rigid posture
- Eye contact
- Hands on the hips
- Sitting with the legs apart

SUMMARY

Patients need time to experience the initial shock of their diagnoses. From shock, they react consistent with stress: flight, freeze, or fight. Recognizing how newly diagnosed patients react, and what it means for coping, can revolutionize the communication process between patients and health-care professionals. Using patient reactions, members of the health-care team can gauge how to present information, how to make recommendations, and how to react when encountering resistance to treatment compliance and lifestyle management.

Flight, Freeze, Fight: The Test

To help you determine whether a patient is having a flight, freeze, or fight reaction, administer the following brief test.

Preparing for the Test

Whether administered verbally or in paper-and-pencil format, this test can help health-care professionals gain insight into how patients are reacting to their diagnoses. Before administering the test, explain the following to the patient:

- These questions are only tools to help the health-care professional and the patient better understand how the patient is reacting to the medical diagnosis.
- This test does not assess knowledge and will in no way affect the patient's treatment.
- This test is not scientifically valid.
- The health-care professional and the patient will review the responses together, and the results will help them to communicate better.

The Test

How are you reacting to your—or your loved one's—diagnosis? Are you or yours having a fight, flight, or freeze reaction? Take the following test, and find out.

For each question, circle *T*, *L*, or *R*.

1. The best thing about having access to medical information is it:
   T   Presents treatment alternatives for my condition
   L   Identifies questions I can ask my doctor
   R   Helps me better understand the treatment my doctor selected

2. I would get a second opinion on a medical diagnosis:
   T   Always, even for common and easily treatable conditions
   R   When my doctor or insurance company recommended it
   L   Upon diagnosis with an unusual condition

3. If a doctor you know and trust recommended a treatment for a medical condition, which of the following most closely approximates how you would view the recommendation?
   L   My local doctor has experience treating this condition and knows me, so she knows what's best.
   T   The recommendation is an important consideration as I decide what I want to do.
   R   The first course of treatment doesn't really matter. If it doesn't go well, I can always try something else.

4. The downside of information on the Web is:

    L   Reading too much about poor prognoses or treatment side effects that may not apply to me can be discouraging.

    R   If you get conflicting information from different Web sites, you can end up not knowing what to believe.

    T   Some Web sites are really for medical professionals and can be hard for the layperson to understand.

5. Assume you are about to receive the results of a medical test. Which of the following best describes how you would prepare?

    R   Go on with my daily routine to keep focused on what matters.

    L   Get support from my family and friends to help me feel emotionally grounded.

    T   Read about treatments for the condition I am being tested for.

6. The treatment for a routine medical diagnosis:

    R   Is relatively standard based on established guidelines

    T   Should be trusted only to a highly regarded specialist

    L   Should be selected by my doctor, whom I have trusted in the past

7. A friend recommends a medication that differs from the one your doctor has prescribed. Which of the following most closely approximates your response?

    T   Do research to locate patients who are using the medication

    L   Ask my doctor to discuss personal experiences with the medication

    R   Listen to the friend but trust my doctor to recommend the best option

8. For someone dealing with a long-term illness, which of the following attitudes toward treatment is most important?

    R   Peace of mind

    T   Skepticism

    L   Optimism

9. If a friend was being treated for a serious medical condition, the first thing you would offer is:

    L   Listening ear

    T   List of medical Web sites

    R   Help around the house

10. If your regular doctor sent you to a specialist for treatment of a serious condition, how would you decide whether this specialist was right for you?

    L   Talk with the specialist to make sure I feel that I can develop a relationship

    T   Talk with the specialist to understand his approach to treating my condition

    R   Talk with the specialist to gain reassurance that she is working closely with my doctor

Count the Number of T, L, and R responses for Questions 1–10.

    T _____

    L _____

    R _____

Mostly T responses: Fight

Mostly L responses: Freeze

Mostly R responses: Flight

Based on the responses, the patient is in _____ reaction.

Following Up the Test

After the patient has answered the questions and the test has been scored, do the following:

1. Briefly review the test, reassuring the patient that it is only a tool to help the health-care professional and the patient communicate better about the patient's diagnosis. Remind the patient that this test is not scientifically valid, that the patient is not being diagnosed in any way, and that the results are not being entered into the patient's chart.

2. Briefly explain the three reactions patients have to diagnoses: flight, freeze, and fight. Be sure to emphasize that these are normal human reactions to stressful events and that, as such, none are good or bad.

3. Share the test results with the patient. Ask the patient to respond based on an understanding of the three reactions.

4. Review the patient's responses, focusing on those that contributed to the determination of the patient's reaction.

5. Discuss what this means going forward. Focus on what the two of you can do together to help the patient cope with the diagnosis and its treatment.

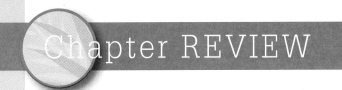

Multiple-Choice Questions

1. The shock patients experience when they are initially diagnosed generally lasts:
   a. Up to 1 hour
   b. 1 to 2 days
   c. Until the patient has had time to process the information emotionally
   d. Until the patient becomes fully informed about the condition

2. Patients who refuse to accept their diagnoses and make treatment decisions are most likely experiencing the _____ reaction.
   a. Freeze   c. Fright
   b. Flight   d. Fight

3. Patients who react to their diagnoses by blindly attaching to their physicians and insisting on thinking positive are most likely in _____ reaction.
   a. Freeze   c. Fright
   b. Flight   d. Fight

4. Patients who react to their diagnoses with determination to be in charge of their own treatment decisions are most likely in _____ reaction.
   a. Freeze   c. Fright
   b. Flight   d. Fight

5. Which of the following is *not* recommended when talking with a patient in flight reaction?
   a. Acknowledge emotions   c. Offer gentle references to reality
   b. Model the use of feeling words   d. Explore treatment expectations

Fill-in-the-Blank Questions

1. Because patients in freeze reaction are most likely avoiding their feelings, it may be useful to begin a conversation using _____ words.

2. Patients in flight reaction will most likely benefit from having their emotions _____ rather than _____.

3. Newly diagnosed patients are more likely to be responsive to an approach that is more _____ than direct.

4. Patients in fight reaction may need _____ to ask for help when they need it.

5. When patients communicate through facial expressions and physical gestures instead of words, they are using _____.

Short-Answer Questions

1. How can the ability to recognize a patient's emotional reaction to a diagnosis be useful when working with newly diagnosed patients?

_____

_____

_____

_____

2. When a patient in flight reaction is experiencing an extreme emotional reaction, what can health-care professionals do to reach them?

_____

_____

_____

_____

3. Patients in fight reaction may resist listening to advice or suggestions from their health-care providers. What is the best way to approach a patient who is resisting?

_____

_____

_____

_____

4. What is the value of reading and understanding a newly diagnosed patient's body language?

_____

_____

_____

5. When a newly diagnosed patient is in freeze reaction, how can enlisting family members be helpful?

_____

_____

_____

_____

Critical-Thinking Questions

1. While body language is an important element in the way newly diagnosed patients communicate their feelings, effective use of body language in communications between health-care professionals and patients requires that the health-care professionals interpret body language correctly. From a multicultural perspective, how can working with patients from other cultures complicate the interpretation of patient body language? What can health-care professionals do to avoid misinterpretation?

_____

_____

_____

_____

_____

2. How does understanding a newly diagnosed patient's reaction potentially enhance communications between health-care professionals and patients? How can misunderstanding patient reactions, for example, assuming patients are in flight reaction when they are fighters, cause communication problems?

_____

_____

_____

_____

_____

Internet Exercise

Consider three patients, each diagnosed with a chronic illness such as diabetes or hypertension.

Find Web sites that include information on each condition. As you review this information, think about the emotional state of each patient. Is the information presented such that the patient would be able to comprehend it, or would it be disturbing? For example, is the information too direct and clinical for a patient in flight reaction? Does it contain enough detail for a patient in fight reaction, or at least have links to additional information? Is there any aspect of the information, such as a case study, that a patient in freeze reaction might find acceptable?

Determine which resources you would recommend to each type of patient.

CHAPTER 3

Acknowledging Emotional Reactions

OVERVIEW

After reading this chapter, you should be able to:

- Define and use the keywords of acknowledging emotional reactions.

- Identify the key emotions of newly diagnosed patients.

- Understand how patients in flight, freeze, and fight reactions experience emotions.

- Know how to approach a patient discussion about emotional issues.

- Discuss the role grief plays in accepting a medical diagnosis.

- Describe how to approach people from other cultures on an emotional level.

- Tell how to make mental-health referrals for patients who are having difficulty coping.

- Name the symptoms of depression, and outline the role of health-care professionals in helping depressed patients.

- Understand how health-care professionals help patients express and cope with their emotions.

KEYWORDS

Anger

Beliefs

Change

Depression

Disappointment

Educational moment

Emotional reaction

Equilibrium

Fear

Fear factor

Frustration

Grief

Healthy grief

Perceptions

Reflective listening

Relief

Roles

Sadness

Self-destructive behavior

Shame

Suppress

Suppressed feelings

Ventilate

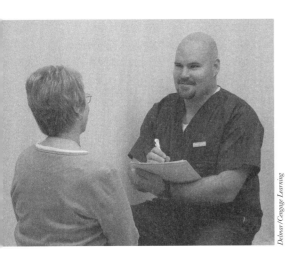

Delmar/Cengage Learning

Case Study

Shana received her diagnosis a few days ago. At that time, her health-care professionals had given her some basic information about her condition and described treatment options. Shana had listened quietly but said little, so her team knew she would need time to react to her diagnosis and begin processing it. Her return visit to the office would provide the opportunity for further discussion.

When Shana returned, Lars, a physician's assistant, immediately noticed that she had been crying. Intent on reviewing what Shana's physician had discussed upon initial diagnosis and answering any of Shana's questions, Lars sat the woman in a chair and took one in front of her.

KEEP IN MIND

When patients exhibit strong emotions, health-care professionals can sometimes feel unsure about what to say. If you were Lars, what would your instinct be in terms of approaching Shana?

Gently, Lars asked the visibly upset Shana if she was ready to talk more about her diagnosis. Shana nodded, but had difficulty saying anything more than, "Yes." Her ability to participate in a discussion and process information seemed dubious at that moment. Given that, instead of starting with a brief description of Shana's treatment plan, Lars reconsidered his approach. He opted instead to pause for a moment.

After the moment had passed, he asked quietly, "Are you okay, Shana?"

Shana slumped forward in her chair. It was clear she would need time to experience her feelings before she would be able to talk further.

"Hey, Shana," Lars continued. "You look really upset. Do you want to talk about it?"

At that, Shana burst into tears. Lars reached for a box of tissues and placed it in front of her. He sat with Shana as she cried, but he did not speak.

Introduction

"I feel so sad."

The reaction to a medical diagnosis—whether flight, freeze, or fight—manifests in a range of emotions, from anger, fear, sadness, and even relief. Patients themselves determine the landscape of these emotions. Patients are individuals with unique sets of life experiences and their own ways of coping with stressful situations.

For their part, health-care professionals are not expected to be psychotherapists, counselors, or mental-health staff. On the contrary, those who try to counsel patients without the benefit of professional training can risk patient safety. Instead of counseling, then, health-care professionals should focus on recognizing the **emotional reactions** of their patients.

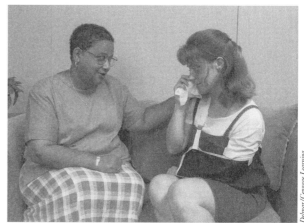

Delmar/Cengage Learning

Foremost, patients who are preoccupied with their emotions can neither listen to nor process information about their diagnoses. As a result, they also cannot ask relevant questions. When health-care professionals fail to acknowledge patients' emotional states, they waste time trying to discuss facts and often confuse and incite the patients in the process. The health-care professionals can become alarmed and frustrated, and further patient resistance and emotional disturbance can ensue.

While some newly diagnosed patients can access their emotions and express them openly, others may withhold or **suppress** them. Much like expressed feelings, **suppressed feelings** erode patient communications. Patients who are struggling with their emotions cannot interact with health-care staff in ways that are productive.

Despite the challenges and limitations of patient interactions, health-care professionals play an important role in helping patients cope with their diagnoses. While most patients develop coping skills and support networks as they move through the process, often encouraged and guided by their health-care partners, at initial diagnosis health-care professionals may be the only form of support some patients have. Patients rely on their health-care providers to give them the words, and strategies, to move forward. Family members may not participate in early diagnosis discussions, or they may simply be unprepared to engage. Chapter 11 covers this topic in greater detail.

Defining the Role of Emotions

The news of a medical diagnosis can unearth a lot of feelings in a newly diagnosed patient, many uncomfortable and, consequently, unacceptable. It is common, for example, for newly diagnosed patients to feel sad, scared, or angry. After all, a medical diagnosis likely imposes **change**—in routine, relationships, or self-image—and human beings are creatures of habit. A medical diagnosis also renders the future uncertain and poses new challenges. In addition to fears about the future, a medical diagnosis can introduce fears about losing finances, relationships, and favorite activities.

Newly diagnosed patients experience their emotions in unique ways according to the following factors:

KEEP IN MIND

Emotional distress is a common reaction to a medical diagnosis. What would your internal reaction be to a patient who is as emotionally distraught as Shana? What would your external reaction be? What would you say? How comfortable would you be remaining silent while the patient experiences strong emotions? At what point would you feel ineffective? At what point would you be concerned that you might be overstepping professional boundaries?

- *Perceptions of the severity of the diagnosis and its potential effect.* **Perceptions** influence patients' emotions. Upon first receiving their diagnoses, patients often have minimal or erroneous information about their conditions, too little to accurately evaluate the implications on their lives. Patients' perceptions and misperceptions may lead them to react inconsistently with reality. In contrast, patients who are well versed in their conditions experience emotions that are both realistic and consistent with the conditions' severity levels.

- *Personal coping style and comfort level expressing emotions.* Some people grow up in families in which emotions are always on the surface, and family members are encouraged to express their feelings. In other families, emotions are less acceptable and kept below the surface. Newly diagnosed patients who have not been comfortable expressing their feelings are likely to have difficulty talking about how they feel.

- *Choice of flight, freeze, or fight reaction.* As discussed in Chapter 2, emotions are closely tied to how patients react to their diagnoses. Patients in flight reaction are likely highly emotional, though they may appear stuck in one emotion, like fear or sadness. The key characteristic of patients in freeze reaction is emotion suppression, which means emotions are not absent, just held down. Patients in fight reaction can think rationally while expressing a range of emotions.

- *Personal experience coping with illness.* Newly diagnosed patients who have been diagnosed before may reexperience negative emotions. On the positive side, the patients' previous diagnoses may have armed them with coping skills they can leverage again. Patients who have helped friends or family members cope with medical conditions usually have knowledge and experience they can apply personally.

Supporting Patients Who Ask, "Why Me?"

Newly diagnosed patients inevitably ask one question: "Why me?" The motivation may be medical: The patient wants to understand the medical reasons behind the diagnosis. In asking, however, patients may feel a sense of self-punishment, wanting to know if they have done something to cause the diagnoses. Patients with conditions like lung cancer and Type II diabetes often feel their lifestyle choices contributed to their diagnoses. Other patients may suspect genetics.

While the "Why me?" question may be medically motivated, it may also be spiritual in nature. Ultimately, "Why me?" is an existential question: a question of greater meaning from a spiritual perspective. Patients with this perspective often examine their religious beliefs and/or issues of fairness and unfairness. Patients may have a sense of guilt and wonder if they even have the right to question why they, and not others, received their diagnoses.

Following is an example of how one patient verbalized this experience:

"My first question was, 'Why me?' I knew it was a question without an answer. But still, I had to ask why this was happening to me. I certainly didn't think I had done anything to deserve it. And in some ways, I felt guilty for even asking it. I mean, bad things can happen to anyone."

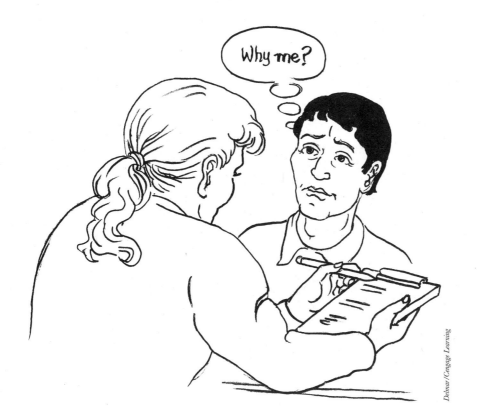

Asking "Why me?" often inspires an emotional reaction: sadness, anger, disappointment. For many patients, emotional floodgates open, because in asking the question they are in a way articulating two core issues patients grapple with postdiagnosis: the basic question of fairness and the role of fate.

Health-care professionals who initiate discussions of the medical reasons for diagnoses help patients start to gain perspective. Those who discourage such exchanges effectively short-circuit the acceptance process. Some of the reasons for medical conditions are simply more palatable than others. Even when a diagnosis has no medical reason, a patient can feel reassured that there is limited personal responsibility for the diagnosis and the "Why me?" question has at least in part been answered. Like the patient in the example, however, patients often conclude that the question of "Why me?" really has no answer.

To ensure "Why me?" and related questions are addressed appropriately, health-care professionals should remind patients of the following:

- Asking "Why me?" is normal for newly diagnosed patients.

- Conditions do arise for medical reasons.

- Patients can discuss guilt or self-blaming in a support group or with trained professionals.

- Members of the clergy are best equipped to handle spiritual questions.

Identifying the Emotions of Newly Diagnosed Patients

A medical diagnosis can lead to a wide range of emotions. The following sections describe some of the key emotions of newly diagnosed patients.

EXPLORING FEAR: YOLANDA'S STORY

"All I could think about was how concerned my doctor was when she told me I was HIV positive. I had never seen this look on her face before, and I just kept thinking that if she was this concerned, I must be in a lot of trouble. Big trouble. I felt like I was on the edge of a cliff, and I needed to hang on to something. But there was nothing to hang on to. At any second, I might go falling into the darkness."

Newly diagnosed patients often identify **fear** as the emotion they feel most strongly, emphasizing that getting beyond the **fear factor** is key to coping. As is examined in depth in Chapter 4, a medical diagnosis can cause fear for varied reasons. One obvious one is the possibility of death. When a diagnosis is life-threatening as Yolanda's was, patients are justified in feeling their lives are at risk. Even when not considered fatal, a diagnosis can challenge a patient's assumptions about life choices

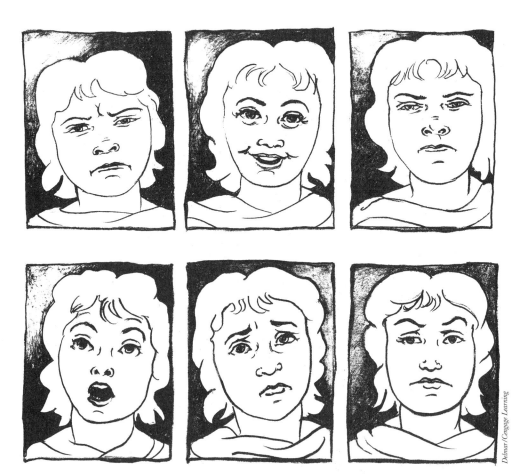

Delmar/Cengage Learning

and the future. At least temporarily, diagnoses may leave patients feeling they have nothing to count on.

TAPPING INTO ANGER: MARK'S STORY

"I said it right from the start: I was really ticked off about this. I was doing great in my career. My fiancée at the time and I had wedding plans. I was actively involved in my community. And then the doctor walked in and basically told me I'd better plan on taking a year off to get medical treatment. I felt like everything I valued in life was being taken from me. The world was laughing at me while I was standing there empty-handed. I wanted to yell and holler. In fact, I did."

Anger is a common reaction to a medical diagnosis. Angry patients describe feeling "backed into a corner with no options" or, as the patient in the example did, "laughed at by the world." Anger is essentially a reaction to feeling powerless. Some patients substitute it for other emotions. In Western culture, for example, men find it easier and more acceptable to express anger than sadness or fear. In further masking, patients may use other terms for anger, such as **frustration**.

LEARNING ABOUT SADNESS: LEAH'S STORY

"I sat and cried for hours. The tears kept coming to the point that I didn't think I had ever cried this hard my whole life. At times, I felt like my body was going to turn itself inside out I was so sad. My diagnosis left me feeling like my whole life had been taken away, and I guess I was grieving for what I thought I had lost."

Like anger, **sadness** commonly follows a medical diagnosis. An emotional reaction to loss, sadness, sometimes called **disappointment** by patients, reflects the devastation patients feel as they consider changes to day-to-day life, relationships, and the future. Patients feeling an extreme level of **grief** appear inconsolable.

UNDERSTANDING SHAME: MARIO'S STORY

"When my doctor handed me the Type II diabetes diagnosis, I said to myself, 'You knew this was coming, and you didn't do a thing to prevent it. You kept eating anything you wanted.' I didn't do a thing to prevent my diabetes, and I knew all along that I was at risk. Now, it's payback time for not taking care of myself. And the people who care about me are going to have to start watching over me like a child."

Messages about health self-determination, especially in regard to factors like diet, exercise, and smoking avoidance, dominate American culture. Through them, we are taught to take responsibility for avoiding chronic illness. While these messages have benefit, the fact is that few people do everything they can to stay as healthy as possible. Reasons include not knowing what to do and lacking willpower. Because few execute all the healthy lifestyle choices, patients diagnosed with preventable conditions like Type II diabetes feel a sense of failure upon diagnosis. Those around the patients, including health-care providers, may reinforce that sense of failure. Patients end up feeling **shame** or guilt.

ADMITTING TO RELIEF: JANA'S STORY

"I don't mean to imply I was happy hearing I had picked up a virus. It was going to mean lots of medicine and some time away from my job. But I'll be honest. I'd been sick for a while, and during that time, many thoughts passed through my head, mostly scary pictures of what could be going on in my body and what they might mean. So when my doctor said it was a virus, I felt like a load had been taken off my shoulders. I told myself, 'This could have been worse.' And then I think I had a good cry, I was so relieved."

In the absence of information, patients who are experiencing symptoms may jump to conclusions about their diagnoses, or they may suspect diagnoses due to lifestyle choices or heredity. When the actual diagnoses are less serious than expectations, patients usually greet them with **relief**.

> **KEEP IN MIND**
>
> Most newly diagnosed patients express the emotions they are most comfortable with based on patterns they have established. What emotions are you most comfortable expressing in challenging situations? Do you tend to get angry? Sad? Or do you avoid your emotions?

Relating Flight, Freeze, and Fight with Emotions

The reactions of newly diagnosed patients to medical diagnoses—flight, freeze, and fight—are primarily functions of how patients handle emotions. Remember that patients may experience any number of emotions as they process their diagnoses. The following sections review how newly diagnosed patients experience and express emotions.

WORKING WITH PATIENTS IN FLIGHT REACTION

Patients in flight reaction may attach to one emotion. For example, they may experience extreme sadness or fear and appear to completely give in to it. Because flight patients are so emotionally focused, health-care professionals may find it difficult to give them information or discuss their diagnoses and treatments with them.

Much like they attach to emotions, patients in flight reaction can attach to physicians or treatments. Then, because they are not thinking rationally, they believe they are going to be cured and express joy or elation. In addition to basing their reactions on possibly invalid reasons, flight patients can set overexpectations for the health-care team.

UNDERSTANDING PATIENTS IN FREEZE REACTION

Patients in freeze reaction have emotional reactions to their diagnoses, but they do not express them as a means of self-protection Some freeze patients are so afraid of their emotions that they suppress them completely, at least temporarily. While health-care professionals are not responsible for getting patients to openly express their feelings, they should remember that patients like these are capable of doing so.

DISCUSSING PATIENTS IN FIGHT REACTION

Unlike patients in freeze reaction, patients in fight reaction express a range of emotions, and they express them strongly. They do not allow their emotions to control them, however. Fight patients experience and express their feelings and then think and act rationally. As treatment progresses, fighters remain in touch with and express their emotions. Accessible emotions are one benefit of the fight reaction, because they help patients cope with the ups and downs of their conditions.

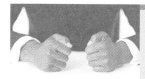

Body Language

As discussed in Chapter 2, body language can reflect emotions. Following are emotion and body language associations:

Fear
- Eyes wide, unblinking
- Arms folded across the chest
- Hands held to the mouth
- Ankles locked

Sadness
- Crying
- Hands held to the face
- Shoulders hunched
- Rubbing eyes

Shame
- Eyes diverted
- Hands held to the face
- Slumping forward
- Arms folded across the chest
- Patting/playing with the hair

Anger
- Standing with the hands on the hips
- Sitting/standing erect or legs crossed
- Hands clasped
- Unblinking eye contact

Relief
- Sitting with the legs apart
- Hands open
- Rubbing hands together
- Relaxed expression

Introducing "Educational Moments"

When interacting with newly diagnosed patients, health-care professionals often have opportunities to identify patients' emotions and to encourage those patients to consider alternative viewpoints or behaviors. For example, a health-care professional might point out that a patient appears sad or angry. For patients who have difficulty acknowledging or discussing their emotions, this is helpful. For a patient who expresses expectations based on faulty information, the health-care provider might provide accurate information and encourage the patient to talk with the physician.

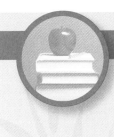

Educational Moment

Overwhelmed by information they are receiving and unprepared to make decisions, newly diagnosed patients may experience unfamiliar and uncomfortable emotions. Because family members have their own reactions to patients' diagnoses, they may be unable to listen to the patients' feelings. Fortunately, during discussions with health-care professionals, patients may directly or indirectly show their feelings. To help patients identify their feelings and questions, and to provide a listening ear, health-care professionals can use techniques like paraphrasing what the patient is saying, to show that you are listening fully. Paraphrasing was described in Chapter 2.

Opportunities like these, called **educational moments**, arise often when health-care professionals and newly diagnosed patients interact. When appropriate, health-care professionals can use moments like these to provide information, help patients express emotions, and deepen the patient connection.

Subsequent chapters highlight educational moments.

Explaining How Medical Diagnoses Challenge Life Beliefs

Human beings have certain basic assumptions about life. Mental-health professionals call these assumptions beliefs. **Beliefs** are our own personal sets of "shoulds" regarding such things as what we owe the world around us, what others should give us, and how others should behave. Beliefs result from our upbringings, personal experiences, and cultures.

A medical diagnosis challenges some of the core expectations of our beliefs. As patients react to the stress of a medical diagnosis, much of it arising from a shift in life expectations, they test their fundamental life beliefs. The emotions patients experience arise from projections about how their conditions will impact their lives.

Patients may share a similar belief yet react differently. For example, a belief that a condition will cause relationships to change drastically might sadden one patient, anger another, and frighten yet another.

While the health-care team is not responsible for working with patients about their beliefs, the roles of beliefs in patient behavior are important for health-care professionals to remember. Emotions arise not only from beliefs, but from patients' interpretations of information and the guidelines they are provided. Table 3.1 outlines the expectations patients may have about life.

> **KEEP IN MIND**
>
> Each human has a unique set of life beliefs. What are your basic assumptions about life? Do you identify with any of the assumptions in Table 3.1? How do your beliefs affect your reactions to stressful events?

TABLE 3.1   Patient Beliefs about Life

I should be able to live my life with a sense of security and certainty.	We expect that our lives will pass day to day according to certain, established routines. Basically, we want to know what we can expect every moment of the current day, as well as the coming one. While minor fluctuations may occur, we assume that the overall flow of life will be maintained. In this scheme, a medical diagnosis is an uncertainty that can affect finances, relationships, and plans for the future.
I should be in control of what happens to me in life.	Humans live with the illusion that they control their lives, that somehow they can be the masters of their destinies. One of the ways we maintain control is by denying that something out of our control could somehow happen. A medical diagnosis introduces a sense of lack of control.
I should be able to be effective in the roles I play in life.	The **roles** we play in life—parent, child, employee, spouse, and so on—have defined sets of responsibilities and benefits. Because these roles define who we are, we risk our identities when we cannot perform them according to our standards.
My life should change only when I want it to (and I usually don't).	Human beings are hardwired to maintain what scientists call **equilibrium**, a sense of balance maintained by avoiding change. Humans value the familiar to the extent that they maintain even unpleasant or boring routines out of a fear of the unknown. In short, it is normal for humans to fear change. A medical diagnosis can be fraught with change, including in diet, daily routine, and work schedule.
If I live a good life, bad things won't happen to me.	A medical diagnosis directly threatens one of the greatest examples of superstitious thinking: the belief that if we live our lives with an attitude of fairness and generosity, we will be treated with fairness and generosity.

Delmar/Cengage Learning

Conducting Healthy Grieving

Newly diagnosed patients, primarily those in fight reaction, often go through a grieving process. Often, patients must complete this process to accept their conditions and move forward with treatment and lifestyle adjustments. Grief is the first step of acceptance. **Healthy grief** is based on accepting that the basic life beliefs are irrational. For many patients, diagnoses inspire belief reevaluations. For some, diagnoses are the first times they look at beliefs and assess how they affect actions and emotional reactions.

One patient described it the following way:

"My attitude toward life was always, 'If I'm positive and caring toward other people, I'm always going to be successful.' I realize I also thought that this attitude would keep me healthy. Kind of like, 'You get what you give.' And then, when I got diagnosed, I had to question all my beliefs, especially this one. At first, I felt like life had betrayed me, and I was really angry. I had to sit with that realization for a while, and I felt really sad. It had been a nice

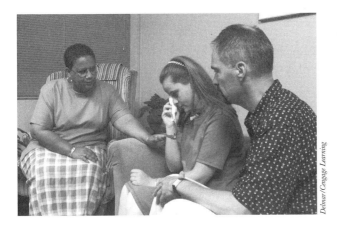

hope, but one I had to let go of. As people around me reached out to see if they could help, I realized that being nice to people wasn't going to keep me from getting sick, but it meant that when I needed people, they would be there for me."

The healthy grieving process, which is generally accompanied by sadness primarily and secondarily by emotions like shame and anger, occurs at various intensity levels. Patients may grieve openly, crying and talking about what they have lost, or they may be more subtle. Grieving patients review their lives, contemplating their accomplishments and regrets. They also contemplate their plans for the future and question how the medical diagnoses will impact those plans. Newly diagnosed patients commonly consider their relationships, especially family ones, in terms of what they may need from caregivers.

While health-care professionals may not necessarily help patients through their grief, knowing the potential for healthy grieving can be useful. Grieving patients may exhibit the following:

- Constant crying, similar to that experienced by someone who has lost a loved one
- Withdrawal into thoughts, lack of responsiveness
- Discussion of past, rather than present concerns or the future
- Concerns about how loved ones will function without their support
- Avoidance of information interpreted as implying an irreversible life change

Healthy grieving helps patients come to grips with the "Why me?" question and identify personally meaningful resolutions. When grieving, patients tend to resist health-care providers with overly positive or optimistic attitudes. This stance makes patients appear overly pessimistic. Grieving is a time when listening ears and gentle encouragement render patients confident that they and their health-care providers are doing all that is possible to treat these patients' conditions and move patients beyond grief.

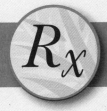 ## Helping Patients to Open Up Emotionally

Chapter 2 case studies provided guidelines for approaching patients in flight, freeze, and fight reactions. Consider reviewing this material before working with patients, both to identify patients accurately and to provide the appropriate emotional support.

Take Shana, for example, the patient at the beginning of this chapter who experienced strong emotions because of her illness, mainly anger. Shana was most likely in flight or fight reaction, as evidenced primarily by her ability to acknowledge and express her emotions. However, patients in freeze reaction might react emotionally, albeit briefly, because patients like this will suppress their emotions as much as possible. Fortunately for Shana, her physician's assistant was trained to help patients cope.

SHANA: I'm sorry for breaking down like that. I let this get the best of me, I guess.

LARS: You don't have to apologize for having feelings, Shana. This is a lot for you to take in at one time. It's normal to feel sad.

SHANA: I am sad.

LARS: Do you want to tell me what you're sad about?

SHANA: This came out of the blue. No symptoms—nothing. A routine checkup and suddenly my life is crashing around me.

LARS: This was totally unexpected, I know. And it feels like a big loss.

SHANA: Yes, it does. Like a part of me got taken away.

LARS: I understand, Shana.

Shana dabbed at her eyes, paused, and looked away, as if considering what she might say next. She looked back at Lars and frowned.

SHANA: And you know what else? I'm also really angry. Up until last Tuesday, I was fine. Just living my life. I had my whole future ahead of me. This isn't fair.

LARS: It seems like you don't have a future right now. Of course you're angry about that.

SHANA: I am angry. I can't believe it.

LARS: You can still have a future. It just means you're going to have to make some changes in your life.

SHANA: Change? That's all you think it is?

LARS: Your diagnosis will mean that you'll need to make some adjustments and take medication regularly, but it doesn't mean you don't have a future.

Shana shook her head.

SHANA: Don't sugarcoat this like I'm a child. I know this is going to change my whole life. I'm going to know I'm not normal, and everyone around me is going to know. How would you like to live your life like this? Would you like it?

LARS: I know this is hard for you. And it's brought up a lot of feelings for you, like sadness and anger. I just want to reassure you that it's normal to have a lot of different feelings when you've been diagnosed with a medical condition. What's important right now is for you to take some time and let yourself have your feelings.

Shana put her hands to her face and sighed.

SHANA: I'm not blaming you, Lars. But I feel awful. I hope you don't think I was yelling at you.

LARS: Not at all, Shana. I know you feel awful right now.

SHANA: I really do.

LARS: Well, I want to reassure you that your health-care team is doing everything possible to treat you and your condition. We'll be with you every step of the way. And as we work together, I'm here to listen to whatever you have to say and to answer any questions you might have. Okay?

SHANA: Okay.

LARS: Now. I do need to talk to you about your treatment plan for the next couple of weeks. Can you have that conversation with me now?

SHANA: Yes, I think I can. I just needed to vent for a couple of minutes.

LARS: I understand.

Helping Patients Talk about Feelings

Following are some guidelines when working with patients who are expressing emotions:

1. *The health-care provider is a listener but not a therapist.* Notice that in the preceding dialogue Lars primarily listened to Shana. He did not try to solve her problems. Newly diagnosed patients can benefit greatly from conversations with a caring person who can listen without judgment. The listener need not resolve the patients' feelings or provide solutions. There are, after all, no easy answers. As Shana and Lars demonstrated, the listening ear of a health-care professional can give the patient a way to **ventilate** and become more receptive to hearing and discussing medical information.

2. *Patients know when they are really being listened to.* Listening is an active process. Newly diagnosed patients may hesitate to open up or fear they will annoy or overextend the listener. The more actively health-care professionals listen, the more open and honest their patients.

   Show you are attuned to patients through physical and verbal cues. Physical cues include direct eye contact, facial expressions, and gestures. Verbal cues include questions and "encouragers" like "Okay" and "Uh huh." In addition, use the patient's name. It makes the conversation personal and can be soothing. Just be sure to ask patients if they prefer to be addressed by their first names or more formally. Often, older patients prefer the latter, especially from younger health-care professionals.

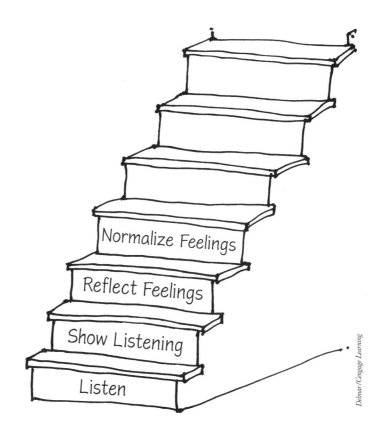

Delmar/Cengage Learning

3. *Reflect feelings to offer support and clarification.* Paraphrasing, and reflecting feelings, as described in Chapter 2, is especially important when newly diagnosed patients describe and/or demonstrate emotions. Paraphrasing and reflecting feelings shows that the health-care professional is **listening reflectively**, and it helps patients clarify their thoughts and feelings. In the preceding dialogue, Lars reflected to Shana that she was angry about her diagnosis. While patients do not need health-care professionals to advise or counsel them, they can benefit from statements that show the health-care professionals are listening and can help them identify their emotions and perceptions.

4. *Conversations about feelings are opportunities to normalize patient emotions.* In the sample dialogue, Lars told Shana that it is normal to have feelings like sadness and anger about a diagnosis. Patients do not always accept their emotions, especially the negative ones like anger, because they may feel they are supposed to think positive or keep their emotions to themselves. When health-care professionals assure patients it is normal to have a range of emotions, patients more easily accept their feelings and talk more.

5. *Listening is a way of honoring another person.* When patients talk about their feelings, health-care professionals can sometimes feel helpless. After all, it is only normal to want to help someone who is suffering. Deeply felt and expressed emotions can be especially difficult to listen to without feeling pressure to take some kind of action. However, the value of listening alone—without judgment, without interpretation, without responsibility—cannot be underestimated. Patients simply need someone to hear and acknowledge their reactions.

Often, patients' families are distracted with their own reactions to the patients' diagnoses and cannot listen to the patients. To try to avoid feeling helpless, family members may tell patients to "think positive," or they may try to reassure the patients that "everything is going to get better" when the patients are unconvinced. The patients are left with a lot of feelings and no outlet for expressing them. Perceived as objective but also caring, health-care providers can bridge the gap between patient and family.

Assessing Depression

When an unfortunate event occurs, it is normal to feel sad for a day or two, or even a few days. The image of **depression** is profound sadness, excessive crying, and the inability to get through the day. Indeed, people who are depressed have trouble maintaining their normal lives—getting up in the morning, getting ready for the day, working around the house, getting together with friends or family. Depression pains the people who are suffering. It also pains the people around them.

UNDERSTANDING DEPRESSION IN HEALTH CARE

Because newly diagnosed patients are at risk for depression, it is critical that their health-care professionals be alert to its signs. Depression can impede compliance with treatment and lifestyle directives (Gary, et al., 2010; van Bastelaar, et al., 2010).

Patients who are highly depressed may be unable to motivate themselves to be compliant, or may feel that the future is so bleak that they don't care whether they get better or not. Experience has shown that patients who are compliant with treatment are more likely to have better treatment outcomes. In addition to recovering more slowly, depressed patients are at risk for such **self-destructive behavior** as suicide (Vannoy, et al.).

In the health-care arena, depression occurs when diagnoses overwhelm patients to the point that they cannot harness the psychological resources they need to cope. While patients in flight reaction are most prone to depression, depression may emotionally disconnect patients in freeze reaction. Fighters, for their part, can fall into depressed states when they experience setbacks like additional diagnoses or treatment failures.

The Depression Mindset

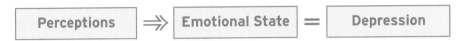

Perceptions ⟹ Emotional State = Depression

Perceptions

"I can't deal with this."

"I'll never be the same again."

"My life is over."

"All my plans for the future are going up in smoke."

"No one is going to want to be around me. I'll just be a burden."

"I'll be useless to the people who count on me."

"I won't be normal again."

Result

Anger Turned Inward = Hopelessness, Helplessness, Shutting Down

IDENTIFYING THE SIGNS OF DEPRESSION

It can be difficult to determine when patients who are grieving healthily over their diagnoses become depressed. Lacking mental-health backgrounds, health-care professionals often feel unqualified to diagnosis depression, but they may need to raise an alarm if its symptoms manifest. Doing so is easier than it might seem. The symptoms of depression are relatively easy to recognize (Table 3.2), and when patients have one or more, the potential is clear.

Because depression can profoundly affect patients and risk their lives, many organizations train health-care professionals to recognize its symptoms. They also institute formal procedures for identifying depressed patients and making mental-health referrals. A number of simple tests and questionnaires simplify the diagnosis process for non-mental-health professionals. Because medications can cause feelings of depression, health-care professionals should conduct their evaluations with this in mind.

KEEP IN MIND

Depression impacts patients and those around them as well. Some health-care professionals feel helpless when they are with depressed people and would prefer to avoid them. Have you interacted with people you thought were depressed? What was the experience like? How do you feel about working with depressed and potentially uncommunicative patients?

TABLE 3.2   Symptoms of Depression

Working with a physician, a mental-health professional can help diagnose depression. A diagnosis is based on symptoms that are common among people with depression. Following are some of the common ways depression manifests. The presence of any of these symptoms does not necessarily confirm a diagnosis of depression. Only a mental-health professional can make that determination.

Sadness

Tiredness, fatigue

Loss of interest in favorite hobbies or other activities

Withdrawal from friends and family

Changes in eating habits, with weight loss or gain

Trouble sleeping at night, sleeping too much, or sleeping during the day

Feeling like a burden to other people

Use of alcohol or other drugs, including prescription types

Thoughts of death or suicide

Anxiety or irritability

Forgetfulness of things like medication or personal hygiene

Feeling that the world would be a better place without you

Delmar/Cengage Learning

Studying the Influence of Culture and Gender

As discussed previously, a range of factors affect how, and whether, individuals express emotions, including personal experience and family background. Knowing that communication differences exist between groups, and trying to be as sensitive as possible to those differences, greatly enhances the communication between patient and health-care professional.

Culture is one factor that can influence the ways in which patients experience emotions and accept mental-health intervention. In some cultures, emotions are on the surface and appear pronounced. In others, expressing uncomfortable feelings is considered a sign of weakness. To learn more about cultural differences, do some research. Talk with people from other cultures to learn more about how they express emotions and to identify the barriers that could interfere with patient discussions. Simply asking patients if they are uncomfortable talking about their emotions can often help prevent discomfort on both sides of the conversation.

Like culture, gender can complicate discussions about emotions. In Western culture, for example, men are traditionally less comfortable than women discussing their feelings, because they view doing so as a sign of weakness. Therefore, as with culture, it is important to be sensitive to gender issues when emotions are involved. Gender roles are rapidly changing in cultures throughout the world. As the world becomes more psychologically sophisticated, men and women will be more able to comfortably articulate their feelings.

Following are guidelines for working with patients from other cultures:

- Avoid stereotyping the patient. Make no assumptions about the patient's comfort level discussing emotional issues.
- Make it clear that you are willing to discuss the patient's issues and concerns.
- Do not try to help the patient talk about emotions through direct and persistent questioning.
- Consider enlisting the assistance of another professional who represents, or is familiar with, the patient's culture.

Making Referrals for Mental-Health Treatment

Generally, health-care organizations offer some form of mental-health services, or they have formal referral processes. When making a mental-health referral, refer to the following guidelines.

- Before making a referral, discuss your concerns with the physician in charge of the patient's case. The physician may want to reevaluate the patient's medications or manage the referral process.
- Tell the patient that you will talk to the treating physician about recommending the patient meet with a mental-health professional. Be prepared to explain why you are making the recommendation. Include examples of the behaviors or symptoms that have raised concerns.
- Explain to the patient the potential benefit of seeing a mental-health professional, and describe what the process of seeing a counselor might be like.
- Ask the patient if talking with a mental-health professional is desirable. Offer encouragement as appropriate, but do not force the issue.
- Review the process of connecting with the mental-health professional, including any costs. Outline all options.
- Encourage the patient to connect with the mental-health professional. If the patient is motivated but unfamiliar with mental-health treatment, consider making the appointment with the patient.
- After the patient's mental-health treatment begins, monitor progress with the patient during office visits and provide ongoing encouragement.

SUMMARY

Patients experience a range of emotions when they are diagnosed with medical conditions. Fighters express their feelings and use them to become empowered patients. Patients in flight reaction likely become stuck in singular emotions and have difficulty moving beyond them. Patients in freeze reaction become stuck because they suppress their emotions. Understanding how emotions affect patients' abilities to understand medical information, make treatment decisions, and cope with treatment and ongoing lifestyle adjustments can only benefit health-care professionals who are working with patients.

Chapter REVIEW

Multiple-Choice Questions

1. Patients who are emotionally overwhelmed by their diagnoses do which of the following?
   a. Focus on learning the facts of their conditions
   b. Find it difficult or impossible to listen to medical information
   c. Become motivated to ask relevant questions
   d. Readily talk about how they feel to gain some relief

2. When working with newly diagnosed patients in emotional crisis, their role is to:
   a. Listen and offer support
   b. Use their mental-health skills
   c. Help patients confront the truth of their diagnoses
   d. Avoid any interaction with the patients

3. It is accurate to say that the "Why me?" question:
   a. Should be avoided because it leads to self-pity
   b. Should be encouraged because it facilitates information-gathering
   c. Wastes time because it is unanswerable
   d. May help patients begin to acknowledge their feelings

4. Newly diagnosed patients will most likely experience which of the following?
   a. Sadness
   b. Anger
   c. Fear
   d. All of the above

5. The health-care professional who encourages a newly diagnosed patient to consider an alternative viewpoint to a self-defeating thought demonstrates which of the following?
   a. Educational interlude
   b. Alternative moment
   c. Educational moment
   d. Thought correction

Fill-in-the-Blank Questions

1. Newly diagnosed patients who consider their senses of loss may experience _____.

2. A health-care professional who is concerned about a patient's emotional state may decide to make a(n) _____ to a community agency.

3. In _____ listening, health-care professionals listen to patients, repeating what the patients are saying while identifying the patients' emotions.

4. _____ feelings are those a patient is attempting to deny and avoid.

5. When patients _____, they release feelings they have held back.

Short-Answer Questions

1. Why would a patient who has been diagnosed with a medical condition experience a sense of relief?

_____

_____

_____

_____

2. What is the benefit of newly diagnosed patients asking "Why me?"

_____

_____

_____

_____

3. Discuss the common body language of newly diagnosed patients who are experiencing fear.

_____

_____

_____

_____

4. Name two basic life beliefs that a medical diagnosis might challenge.

_____

_____

_____

_____

5. Why is it beneficial for health-care professionals to acknowledge and normalize patients' feelings?

_____

_____

_____

_____

Critical-Thinking Questions

1. Health-care professionals can help newly diagnosed patients cope with their diagnoses by providing listening ears. What are the likely mental and physical health benefits of listening? When does listening become counseling, and how can health-care professionals know when they are crossing that boundary?

_____

_____

_____

_____

_____

_____

2. While newly diagnosed patients can grow from experiencing sadness and hopelessness while coping, they are at risk for depression. At what point do feelings of sadness and hopelessness turn into depression?

_____

_____

_____

_____

_____

_____

3. Factors like gender, age, socioeconomic status, race, and cultural background impact how patients experience and express emotions. Give some examples of how from your own experiences. How can health-care professionals best accommodate individual communication differences in day-to-day interactions with patients?

_____

_____

_____

_____

_____

_____

Internet Exercise

Consider some of the key emotions that newly diagnosed patients experience (e.g., sadness, anger, disappointment, hopelessness, fear). Choose Web sites that would most help patients understand, and cope with, the emotions you identified. Contrast the level of information in each site, and identify how the information might benefit patients from different educational and cultural backgrounds.

_____

_____

_____

_____

_____

_____

_____

_____

CHAPTER 4

Acknowledging and Confronting the Fear Factor

OVERVIEW

After reading this chapter, you should be able to:

- Define and use the keywords of acknowledging and confronting the fear factor.

- Understand the importance of the "What if?" question as opening discussions to both the initial fears of a diagnosis and realistic expectations for the future.

- Specify patients' fears for the future.

- Discuss how fear may impact important patient discussions.

- Explain how to start patient discussions about fear nonconfrontationally.

- Recognize when fear has led to helplessness and additional intervention is needed.

- Know how to use both rational- and emotional-based techniques for helping patients cope with fear.

- Describe how to conduct the "What if?" discussion with a patient.

KEYWORDS

Antidote   Counterevidence   Negative self-talk

Bibliotherapy   Denial   Resistance

Counterargument   Meditation

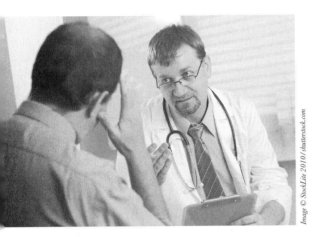

Image © StockLite 2010 / shutterstock.com

Case Study

Amar thought he knew just about everything about HIV. As a volunteer for a local HIV organization, he had passed out literature at community events and participated in fund-raising events. Amar even had a few friends who were HIV positive, and he talked with them often about their treatments and how the virus had affected their day-to-day routines. He certainly thought he knew how to avoid infection himself.

Looking back, Amar described his attitude toward HIV infection as "enlightened." While he knew that HIV required lifestyle changes, and that medications could have numerous side effects, his friends with the condition seemed to be leading full lives with promising futures. Amar did not view HIV as a condition that would keep a patient from a full life. Instead, he viewed the condition as an inconvenience, like other chronic illnesses.

An unexpected turn would change Amar's perspective, however. During his annual physical, Amar's physician informed him that he had become HIV positive.

> **KEEP IN MIND**
>
> The personal experiences of health-care professionals dictate which diagnoses they find easy to discuss with patients. Life-threatening conditions like cancer, and lifestyle-related conditions like Type II diabetes, might raise concerns. HIV is a diagnosis that can cause health-care providers both to question their values and to feel concern. If you were on Amar's health-care team, would you have taken time to identify your own fears and prejudices around this diagnosis? Would you have taken time to be educated?

Immediately after his diagnosis, Amar, like most newly diagnosed patients, felt shock. He could not believe he was being told he was HIV positive. It just did not seem possible. To someone else, yes. But not to him.

As he moved beyond his initial shock, Amar was overcome by fear. He admitted that he thought his life might be slipping away. He imagined himself with a weakened immune system, then with symptoms of AIDS progressing to the point that he needed hospitalization. He worried that he would become debilitated to the point that he would be unable to work, which would leave him financially dependent on others. He also wondered how his friends and family might react to his diagnosis, whether they might think less of him and even reject him. As Amar struggled with these thoughts and images, he was at times left in, in his own words, "a state of terror."

"Everything I thought I knew about HIV got thrown back in my face when I received my own HIV diagnosis," Amar confessed to Jason, the nurse practitioner at Amar's clinic. "At this moment, it doesn't matter how much I know about HIV. I'm still terrified about what might happen to me."

KEEP IN MIND

The objectivity of health-care professionals should start with an awareness of personal responsibilities and boundaries. How would you react initially to Amar's fear? Could you listen objectively, or would you share your own feelings of helplessness to try to fix the situation?

Jason had worked with many patients facing HIV and other chronic conditions, so he understood the fear they often experience when initially diagnosed. He knew that newly diagnosed patients, regardless of their knowledge about their conditions, fear the future—not only the possibility of death, but how they will appear and whether they will be able to maintain their responsibilities as employees or parents. As a health-care professional, Jason knew that it was important for patients to have an opportunity to acknowledge, and talk about, their fears for the future. As Jason knew, patients who address their fears are more able to work with their health-care teams.

While Amar had tried to remind himself he was armed with knowledge, including that HIV is not a death sentence, his fear did not seem to be subsiding. "This is ridiculous," he muttered to himself as he sat in his doctor's office. "I shouldn't be so scared. But I am."

KEEP IN MIND

Amar felt that he should not be scared. Reassuring fearful patients like Amar that they should or should not experience fear might be counterproductive. As a health-care professional, what would be your first response to Amar's contention? Why?

Introduction

"I'm so afraid."

With those few words, newly diagnosed patients describe what may be a temporary emotional state, and one emotion among a range, as they adjust to the news of their diagnoses. Patients who are fighters, for example, may experience fear, but they will recognize it as valid, consider the relevant medical information, and allow no emotion, including fear, to overcome them. Patients in flight reaction, in contrast, may attach to their fear to the point that they commit unwaveringly to uninformed treatment decisions or become engulfed in terror. For their part, patients in freeze reaction shut down emotionally because they are afraid of being afraid, and they fear the loss of emotional control that might result from acknowledging their terror.

Fear has numerous implications for health-care professionals. First, fearful patients cannot process medical information, because they cannot listen. They either want to avoid more fear, or they evaluate information in a way that only increases their terror. Second, fearful patients may try to avoid making treatment decisions. They may fail to trust that they are sufficiently informed or they may fear the alternatives. Fear can keep patients stuck emotionally and unable to communicate with their caregivers at a time when interaction is crucial. In short, patients who have not yet worked through their fear lack the optimism and flexibility needed to cope with their conditions.

Educational Moment

Newly diagnosed patients who are experiencing the fear factor can easily fall into negative thinking. Signs of fear and hopelessness, such as doubting whether treatment is worthwhile, will often enter into conversations with health-care professionals. Health-care professionals can help patients during these moments by acknowledging that it is normal to be afraid when first diagnosed with a medical condition and encouraging patients to discuss their fears and become educated.

Health-care professionals are not responsible for treating fear from a mental-health perspective. However, those who recognize the fear factor in newly diagnosed patients and know how to address it are more sensitive to their patients and help counter reactions like **resistance** and indecision.

Asking "What If?" to Open the Door to Fear

It is human nature to question. Chapter 3 revealed that most newly diagnosed patients ask "Why me?" even as they realize no answer exists. The motivation of "Why me?" may be psychological: Patients may be concerned how past attitudes and behaviors might have factored into their diagnoses. The motivation may also be spiritual: Patients may seek the greater meanings of their diagnoses.

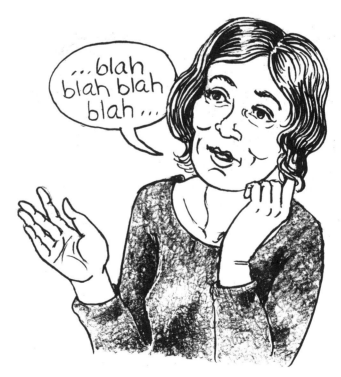

Delmar/Cengage Learning

KEEP IN MIND

A difficult and unanswerable question like "Why me?" can make health-care professionals feel helpless. What initial concerns would you have if your patient asked, "What if?" How would you see your role as a health-care professional, and how would your role relate to those of other professionals like the attending physician? Overall, how do you think you would react?

Often as newly diagnosed patients adjust to their diagnoses, "Why me?" gives way to "What if?" As the following sections discuss, "What if?" reflects patients' fears about the future. Instead of allaying those fears, unfortunately, the question tends to amplify patients' concerns. Images of the worst scenarios tend only to increase feelings of fear and dread.

ACCEPTING MORTALITY

Despite assurances from the health-care team, conditions like cancer can raise concerns about death. Patients may have lost friends or relatives to the disease, so images of death can be very specific. Patients may imagine their bodies shutting down and saying good-bye to loved ones. Some patients visualize their homes or workplaces after they are gone and their loved ones are adjusting to their absences. Even chronic diseases like diabetes can inspire fears of death, as patients imagine their declines over time.

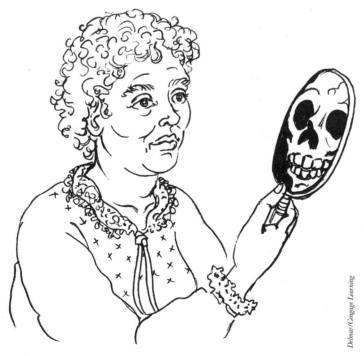

Delmar/Cengage Learning

"I keep wondering if this is going to mean the end of my life.
Do I need to start preparing myself?"

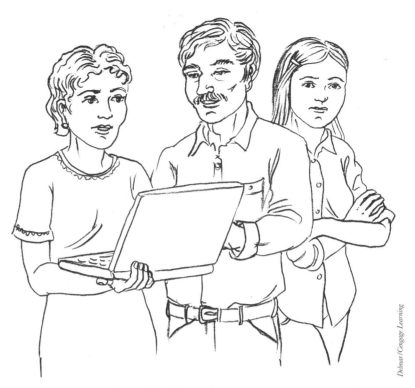

Delmar/Cengage Learning

"Sometimes I feel like I am just in the way. Is everyone going to get tired of me if I can't keep up with them?"

PROTECTING RELATIONSHIPS

Humans are social beings, so medical diagnoses invariably introduce the fear that important relationships may change. Patients who are partnered fear they will be less attractive, that they will be unable to handle their household responsibilities, that they will somehow be embarrassing, or burdensome, to those they love. Parents worry they will be unable to care for and guide their children. For all patients, concerns about losing friends and activities or needing help are common. Other concerns include changes in workplace relationships, such as needing to accept reduced roles or forego promotions. All these concerns can erode patients' self-esteem.

Inevitably, relationship fears lead to the fear of abandonment. Conditions that require extensive periods of recovery, and potentially extensive caregiving, are especially likely to raise concerns. Not even simple diagnoses, or ones that may require treatment but will most likely result in full recoveries, are immune. Patients still tend to question how others will be impacted and whether loved ones will reject them.

SAFEGUARDING FINANCES

Because health care has distinct financial implications, concerns about finances are among those newly diagnosed patients are likely to consider. There are managed-care deductibles, co-insurance, and co-payments to consider, as well as costs for transportation, lodging, and special diets. Even lifestyle changes like exercise come at a cost. Medical conditions often require time off from work, a particularly daunting prospect when the newly diagnosed patients are the primary income providers.

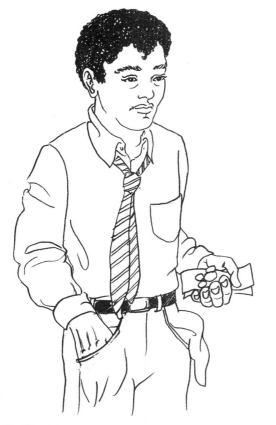

*"I am getting hit with one expense after another. If I can't get back to my
job right away, what's going to happen to my finances?"*

Because financial concerns are both immediate and ongoing, patients continually struggle with them. Even understanding insurance benefits can be an ongoing
struggle. Compounding the problem, patients often lack the physical and emotional
energy to effectively advocate for themselves when financial and other pressures do
arise.

LOSING TRADITIONAL ROLES

Roles provide a measure of comfort, reliability, and routine in daily life. We are expected to behave in certain ways, and people tend to respond to us in prescribed ways.
It is no surprise then that people identify themselves by their roles—professional, parent, spouse, son/daughter, boyfriend/girlfriend, community member, church/syna-
gogue member, volunteer—each associated with a set of responsibilities and, to some
extent, status.

Newly diagnosed patients often fear that the roles they value will somehow be lost
or denied. For example, patients who tie their value to their job titles will likely experience a great deal of fear upon considering losing their roles in the workplace. While
job losses affect finances, they also affect self-esteem. Similarly, an older person who
gains self-esteem from volunteering will likely view the inability to continue doing so
as a major loss.

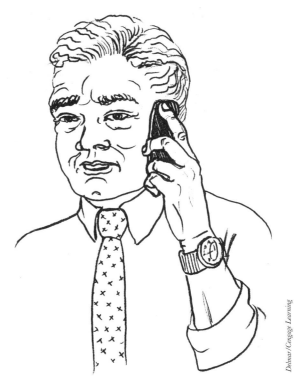

"I'm going to have to drop off the committee for awhile.
I'll let you know when I feel well enough again."

CHANGING ROUTINES

Routines give our lives structure, security, and a sense of normalcy. The familiarity of day-to-day routines is soothing. Often, though, we take the basic elements of our daily routines—waking up, making coffee, going to work, coming home—for granted. Yet the prospect of having to make even the smallest changes to our routines can be fear inducing. To a newly diagnosed patient, the prospect of having to take a medication in the morning and delay breakfast can feel drastic.

Facing Overarching Fears: Uncertainty and Change

As human beings, we want to feel we know what is going to happen tomorrow, next week, next month, and beyond. We do poorly with uncertainty. Uncertainty can lead to change, something we are hardwired to avoid. A medical diagnosis, with its potential to affect things like routines, relationships, and finances, introduces the possibility that life may never be the same. For the first time, newly diagnosed patients may have to consider that they do not control their lives, and that prospect can be terrifying.

Coupled with the fear of uncertainty and change is the fear associated with the loss of normalcy. Medical diagnoses cause many patients to ask, "Will I ever be normal again?" Being normal means not only performing basic tasks and maintaining relationships, as discussed previously, but appearing normal to others. Somehow, we never outgrow the need to feel like everyone else.

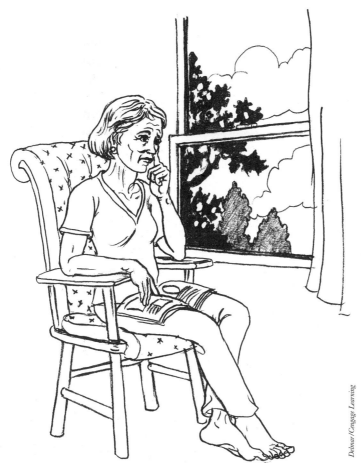

"I love walking to work in the morning, it's one of my favorite parts of the day. How could I possibly replace it?"

Approaching Patients Overwhelmed by Fear

As discussed previously, newly diagnosed patients who are caught up in fear will challenge health-care professionals. Health-care professionals should use the following guidelines when interacting with fearful patients:

- Be sensitive to the patient's fear. As irrational as it may seem to the health-care professional, it is real to the patient.

- Remember that fear may be temporary. A patient may experience fear as part of a range of emotions, such as sadness and anger. Consider delaying discussions that patients are not ready to have.

- Be gentle and tentative when approaching the patient. Fearful patients may overreact and feel that their health-care professionals are confronting them.

- Suggest information and experiences that are contrary to the patient's perceptions, but do so tentatively and nonconfrontationally.

The following sections give examples of how fear may enter into patient interactions.

> **KEEP IN MIND**
>
> Patient fear is a multifaceted challenge with widespread health-care impact. In what areas would you see the fear factor to be of greatest concern in patient interactions? Patient education? Treatment decisions? Ongoing compliance? Why would you choose these areas?

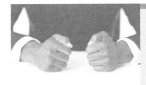

Body Language

Newly diagnosed patients experiencing fear might exhibit such body language as:

- Hunched-over posture, arms folded tightly across the chest
- Frowning, anguished expression
- Eyes wide open
- Rapid breathing
- Hands up to mouth
- Nervous movements
- Expressionless, looking away

UNDERSTANDING THE FEAR CONDITION

Patients who are overwhelmed by fear, even temporarily, will have difficulty listening to and processing information regarding their conditions. Often, such patients listen selectively: They hear only negative information. They then process that information in a manner that further contributes to their fear. The following conversation between Marla, a nurse, and Saundra, a patient, demonstrates this difficulty.

> MARLA: I want to review what the doctor told you about your condition. First, I'd like to talk to you about what it means to have sickle cell anemia.
>
> SAUNDRA: I know what it means. It means I'm going to die.

At this point, Saundra is demonstrating extreme fear about her condition. In her mind, her diagnosis means death. While she may be open to information, she may also be likely to interpret it from this viewpoint.

What not to do:

> MARLA: That's not true at all. Who told you that?
>
> SAUNDRA: I don't need anybody to tell me. I've heard all the stories.
>
> MARLA: Well, you need to update your information.

The optimal approach:

> MARLA: Saundra, it sounds like you're really scared about this.
>
> SAUNDRA: I *am* really scared. I feel like my life is going to be over, and I can't think about anything else right now.
>
> MARLA: Would you like me to talk to you about some of my experiences in working with patients with sickle cell anemia? I can tell you that I know a lot of patients with sickle cell who are leading happy and productive lives.
>
> SAUNDRA: I'm not sure if I can listen to anything else about it.
>
> MARLA: It's up to you. But I'm going to leave you with some literature and my number here at the office if you have questions.

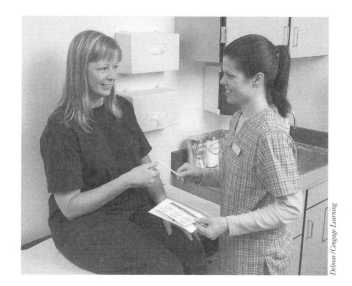

Delmar/Cengage Learning

Marla could have confronted Saundra with rational knowledge or spoken with her from an emotional perspective. Given that Saundra was viewing her situation from an emotional perspective, she was more receptive when Marla also communicated emotionally.

MAKING TREATMENT DECISIONS

Patients must often make treatment decisions soon, if not immediately, after being informed of their diagnoses. While some patients are able to do so, others must rely on the recommendations of their health-care providers and/or families. When patients must be actively involved in treatment decisions, the prospect of the condition itself, as well as the treatment, may render the patients unable to consider treatment options.

In the following example, Jack has been presented with options for a back problem, and his medical assistant, Tanya, has been tasked with offering assistance as he makes his decision.

> **TANYA:** Jack, the doctor talked with you about surgery as taking a wait-and-see approach with physical therapy. Any thoughts about what you're considering?
>
> **JACK:** What I can tell you is that I have a family to support, and if I'm not able to do my job, a lot of people are going to be suffering. I can miss work while I recover from surgery, or I can miss work while I go to physical therapy. I don't see any upside to either option.

Jack's response tells Tanya that he is afraid about how his condition is going to affect his finances. His fear of economic distress is so strong that both options are being considered only in relation to his fears around loss of income.

What not to do:

> **TANYA:** Jack, your income is not the issue here. You've got to decide what you want to do about your back and get started on getting better.
>
> **JACK:** Don't you understand that this may break my family? How are we going to pay the bills if I'm laid up?

The optimal approach:

TANYA: You're really concerned about your finances right now.

JACK: Yes, I am. And so I'm afraid to make this decision. Either way, I lose.

TANYA: Is there any information I could give you that would help you to look at your treatment from the financial perspective?

JACK: Well, I'm still not sure how much time I might be out of work after the surgery. And I didn't get much of an idea what the time commitment would be with the physical therapy.

TANYA: Okay. Let's talk to the doctor, and ask her to make some projections for you.

Tanya recognized that Jack needed to move beyond his financial concerns and focus on getting better. However, had she focused on Jack's decision, and not his fears, she risked more resistance. Because Jack did not want to launch into a decision until he had dealt with his fears, Tanya acknowledged Jack's fear and offered to facilitate the information-gathering that would help him make a more educated decision.

INSTITUTING LIFESTYLE CHANGES

Fearful patients can resist discussions about lifestyle changes—diet, exercise, daily activities—for two reasons. First, lifestyle changes force patients to assess how their conditions will impact their lives. Second, lifestyle changes force patients to consider how their conditions will impact others.

Donna, recently diagnosed with high cholesterol and high blood pressure, discusses lifestyle changes with her nurse, Alberto, in the following.

ALBERTO: Donna, I know you met with the dietician and the fitness coach about having a healthier lifestyle. How did that go?

DONNA: How did it go? I can have food with no salt, no fat, and no taste. My husband and I used to enjoy cooking and eating together, but they're telling me that has to end. And I'm supposed to become a fitness nut instead of sitting with my husband and watching TV. How long do you think it's going to be before he decides to find someone more fun to spend time with?

Like many patients, Donna fears her lifestyle changes will affect her relationship with her husband. Indirectly, she is expressing the fear of abandonment. At this point, she cannot have a productive discussion about lifestyle changes. Alberto knows that emphasizing the importance of these lifestyle changes, without acknowledging her fears, may increase Donna's resistance.

What not to do:

ALBERTO: We can't worry about what your husband is going to do right now, Donna. What's important is that you focus on your health and get started right away with a healthy diet. I recommend that you plan on starting tonight by cooking a healthy meal for the two of you.

DONNA: So, I'm supposed to just drop this on him? Either he gives up the food that he loves or we eat separately? That's like telling him he isn't good enough for me anymore. What do you think he's going to do with that message?

The optimal approach:

ALBERTO: I know the diet feels really drastic to you. And I can see you're worried about how this is going to affect your husband, too.

DONNA: You bet I am. This isn't going to be fair to either one of us. How would you like it if the person who cooks for you suddenly changed the rules?

ALBERTO: I know this is frustrating. Can I ask if you have talked to your husband about your diagnosis?

DONNA: Just a little bit. I didn't want to upset him.

ALBERTO: I'm wondering if it might help to have a conversation with him about what's going on with you and what your health-care team has recommended. Do you think that might help?

DONNA: Maybe. I'll think about it.

ALBERTO: And let's talk about how we can all work together on this end to help you get started on keeping you as healthy as possible. Can we do that?

Rather than confronting Donna with the rational argument for changing her diet, Alberto instead talked to her on a feeling level, beginning with reflecting that she is worried. Donna responded to that approach, being more open to what Alberto had to say. Notice that he offered the beginning of a solution by suggesting that Donna educate her husband. Given her resistance to change, Alberto offers the assistance of the health-care team in implementing the change. Actions like these reassure fearful patients.

KNOWING WHEN FEAR LEADS TO HELPLESSNESS

The fear of newly diagnosed patients can be so strong as to be immobilizing. Thoughts and images become overwhelming, and patients come to believe they cannot control their outcomes. Often, the cycle is self-fulfilling: Patients' fear is driven by lack of information, but they are so fearful, they cannot process the information that would benefit them. At this point, patients begin to feel helpless. Patients who feel helpless may be unable or unwilling to address their diagnoses.

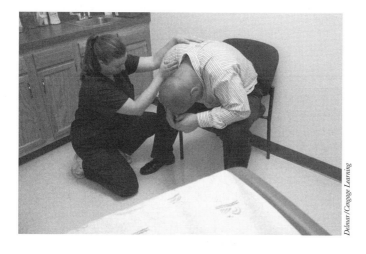

The symptoms of helplessness are similar to those for depression. Patients in flight reaction are likely to appear distraught, while those in freeze reaction may exhibit no emotions. When patients appear to have fallen into states of helplessness, health-care professionals should refer them to mental-health professionals as described in Chapter 3.

Appreciating the Upside of Fear

Like stress, fear can be motivating. Stage fright, for example, can motivate a presenter to carefully prepare and practice a presentation. When balanced by rational understanding, fear can empower newly diagnosed patients to do what they need to remain healthy.

Patient fear may result from a lack of information about consequences. Patients who lack information may fill the gaps with their own projections and inadvertently create more fear. By providing realistic information, including consequences of non-compliance, health-care professionals can dispel irrational fear and use rational fear as a motivator. For example, smokers are often heavily influenced to quit by the prospect of lung cancer, and diabetics are motivated to remain compliant by the potential consequences of kidney failure and amputation.

To avoid triggering a fear response, when relaying realistic consequences health-care professionals should focus on benefits to the patient rather than risks. Appropriate phrases include the following:

- "Do you want to talk about why it's important to start treatment as soon as possible?"

- "I'd like to go over some of the reasons you can benefit from a healthier diet."

- "Let's talk about why making these changes can help you avoid certain conditions."

- "You have a lot of choices here, and the choices have consequences, some good, some not so good. I'll go through them with you."

Patients in fight reaction are most likely to be naturally motivated by fear. They acknowledge fear as a valid emotion and, rather than being defeated by it, use it to empower themselves to perform tasks like information-gathering. These patients have essentially faced their fears, understand what they fear most, and have concluded what they can and should reasonably be afraid of in regard to their conditions. Fighters are motivated most by the fears of making uninformed decisions and not doing everything possible to maintain their optimal health.

KEEP IN MIND

In the health-care arena, fear can be a particularly useful motivator. When are some of those times? Have you witnessed another health-care professional use fear as part of a pep talk with a newly diagnosed patient? Have you witnessed fear used to force compliance? How do you personally view the role of fear as a motivator? What is your comfort level in using fear to motivate patients? What do you see as the risks?

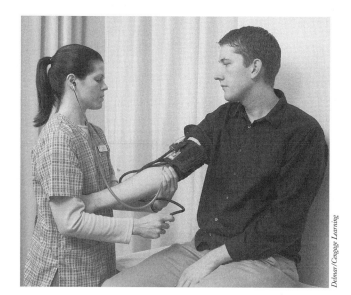

Delmar/Cengage Learning

Using Techniques for Coping with Fear's Emotional Effects

A number of techniques can help newly diagnosed patients cope with their fears, and they run the gamut. Some are rationally based, while some approach issues from an emotional perspective. Some require active involvement of health-care professionals, while others can be executed through recommendation or referral. Descriptions of the techniques follow.

ENGAGING THE PATIENT'S RATIONAL SIDE

Presenting Counterevidence

Patients who are overwhelmed by fear respond poorly to confrontation. With these patients, a better approach is to gently suggest evidence that is contrary to the patient's information. Because the patients are highly emotional, a straightforward presentation of facts is less effective than a discussion with feeling words. The latter gains patients' trust and lowers their resistance. Health-care professionals should introduce all information tentatively. If patients remain resistant, this approach may be more useful at another time.

Used appropriately, however, information contrary to the patients', or **counterevidence**, can help reduce patients' fear factor. Counterevidence can be based on the health-care professional's knowledge or on the professional's experience working with patients with a similar diagnosis.

The following conversation between a nurse, Charlene, and a patient, Ashweeta, uses a counterargument.

CHARLENE: How are you doing today, Ashweeta?

ASHWEETA: I'm terrified of what's ahead of me. I don't see any future for myself right now.

CHARLENE: Why no future?

ASHWEETA: Because I know that with this diagnosis, my life is going to go on a downward spiral. The medications are only going to help a little but not enough. It won't be long before I won't be able to do much of anything.

CHARLENE: I've worked with a lot of patients who were diagnosed with MS. And we've been treating many of the same patients for years in this practice, so I've witnessed their success stories firsthand. Would you be interested in hearing some of their experiences?

ASHWEETA: I don't know how that's going to help me. I'm not them.

CHARLENE: You're right about that. But I've learned that people with your diagnosis have a lot of different experiences. I was thinking that hearing about some other experiences might suggest some alternative outcomes. What do you think?

ASHWEETA: I guess that might be interesting, sure.

Note that Charlene began by acknowledging Ashweeta's feelings without judgment and without directly arguing the point that she could be looking at her future differently. This gentle approach encouraged Ashweeta to be open to talking more, as well as listening better. Charlene then suggested that she could impart further information, but she left the decision to Ashweeta.

Applying Bibliotherapy

The term **bibliotherapy** refers to the therapeutic value of information. Being exposed to valid information can be especially helpful for patients experiencing fear, because while it may confirm some of the patients' suspicions regarding their conditions and treatments, it may dispel some fears.

Some patients, like those in fight reaction, are natural information gatherers. However, even fighters may need some encouragement to expose themselves to information when they are feeling the most overwhelmed by fear. Patients in flight and freeze reactions are most likely to need encouragement to gather information.

Generally, hospitals, clinics, and physicians' offices stock information pamphlets that are available through nonprofit organizations and pharmaceutical companies. The World Wide Web also has an abundance of information, but not all is reliable or helpful. When carefully selected and presented by a health-care professional, information given to patients can be helpful.

In the following, Jeanine, a recently diagnosed patient, mentions the fears of her treatment to her nurse practitioner, Alicia.

ALICIA: Any questions you want to ask me about your treatment regimen?

JEANINE: Yeah. How am I supposed to survive it? I know I'm probably going to feel awful. Nausea, headaches. . . . I'm going to be tired. Sounds like fun, doesn't it?

ALICIA: I know this is scary, Jeanine. Where did you hear about all of these side effects?

JEANINE: Everybody knows what you go through with chemotherapy.

ALICIA: You know, Jeanine, we have some really good pamphlets here that you might want to take a look at. They are written in layperson's terms, so can give you a clear picture of what you might expect. Chemotherapy treatment has really improved over the past few years, and you may find that a lot of the side effects have been greatly reduced. Would you like to take a look at a little bit of this information?

JEANINE: I don't want to be even more scared.

ALICIA: If you want, I can go over one of them with you and point out a few things you might want to consider. How would that be?

JEANINE: Okay. I'll give it a try. But not scare tactics like telling me all the bad things that might happen!

ALICIA: Absolutely not. Just some information.

As in the preceding conversations, Alicia, the health-care professional, began the exchange by acknowledging her patient's emotional state. Rather than confronting Jeanine with the need to update her knowledge and not create stories, she suggested that she might want to read some valid information to update her knowledge. To help Jeanine take this first step, Alicia offered to review some of the information with her. This way, she could be assured that Jeanine read the information thoroughly, not selectively, which would help prevent added fears. In addition, she could answer any of Jeanine's questions as they came up.

Tapping into Support Groups

Support groups can greatly benefit newly diagnosed patients in that the experiences of other, established patients can neutralize some of the new patients' less rational fears about conditions and treatments. It is important to keep in mind, however, that newly diagnosed patients may be unprepared for support groups initially. The stories of other patients may increase, rather than decrease, their fears. Consequently, the health-care professional may consider postponing support-group recommendations and instead suggest that patients talk individually with other patients who can be trusted to project upbeat, positive attitudes.

Combating Negative Self-Talk

Patients who are feeling afraid often focus on the worst possible outcomes and then repeatedly remind themselves of what might be in their future with phrases like, "This will happen to you," "You'll feel that way," or "You'll end up like this." Mental-health professionals call this **negative self-talk**, because patients talk to themselves about all the possible negative outcomes, and often with too little information to know if the possibilities are realistic or not. When patients bombard themselves with negative messages, they simply reinforce their fears.

Because they fuel fear, negative thoughts are like poison, but poison can be cured with an **antidote**. For negative self-talk, the antidote is a **counterargument** that counteracts the negative self-talk and turns it positive. Before using this technique, health-care professionals should first listen to patients, to specify the outcomes they are envisioning. Then, they should gently introduce antidotes into patient conversations.

In the following example, Tyrone discusses his lung condition with his nurse, Albert.

ALBERT: You seem upset, Tyrone. What's going on?

TYRONE: I'm upset. I can't help but see where I might be in another year or less. I might not be able to take care of myself. I'll be a burden to my wife. I won't be able to work. Who knows? I might be bedridden by then. I have to be realistic here.

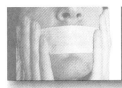

SELF • talk

The fear factor can result in self-talk that includes the following statements:

I'm not going to come out of this alive.

My God! What's going to happen to me? I know it's going to be awful.

Why have any hope when I'm just going to be disappointed anyway?

Maybe the best thing to do is give up and let my life fall apart.

I'm so afraid, I can't even think about this.

Antidotes to fear-related self-talk include the following:

I have a great team of health-care professionals around me, and they are doing everything possible.

I can't predict the future, but I have a lot to live for right now.

I'm going to focus on being calm and focused and not give in to fear.

My family will be with me as I face the future, and I'll be there for them.

The evidence shows that many people go on with their lives with my condition, even though they have to make changes. I'm ready to face the future.

ALBERT: You're really thinking a lot about what could happen.

TYRONE: Yes, I am. I need to prepare myself for the worst, and the worst is about all I see right now.

ALBERT: Maybe I could make a suggestion, Tyrone. Would that be okay?

TYRONE: Okay.

ALBERT: It seems like you're being hard on yourself by reminding yourself of all the bad things that can happen. I'm thinking you might want to also say some positive words to yourself.

TYRONE: Like what?

ALBERT: We really don't have all the information yet in terms of what your treatment is going to be, and we don't know how you'll do on whatever treatment you and your doctor decide on. So maybe you could also remind yourself that you don't know what the future holds but that you and your doctors are doing everything possible to treat your condition. Do you believe that?

TYRONE: Yeah, I believe it. But it's hard not to look on that scary side when you have this diagnosis staring at you.

ALBERT: I know, Tyrone. Let's work together on standing up to the fear with some positive thinking. Maybe every time you have one of those scary thoughts you could come back at it with a reminder that you're doing all the right stuff. Want to try it?

TYRONE: Okay, I'll give it a try.

Albert heard how Tyrone was inundating himself with repeated messages about fearful outcomes and suggested antidotes of more hopeful messages. Notice that Albert

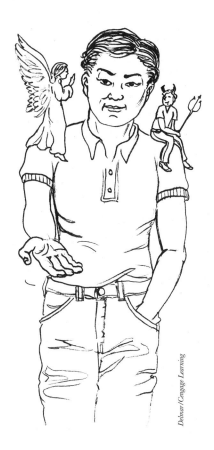

Delmar/Cengage Learning

did this by suggesting a positive thought. He also did a reality check with Tyrone in terms of whether he believed the message. Once Albert had Tyrone's agreement, he suggested how Tyrone could use the message to counteract his fear.

WORKING DIRECTLY WITH THE PATIENT'S EMOTIONS

Instead of talking, patients overwhelmed by fear may respond better to techniques that engage their emotions, and directly. Such experiential techniques help patients achieve a sense of relaxation and inner peace. Research has shown that complementary therapies like meditation and visualization can be highly effective in helping fearful patients move beyond their fear (Dane, 2000; Johnson et al., 2009; Lykins & Baer, 2009). While health-care professionals may not deliver these services, they should suggest them as appropriate.

Demonstrating Meditation

The fear factor is accompanied by a rush of adrenaline and other hormones that increase blood flow to the muscles and feelings of stress. Newly diagnosed patients can benefit from **meditation**, because it helps release feelings of fear and anxiety. In addition to easing stress, meditation has the following benefits:

- Enhanced sense of self-confidence
- Increased restfulness
- Decreased anxiety
- State of relaxation and feeling of well-being

Jon Kabat-Zinn, PhD, is a pioneer in using meditation and related wellness techniques with patients facing catastrophic illness. His research has shown that meditation not only reduces anxiety, it can greatly benefit patient treatment because it reduces fear and creates a sense of well-being that renders patients more receptive to treatment (Kabat-Zinn, 1990 and 2006).

While some patients are familiar with mind/body practices like meditation, others who are less familiar are usually receptive provided they experience the technique in ways that are consistent with their religious beliefs and overall comfort levels. Among the range of meditation techniques available, some are based in Eastern religions like Buddhism while others have been adapted for Westerners.

Encouraging Activity

Active patients may have reduced anxiety levels. Activity, especially in some form of exercise, can release hormones that contribute to a sense of well-being and peace of mind. The increased circulation that results from exercise is also beneficial. Exercise has reduced depression and helped to create more positive moods (Dalgas et al., 2010; Derelli & Yaliman, 2010; Harvard Mental Health Letter, 2010). Active patients often feel self-confident and enjoy a sense of empowerment. Group activities give patients an opportunity to receive emotional support.

Obviously, patients are not always able to engage in vigorous aerobic exercise. However, in consultation with physicians, patients can be encouraged to try some form of activity, whether mild exercise, yoga, or a hobby.

Facing Fear with "What If?"

While it is important for newly diagnosed patients to remain focused on maintaining their health, they can benefit from frank discussions about the future. Some patient fears are identifiable and concrete and must be discussed with health-care professionals. Among these fears are the side effects of medication, loss of work and maybe even medical benefits, and the need for increased assistance from caregivers.

Asking "What if?" gives patients an opportunity to both confront their greatest fears as well as obtain useful information that might help dispel those fears. However, there is a fine line between encouraging patients to remain optimistic and not give in to irrational fear and encouraging those patients to deny their conditions. For patients in flight reaction, the potential for **denial** is especially strong because their emotions may be uncontrolled. The key is to remember that some fears are realistic and some are not. To make the distinction, patients should talk with their health-care professionals and become informed about their conditions and treatments. The "What if" discussion is most productive when health-care professionals use rational and emotional-based techniques to expose and dissipate patient fears. Patients can then make informed, rational treatment and lifestyle management decisions. Fighters will insist on having this discussion, while patients in flight and freeze reaction will likely need help coming to terms with their emotions first.

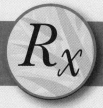

Helping a Patient Cope with the Fear Factor

Amar, the patient from the beginning of this chapter who had recently received an HIV diagnosis, discussed his diagnosis with Jason, his nurse practitioner. In the following scenario, Jason gives Amar an opportunity to discuss his fears in more depth and attempts to help Amar to resolve some of his feelings.

JASON: It's normal to have a lot of fear when you receive a medical diagnosis like HIV. You weren't feeling sick, so this diagnosis is totally unexpected.

AMAR: Totally unexpected is right! I feel like I'm standing on the edge of a cliff, and I'm not sure when I might fall over.

JASON: That's a scary feeling.

AMAR: Yes, it is.

JASON: I know you've talked about your feelings with some of the other members of the team. Any ideas that were helpful to you?

AMAR: Terry suggested I might try a meditation group to help me to relax and sleep better. They have one here at the center that meets every week, and I'm going to give that a try. I've been thinking about trying meditation, and I guess now I finally have a good reason to.

JASON: Great. Anything else?

AMAR: I was really down in the dumps about a week ago when I stopped in for a blood draw. Tony mentioned using more positive thinking, starting with telling myself that I have excellent health care and am doing all the right things to keep the upper hand with my health. So I'm doing that, too. And, of course, I've picked up a few pamphlets.

JASON: Fantastic. Have those things been helping?

AMAR: I would say they have. But let's be honest. I still have a lot to be scared about.

JASON: I understand. Why don't you tell me what's scaring you the most?

AMAR: How about dying, to start with? I mean, I do have a fatal illness.

JASON: Do you mind if I offer you a couple of thoughts here?

AMAR: Okay.

JASON: You're familiar with the recent advances in HIV treatment, right?

AMAR: Yes, I am.

JASON: So you know that medical science has made incredible advances. People are living longer, much longer, as long as they work closely with their physicians and comply with their medication schedules.

AMAR: But what if I'm put on the meds and they don't work? If that happens, I'm outta here.

JASON: Did you know that if one treatment regimen doesn't work, there are other options available?

AMAR: I guess I hadn't thought much about different treatment options being available. I can accept that possibility. Still, I don't want to hear that people don't ever die of AIDS. I read about a case in the paper just last week.

JASON: I can't tell you people don't die of this condition. A lot of factors are involved, including adopting the best regimen, maintaining a healthy lifestyle, and being compliant. But you're right: There aren't any guarantees.

AMAR: So you're being honest with me here.

JASON: I am, Amar. And you're working with a really experienced team of professionals here.

AMAR: Okay. That's reassuring anyway.

JASON: I have a chart in one of the treatment rooms that shows all the current medications and how they can be combined in various ways so that patients have the best regimens available to them at the time. Can we take a quick look at that together?

AMAR: If you think it might help. I'd be willing to try anything that would help me not be so scared about this.

JASON: I can't promise you will feel any less scared. But I can certainly give you some education.

AMAR: Okay, thanks.

Guidelines for Addressing Fear and the "What If?" Question

Following are some guidelines to keep in mind when working with patients who are experiencing fear:

1. *Use emotional words to reduce resistance.*   As discussed in Chapter 3, patients who are acting and reacting from an emotional perspective are more open to emotional words. Jason began the conversation by acknowledging and showing empathy for Amar's feelings of fear. In so doing, he honored Amar and rendered him more open to talking. He also increased his trustworthiness.

2. *Reinforce progress in actively overcoming fear.*   Patients like to feel they are making progress, even when they are initially diagnosed and may not have yet begun treatment. Health-care professionals can help by linking progress in coping with specific actions. Professionals' praise encourages more patient action. When Jason responded enthusiastically to Amar's interest in meditation and use of positive thinking, he helped to ensure that Amar will continue his efforts.

3. *Ask the patient to articulate specific fears.*   When speaking with health-care professionals about fear, patients may feel a need to please or to avoid. As a result, they may admit to fears they do not have, or they may mask ones they do have. Health-care professionals can even inadvertently introduce new concerns. To circumvent assumptions and avoidance, invite patients to start conversations. Ask them to identify their fears, perhaps starting with the greatest ones, as Jason did by asking, "Why don't you tell me what's scaring you the most?"

    This approach gives patients an opportunity to attain some emotional relief by identifying their fears and provides a starting place for helping the patients view their fears realistically.

4. *Approach the discussion of information tentatively.*   As discussed previously, patients who are experiencing strong fear are sensitive to aggressive behavior or any suggestion that they should be feeling or behaving in certain ways. Similarly, they will likely reject any information perceived as forced on them. Jason started his conversation by inviting Amar to discuss his fears. He then followed with a tentative offer of information, which Amar could accept or reject.

5. *Realize that patients may react to the word* **fear**.   Even when newly diagnosed patients appear to be experiencing fear, health-care professionals should use the "fear" label carefully for two reasons. First, directly addressing fear may imply to patients that they have reason to be fearful. They may take the word as a cue for alarm. Second, patients may assume that their health-care professionals are implying they are overreacting, or somehow weak, if they are experiencing fear. Instead of *fear*, then, health-care professionals should use softer phrase like "concerned about" and let patients be the first to use stronger terms like *fear* and *scared*. The health-care professionals can then follow up using the same language.

6. *Be prepared to make a mental-health referral.*   Fear can be crippling if it leads to helplessness and depression. Therefore, health-care professionals should always be on the lookout for symptoms of depression, as described in Chapter 3, and prepared to make mental-health referrals as needed.

Outlining the Role of Superstitious Thinking

The fear newly diagnosed patients have for their conditions can be related to superstitious thinking—imagining the worst in the hope that the situation will be better. The following quote illustrates superstitious thinking in regard to medical diagnosis:

> *"If I think it's going to be awful, then maybe it won't be quite as bad and I won't be disappointed. In fact, I might be pleasantly surprised."*

Patients who cope with their diagnoses through superstitious thinking create and express irrational fears. For example, they may express the belief that they are going to die from their conditions, regardless of the evidence to the contrary. They may talk about expecting to lose their jobs or families or having to give up the activities they enjoy most. Superstitious thinking is a way of avoiding disappointment

Patients who derive fear from superstitious thinking can challenge health-care professionals, because they have a stake in believing, or at least professing to believe, the worst. They can refuse to listen to recommendations and information and/or insist on interpreting the information in ways that support their superstitions. Patients in flight and freeze reactions are susceptible.

Health-care professionals who suspect that patients are basing their fears on superstitious thinking should gently encourage the patients to consider the facts as well as their own positive experiences with their diagnoses. Repeated discussions may be needed to help patients move away from this attitude.

SUMMARY

Fear, a normal response to a new medical diagnosis, is experienced at varying levels of intensity and duration. Patients experiencing fear may have difficulty processing information or making decisions about their treatment. Health-care professionals can help fearful patients by being sensitive to their fears and preventing those fears from becoming barriers to communication.

Chapter Review

Multiple-Choice Questions

1. Health-care professionals should offer fearful, newly diagnosed patients pamphlets on their diagnoses because the patients:
   a. Must be fearful enough to comply with treatment
   b. Can identify new fears
   c. Should be distracted
   d. Can confirm accurate information

2. Health-care professionals should encourage patients experiencing fear to:
   a. Talk about their fears and delay treatment indefinitely
   b. Make their decisions as soon as possible despite their fears
   c. Identify family members to make their decisions
   d. Talk about their fears and become better informed

3. How should health-care professionals use the fear of newly diagnosed patients to encourage compliance?
   a. Describe the worst possible outcomes followed by what they can do to avoid them
   b. Identify the worst possible outcomes and ask the patients to create avoidance strategies
   c. Focus on the benefits of compliance
   d. Avoid any discussion of the future

4. The value of encouraging newly diagnosed patients to try techniques like meditation and yoga is:
   a. Patients may experience relief from their fear by learning to relax.
   b. Patients may experience relief from their fear by finding things to do on their own.
   c. Driving to a class can be a good way to maintain mental abilities.
   d. None of the above

5. The ability to cope with fear benefits newly diagnosed patients by making them:
   a. More open to listening to information about their conditions
   b. Better able to evaluate treatment alternatives
   c. More optimistic and flexible when facing lifestyle changes
   d. All of the above

Fill-in-the-Blank Questions

1. Newly diagnosed patients who constantly remind themselves of the worst possible outcomes demonstrate the concept called _____ _____.

2. Patients who are experiencing a feeling of helplessness often exhibit symptoms similar to _____.

3. Information that proves the inaccuracy of other information is called _____.

4. Positive _____ -talk, also called _____, can help patients who constantly remind themselves of the potential negative outcomes of their conditions.

5. Because information-gathering can help patients face the fear factor, it is called _____.

Short-Answer Questions

1. What key, relationship-related concerns do newly diagnosed patients have?

_____

_____

_____

2. Why can fear sometimes motivate patients to make needed lifestyle changes? With fear as a motivator, are these changes long-lasting? Why?

_____

_____

_____

3. What are some of the life roles newly diagnosed patients fear may be changed dramatically, if not lost, as a result of their conditions?

_____

_____

_____

4. What is the value of counterevidence for newly diagnosed patients who have misperceptions about their conditions?

_____

_____

_____

5. What, if any, value does activity have for newly diagnosed patients?

_____

_____

_____

Critical-Thinking Questions

1. As a health-care professional, what would you like to see the health-care system do for newly diagnosed patients concerned about finances?

_____

_____

_____

_____

_____

_____

2. Health-care professionals know the importance of coping with medical diagnoses and getting treatment under way. Patients, in contrast, may be so overwhelmed by their fear that they place themselves at further risk by delaying treatment. Is there a point at which newly diagnosed patients can benefit from a more direct approach to encourage them to address their diagnoses? What is that point? Who should deliver the message?

_____

_____

_____

_____

_____

_____

3. Health-care professionals may feel most comfortable focusing on facts when working through the fear of newly diagnosed patients. Others may be comfortable using feeling words with patients. What is the value of both approaches? Is it possible to acknowledge fear while helping patients to accept reality? If so, how is this done?

_____

_____

_____

_____

_____

Internet Exercise

Imagine that you are working with a patient who is experiencing a high degree of fear about a diagnosis and its treatment.

Develop a strategy for helping the patient to begin using Web-based resources. After choosing a diagnosis, identify Web sites that provide basic facts about the patient's condition, descriptions of recommended treatments, success stories, coping information, and community resources.

Given that it is not advisable to overload the patient with too many Web sites or recommend sites with information that is too detailed or direct, where would your starting place be? What additional sites would you recommend after initial information-gathering? Consider how you might encourage information-gathering in phases.

_____

_____

_____

_____

_____

_____

_____

_____

CHAPTER 5

Emotions and Health-Care Decision Making

OVERVIEW

After reading this chapter, you should be able to:

- Define and use the keywords related to emotions and health-care decision making.

- Understand the role emotional and cognitive perspectives play in treatment decisions.

- Know how to assess when patients are ready to make treatment decisions.

- Recognize when patients may be overestimating their abilities to make treatment decisions.

- Describe the importance of establishing trust with patients and use trust to help patients make decisions.

- Identify the role patients' families play in treatment decision making.

- List the steps in decision making and take patients through these steps to evaluate treatment options.

KEYWORDS

Bias

Bond

Cognitive

Cognitive exhaustion

Cognitive skills

Faith

Goals

Nuance

Objective

Prejudices

Self-efficacy

Subconscious

Teamwork

Trust

Unemotional

Wishful thinking

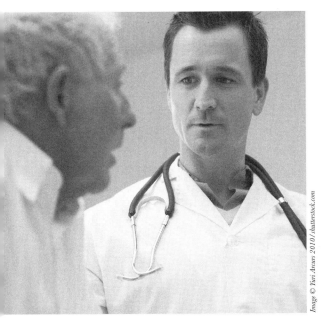

Image © Yuri Arcurs 2010/Shutterstock.com

Case Study

Walter thought his prostate cancer diagnosis, delivered only a month ago, was the worst thing that could happen. At 61, he felt his future was suddenly cut short when his urologist "signed, sealed, and delivered" the news. With few symptoms, other than some difficulty urinating, he had had little reason to prepare to face a serious illness.

A week after his diagnosis, Walter sat down with Dr. Shapiro, his new oncologist, to discuss treatment. If the situation had been less serious, Walter had told his wife, Betty, he would have been tempted to laugh as the doctor tried to sound positive. "You've got a lot of options," Dr. Shapiro had told Walter, "not just one like in the old days. And while each option has a downside, we can work together to decide which one is going to be best for you."

"Yeah," Walter had said to Betty. "Lots of options: Surgery, radiation, radioactive seeds. How lucky am *I*?"

Dr. Shapiro had reviewed each treatment option thoroughly with Walter, explaining its process, recovery, side effects, and risks. When Walter thought about this conversation later, he realized he had focused on risks and side effects and missed a lot of other details. For each option, he really had only two questions: "Will I be able to function fully at my job?" and "Will I be able to have a sex life again?"

Dr. Shapiro had addressed each concern honestly with Walter. He told him that while many patients completed treatment and returned to their lives, they had had to

---

KEEP IN MIND

In some health-care situations, multiple options can feel overwhelming. For patients facing complicated treatment decisions, sensitivity begins with identifying our own fears. What kinds of concerns would you have in a situation like Walter's? What would you feel? Confident? Insecure? Confused? Overwhelmed?

make adjustments, at least temporarily, in their sex lives. He told Walter he could give him no guarantees. While Walter knew his wife was probably less concerned about their sex life than he was, it comforted him little.

After considering Dr. Shapiro's statement, Walter had said, "This is a lot to think about. I've hardly even taken a sick day in over 30 years, and now you're telling me that I'm a very sick man with life-and-death decisions to make. And these decisions will affect the rest of my life, whatever *that* is going to be."

"You don't have to decide on treatment today," Dr. Shapiro had responded. "Your cancer is growing slowly, and there is no bone involvement. But I'd like to get treatment under way in the next month."

"I understand," Walter had returned. "I get a little reprieve. But maybe not a sex life after next month."

"We'll keep talking about the best way to treat your cancer," Dr. Shapiro answered. "The health-care team is also available to talk to you about your treatment and answer questions. They've worked with a lot of patients in your situation."

> **KEEP IN MIND**
>
> Walter described the time he had to make a treatment decision as a "reprieve," as if he had been freed temporarily from a type of punishment. This is a valuable insight into Walter's fear about this decision. As a health-care professional, how would you have reacted if Walter had said this to you?

> **KEEP IN MIND**
>
> When discussing treatment options and impacts, health-care professionals should tailor their approaches to patients' mindsets. If you were talking with Walter about the return of his sexual function after prostate cancer treatment, what would be your goal? Honesty? Reassurance? Optimism? Acceptance?

Introduction

"We need to get started on a treatment right away."

These words can alarm newly diagnosed patients, because they mean that decisions, large and small, must be made, decisions that most likely the patients are neither emotionally nor intellectually prepared to make. In addition to understanding the diagnosis and considering a second opinion, patients must make the following choices:

- Short-term treatment options (e.g., surgical or nonsurgical alternatives)
- Long-term treatment options, including medication use
- Options for lifestyle modification
- Alternative medications and treatments

Fighter patients decide to become educated and to work with their health-care professionals to make decisions. Other types of patients resist making decisions, instead leaving the task to their physicians or families. Assertive patients can challenge the health-care team, because they may question their information and recommendations. In contrast, patients who cannot or will not participate in decisions are less likely to be compliant because they may realize that they have ceded control of their decisions and change direction at some point to try to regain some of that control.

As facilitators, health-care professionals play an important role in decision making. They recognize and acknowledge the patient emotions that are interfering with the process, help educate patients, and subsequently evaluate options.

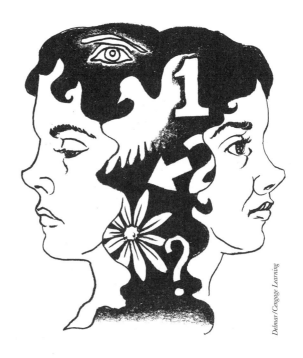

Delmar/Cengage Learning

Identifying the Facets of Decision Making

Ideally, emotional and thinking or **cognitive** perspectives work in tandem as newly diagnosed patients make decisions. The emotional perspective focuses on how patients' needs, personal values, and emotions affect how they make decisions. From the cognitive perspective decision making includes seeking and evaluating information, weighing alternatives, and coming to final decisions.

Patients in flight, freeze, or fight reaction will experience their emotional and cognitive perspectives in ways that are consistent with their reaction types. Fighters are more likely to balance the emotional and the cognitive perspectives as they make decisions. Depending on the situation, fighters are comfortable experiencing their emotions fully or relying on a more **objective**, cognitive perspective. Patients in flight reaction are more likely to view the decision-making process from a primarily emotional perspective, which may render them unable to evaluate information effectively or view decisions from a cognitive perspective. Because they are shut down emotionally, patients in freeze reaction may be unable to harness the optimism and hopefulness that can energize the decision-making process.

TAKING THE EMOTIONAL PERSPECTIVE

Often, newly diagnosed patients must make decisions in the face of uncertainty. As Chapter 4 discussed, uncertainty about the future and fear are closely tied. Uncertainty can cause patients to resist information, and fear-based resistance fuels cycle of fear. In the absence of rational information, it is human nature to fill in the gaps with assumptions that work counter to cognition and make it even more difficult to make sound decisions.

Fear is not the only emotion that colors the decision-making process. Especially under time pressure, decision making can be frustrating, and it is human nature to react to frustration with anger. The question "Why me?" may again emerge, prompting yet more patient anger. Lifestyle-related decisions, especially those equated to loss, may cause feelings of sadness. Happiness, ironically, can negatively impact decision making. Patients who are enthusiastic over treatments that are not necessarily optimal or realistic may refuse to consider other options.

ADOPTING THE COGNITIVE PERSPECTIVE

When making decisions about medical treatment, **cognitive skills** include being able to process information objectively and weigh alternatives. This is seldom an easy process for patients. First, emotions can interfere and impact outcomes. Second, because newly diagnosed patients most likely have no experience with their conditions, and little or no experience with any other medical conditions, they tend to have little cognitive decision-making experience to rely on.

Overall, in the optimal decision-making situation newly diagnosed patients can do the following:

- Discuss their diagnoses and suggested treatments with their health-care providers

- Read the information suggested by their health-care providers and gather their own

- Weigh treatment options, including benefits, risks, and inconveniences

- Consult with family members to discuss a treatment's impact on relationships and caregiving needs

- With health-care professionals, identify and consent to final decisions

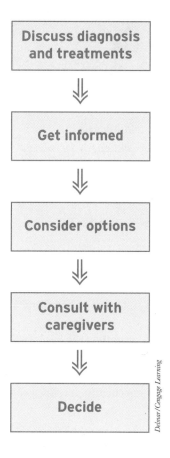

Ideally, newly diagnosed patients work with their health-care professionals, as well as their own resources, to reach decisions about their treatments. Unfortunately, human nature can intervene in the process. For example, patients may have biases about treatments based on experience with friends or relatives or something they read. A patient with a relative who underwent radiation may enter cancer treatment. When presented with other options, like surgery, the patient may listen selectively to the nonradiation options and disregard the rest, considering them less important or confusing. Similarly, patients commonly choose the first option presented to them simply to put the decision behind them or avoid the stress of having to choose.

Wishful thinking can play a role in decision making. Newly diagnosed patients may be so focused on positive outcomes that they downplay the seriousness of treatment decisions and any information they find too uncomfortable to consider. Superstitious thinking, discussed in Chapter 3, may cause patients to avoid questioning treatments and therefore "jinxing" themselves. Wishful thinking, which goes hand in hand with superstitious thinking, can be difficult for health-care professionals to counteract. Wishful thinking tends to be associated more with patients in flight reaction, while those in flight and freeze reactions tend to demonstrate superstitious thinking. Claims of "intuition" and "gut reaction" may be ways to defend both stances

Ideally, patients will ask questions to be able to weigh treatment options appropriately. Unfortunately, experience with health-related information can influence treatment decision making productively and unproductively. Some patients are easily swayed by what they heard initially, others by the most recent argument they heard

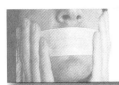

SELF • talk

Following are examples of the negative self-talk that newly diagnosed patients might use when faced with treatment decisions.

Why bother? I'm probably going to die anyway.

I can't know enough to make a life-and-death decision.

Now this is all on my shoulders. I guess nobody wants to take any responsibility for what's going to happen to me.

All I see ahead of me is uncertainty.

My life is never going to be the same, any way I look at it. So why should I care about making decisions?

Antidotes to negative self-talk about decision making include the following:

I don't have to make this decision today. I can take time to get informed.

My health-care team has my best interests at heart, and they can help me make the right decision.

The road ahead is uncertain, but I'm getting the best possible support from my health-care team.

I'm facing change, but I'm taking it one step at a time.

I have access to accurate information and supportive people as I make decisions about my health care.

from other health-care providers or patients. Patients may also pay attention to information that is presented repeatedly, even if it is not the most accurate. Information sources can affect patients' willingness to listen to, and accept, information. Some newly diagnosed patients weigh the opinions of respected companies, favored organizations, or choice Web sites most heavily when making medical decisions.

Basically, when decision making appears to be relatively clear cut, the **nuances** of human nature interfere with patients' ability to navigate this process linearly. That these nuances are primarily **subconscious**, or below the level of awareness, presents further challenges.

Melding the Emotional and Cognitive Perspectives

The emotional and cognitive perspectives need not work against each other, nor must they work separately. Instead, emotion can empower the cognitive side of decision making. As discussed previously, the struggle against unacceptable and uncomfortable emotions is more debilitating than experiencing the emotions. Patients who are able to fully express their emotions tend to gain a sense of calm and acceptance and are able to clear their minds to focus on the present. They face what they have ahead and begin making rational decisions.

KEEP IN MIND

Health-care professionals can support patients by being sensitive to the challenges patients face as they make monumental medical decisions. Have you ever felt so overcome by emotion that you could not think? In contrast, have you ever made a decision motivated out of fear or anger?

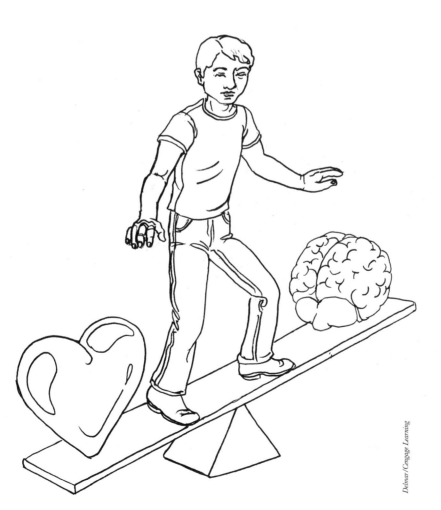

Delmar/Cengage Learning

The interplay of emotions and rational thought distinguishes patients in fight reaction from those in the flight and freeze reactions. Because they have balanced emotions and cognitive thought, fighters are able to work effectively with their health-care providers, listening to and evaluating information, asking questions, and, ultimately, participating in the decision-making process. Patients who feel part of the decision-making process are more likely to also accept risks, cope with side effects and other inconveniences, and comply with treatment (Holme, 2009; Lantz et al., 2005; Pellat, 2004).

Assessing When Patients Are Ready to Make Decisions

Newly diagnosed patients may directly indicate their readiness to make treatment or other decisions, either by enthusiastically embracing the decision or refusing to participate. Following are factors to consider when assessing whether patients are ready to cooperate with health-care professionals in making medically based decisions.

EXPRESSING EMOTIONS DIRECTLY

Patient Readiness Indicators

- Expressing emotions directly
- Failing to emote
- Having numerous questions
- Having no questions

What patients say:

> "I can't face this! I'm so angry that I have to go through this!"

> "What choice do I have? Take some kind of harsh treatment that is going to make me even sicker?"

> "I have about three options, and they're all bad. I feel so awful I can't even think about all this."

> "Leave me alone!"

Body language: Patients react consistent with extreme emotional expression, including slumping, crying, crossing the arms defiantly, and turning away.

What's going on with these patients: Patients cannot think rationally due to a rush of emotions that are at least temporarily interfering with the ability to take in and evaluate information.

FAILING TO EMOTE

What patients say:

> "Just tell me what I need to do. Let's get it over with."

> "I'm sick, and I have to get treated. What's there to talk about?"

> "I can't sit here and wring my hands."

> "Just give me the facts, and I'll decide."

Body language: Patients react consistent with being emotionally shut down, including staring into space, lack of expression, and attentive but with no emotional response.

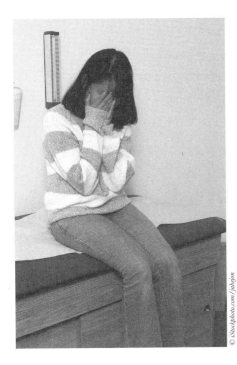

© iStockphoto.com / jabejon

What's going on with these patients: Patients like these may be temporarily disconnected from their emotions, which can be productive when objectivity is needed to evaluate information. Newly diagnosed patients, particularly those in fight reaction, may alternate between being emotional and **unemotional** as they consider the facts and then respond. The alternation is a means of balancing logic and emotions.

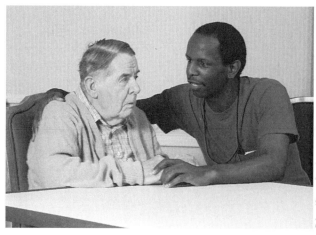

Some patients remain disconnected emotionally during diagnosis, which is not to say that they cannot emote, simply that they may have unemotional approaches to decision making. In general, patients who have prepared for their diagnoses by doing things like recognizing symptoms or heeding physician warnings are more likely to have experienced at least some of the common emotions around their conditions. Unfortunately, patients in freeze reaction have tended to disconnect to the point they both experience no feelings and fail to be able to process information.

HAVING QUESTIONS—OR NOT

What patients say:

"Can you define . . . ?"

"What are the side effects of . . . ?"

"What experiences have you had treating other patients with this approach?"

Body language: Patients who are engaged and asking questions demonstrate active listening, including eye contact and nodding. Patients who are avoiding questions look away and appear either disinterested or overly compliant.

What's going on with these patients: Patients' willingness to ask questions is one of the most telling ways to gauge their willingness to consider the facts and make decisions. While excessive questioning can begin to feel like skepticism and second-guessing to a health-care professional, patients who ask questions are willing to hear information and want to learn as much as possible as they move toward decisions.

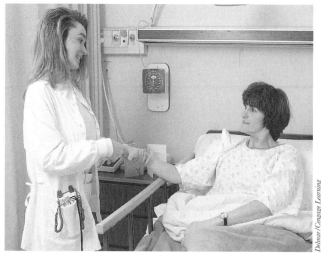

Clearly, some patients are better able than others to articulate questions and provide responses that deepen the discussion. Patients who have not educated themselves, for example, or are unaccustomed to communicating with medical professionals, may need their health-care professionals to help them better articulate their questions. Patients may express fear about the answers they might receive or ambivalence at receiving the "whole truth." Some sensitivity to answer delivery, in terms of being more tentative and hopeful than blunt within the confines of being honest, will encourage patients to continue asking questions.

Supporting Patients Who Overestimate Their Readiness

At times, newly diagnosed patients may assume they are ready to make medical decisions when they are not. This occurs for a range of reasons.

FEELING A SENSE OF URGENCY

Patients often feel a sense of urgency around their medical conditions. Patients with cancer diagnoses, for example, often want to start treatment as soon as possible. For diabetic patients, the fear of sight loss or amputation may inspire urgency on the patients' part. Driven by this sense of urgency, and impatience to move forward with treatment, patients may profess comfort levels with the recommended course of treatment and/or impatience with multiple treatment options. While a sense of urgency may support treatment compliance, it may also render patients unprepared for their treatments and equip them with unrealistic expectations regarding effectiveness.

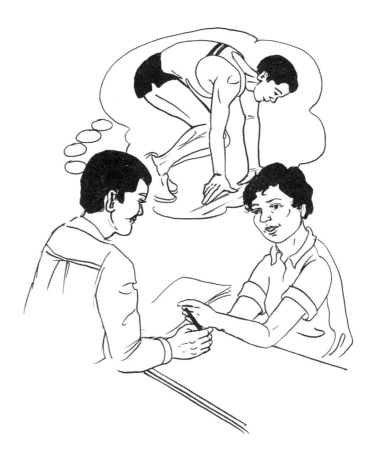

Delmar/Cengage Learning

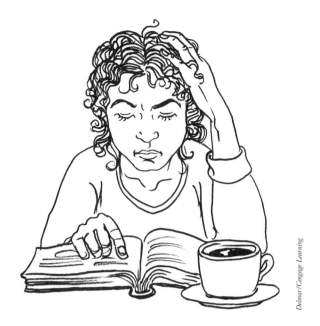

Delmar/Cengage Learning

OVERLOADING ON INFORMATION

Newly diagnosed patients may feel so overwhelmed with their diagnoses, and the information they have had to try to process, that they reach information overload. The result of information overload is **cognitive exhaustion**. Patients may feel that their minds can hold no more information and that they cannot take in, or process, any more facts. The risk is that the patients may grasp at the alternatives that seem most understandable and proclaim that they have made decisions. Information overload can become so uncomfortable that patients may decide against seeking additional information, even from sources that might prove both reliable and helpful, such as the experiences of another patient.

PLEASING THE HEALTH-CARE PROFESSIONAL

Due possibly in part to superstitious thinking, newly diagnosed patients often feel, or want to establish, strong **bonds** with their diagnosing physicians, the professionals they anticipate working with through treatment and possibly beyond. Patients consciously and subconsciously want to believe that their physicians perform some kind of magic to ensure their recoveries. Consequently, they often feel that they need to do whatever possible to show their **faith** in their physicians, whether that means professing their loyalty or pleasing the physicians in some way.

Patients who are experiencing fear and uncertainty are especially likely to want to demonstrate faith in, and believe unconditionally in, their physicians. One way in which patients feel they can please their physicians is by professing immediate faith in the recommended course of treatment and demonstrating a positive attitude. Patients in flight reaction, for example, are likely to do this. While this enthusiasm may streamline the pathway from diagnosis to treatment initialization, patients may have unrealistically high expectations of their health-care teams and treatments. In return for their faith and admiration, patients may expect their teams to be flattered and form reciprocal emotional bonds. Unfortunately, patients who are focused on pleasing their

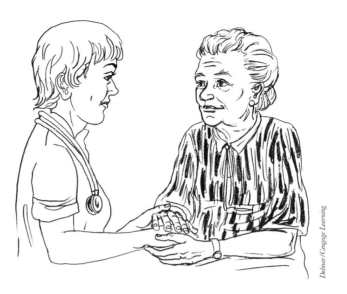

Delmar/Cengage Learning

physicians through premature treatment adoption may fail to embrace information about the less positive aspects of their treatments, like timing and side effects. In short, patients may try to pacify their health-care professionals as a means of avoiding negative information.

RESOLVING DISCOMFORT

When faced with multiple options, newly diagnosed patients can be ambivalent, lulled into inaction by the pluses and minuses of each alternative. The discomfort that comes from allowing ambivalence to persist may become so strong that the patient decides to either give in to the health-care professional who makes the strongest recommendation or flip a coin between two options merely to make a decision.

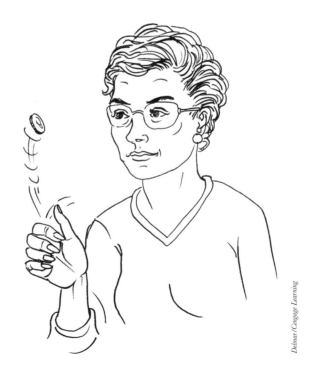

Delmar/Cengage Learning

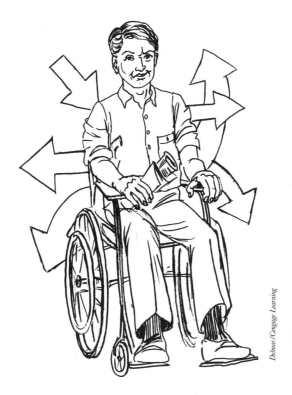

Delmar/Cengage Learning

Facilitating the Medical Decision-Making Process

Health-care professionals play many roles for newly diagnosed patients facing treatment decisions, including educator and assessor. Health-care professionals may recommend resources for second opinions or recommend treatment routes. As patients move forward with their decisions, completing treatment and subsequently recovering, those professionals will inevitably play supporting roles.

> **KEEP IN MIND**
>
> Whatever our role, most of us need support when making difficult decisions. Have you ever looked to someone to help you to make a difficult decision? How did the person help? Would something else have been more helpful?

REACHING THE OVERARCHING GOAL: TRUST

Health-care professionals can be most helpful in facilitating the decision-making process for their patients when they build patient relationships on **trust**. A high level of trust may or may not mean that patients will trust their health-care professionals to recommend the optimal courses of treatment and, in turn, pursue the treatments without question. Actually, most health-care professionals prefer that patients only make treatment decisions after carefully considering the options.

Nevertheless, patients who trust their health-care professionals have faith that their health-care professionals will do the following:

- Ask the right questions and understand how to competently use medical equipment and understand test results.

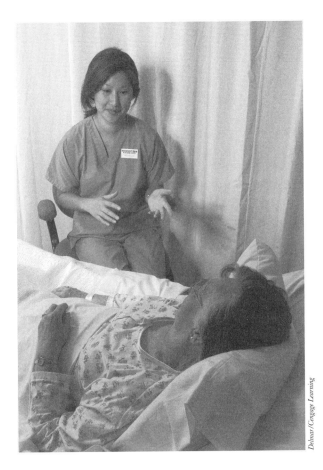

Delmar/Cengage Learning

- Know the latest treatments and provide a balanced discussion of each treatment's benefits and risks.

- Listen to their concerns and answer their questions honestly and in terms they can understand.

- Consider their opinions, including those based on their personal research and those of other health-care professionals.

While health-care professionals participate in the trust-building process, they do not control it. As discussed in previous chapters, newly diagnosed patients bring their own experiences and **prejudices** to health-care relationships and may erect barriers that are difficult, if not impossible, to overcome.

Building a Decision-Making Toolkit for Health-Care Professionals

The following sections outline some basic techniques for creating an environment in which patients are more likely to lower their defenses, accept the information their health-care professionals provide, and make sound medical decisions.

LISTENING AND BEING SUPPORTIVE

Listening to other human beings is the greatest way to honor them. Newly diagnosed patients can greatly benefit from being with health-care professionals who are willing to simply listen to their concerns, gently probing into areas that, if illuminated, might help the patients make more informed decisions. Being a good listener means being nonjudgmental, open, and receptive, without showing disapproval or otherwise directing patients toward or against treatment choices. When patients feel that their health-care professionals are listening to them, they are more likely to feel as if their needs are being acknowledged and considered in the information they receive. Essentially, patients are more likely to feel that their health-care professionals care about them. For newly diagnosed patients, reassurance can be invaluable.

Educational Moment

Newly diagnosed patients who are facing treatment decisions may express their fears and doubts in conversations with their health-care professionals. When patients make comments like, "I don't know how I'm going to make this decision," the health-care team has opportunities to reassure them that the team is available to answer questions, provide information, and offer support. Patients need reassurance that they are not facing these decisions alone.

Sample Dialogue

PATIENT: I'm being hit with a lot of options right now, and I don't think I'm qualified to make a decision.

HEALTH-CARE PROFESSIONAL: Let's go through each option, starting with surgery. Why don't you tell me what you're thinking about each one in terms of its advantages and what you're worried about?

PATIENT: I told you—I'm not an expert. You're not going to get much out of listening to what I have to say.

HEALTH-CARE PROFESSIONAL: Actually, I think I'd get a lot out of it. I'm really interested in knowing how you view each option. For example, you mentioned that you had heard that surgery would provide the quickest route to recovery. Tell me more about what you know about the surgical option, as well as what you aren't so sure about.

Reflective Listening Reminders

- Lean toward the patient, and make eye contact.

- Nod as the patient talks.

- Maintain open body language (e.g., avoid crossing the arms or legs).

- Reinforce your listening with phrases like "Okay" and "Got it."

- Encourage the patient to delve into concerns that will impact the decision, including the ambivalence between two or more treatment options.

- Reinforce a nonjudgmental attitude by identifying the patient's concerns and repeating them to the patient.

- Help the patient identify the questions that must be answered before a decision can be made.

EDUCATING THE PATIENT

Newly diagnosed patients are most receptive to information presented as educational. For patients of all kinds, the teacher-student relationship is a familiar one, and for most it carries positive connotations. Consequently, patients may relax their defenses when health-care professionals present themselves as teachers. Further, the teacher-student relationship is certainly positive when patients are trying to gain and process the information needed to make informed medical decisions.

The difference between lecturing a patient and educating a patient is distinct, however. When a patient is lectured, facts are presented in a one-size-fits-all format, and the patient is left to digest what was clear and what was not so clear. Educating a patient, in contrast, is a step-by-step process that begins by assessing the patient's knowledge. The next step is expanding the patient's knowledge, an activity that is supplemented by periodic check-ins both to ensure that the patient is understanding the discussion and to gauge the patient's reaction. Patient education requires patient interaction on both cognitive and emotional levels.

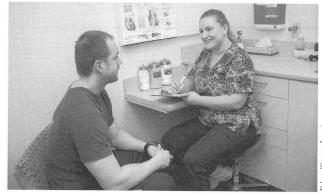

Delmar/Cengage Learning

Patients tend to appreciate learning the treatment experiences of other, similarly diagnosed patients through anecdotes, printed information, and Web site links. They also respond well to third-party information published through independent organizations like the American Heart Association or the American Cancer Society and the brochures provided by pharmaceutical companies. Health-care professionals who provide information from various sources reinforce their objectivity and their credibility.

Sample Dialogue

PATIENT: I'm kind of lost right now on what to do next.

HEALTH-CARE PROFESSIONAL: Would you like to sit down and go over the facts about your condition and the ways it can be treated?

PATIENT: I have a feeling most of this medical jargon is going to be lost on me.

HEALTH-CARE PROFESSIONAL: I'd be happy to go through it step-by-step. We'll start by talking about what you already know, and then move forward from there.

PATIENT: Okay.

HEALTH-CARE PROFESSIONAL: Great. Now, your doctor has recommended making some changes in your day-to-day life. What did she tell you about that?

PATIENT: I can tell you that I know I'm going to need to go on a diet that I'm not going to be very happy about. No salt, no sugar, no taste.

HEALTH-CARE PROFESSIONAL: I can see why that wouldn't seem like anything to look forward to. I don't blame you for not looking forward to it. But I have some brochures from an independent medical organization to give you, and they include some simple and healthy recipes. And I can recommend a great dietician to talk to. Does that sound like a plan?

Tips for Educating Patients

- Offer to educate patients so they feel in control of the situation.

- Start by understanding what patients currently know about treatment options.

- Acknowledge patients' feelings.

- Gradually build on the patients' knowledge, taking time to ensure that the patients understand what they have been presented and seeing if they have any questions or reactions before moving on.

- Reference third-party resources in discussions to enhance credibility and reassure patients that they are being given state-of-the-art information.

PROMOTING TEAMWORK

Patients want to feel like they are working *with* their health-care professionals—as a team. The term **teamwork** implies that the health-care professionals care about the patients' welfare. The emphasis on teamwork is also important because health-care professionals have a stake in seeing patients get better, in terms of adherence to best practices and quality of care standards. Teamwork is especially important when patients are making decisions about their treatments, because teamwork enhances a sense of security and facilitates communication. Health-care professionals can encourage a sense of teamwork through direct measures, such as referring to themselves as members of the patients' team, as well as through more indirect methods, like sharing information, checking in with patients regarding concerns and feelings, and answering questions honestly.

Sample Dialogue

HEALTH-CARE PROFESSIONAL: I want to reassure you that we view our relationship as a team. Your doctors and nurses and other health-care professionals you work with are members of that team, and you're also a team member. We're going to be working together as you go through your treatment and recovery. How does that sound?

PATIENT: It sounds good.

HEALTH-CARE PROFESSIONAL: One of the things *teamwork* means is that we are going to be sharing our knowledge of the options for treating your condition. We want to make sure you're well-informed, and we want to answer any questions you have. We'll also share our experiences with treating other patients with your condition.

PATIENT: What does that mean for the next steps?

HEALTH-CARE PROFESSIONAL: As a team, we'll work together to decide the best option for treatment. We'll work together to make the best decision, but you'll always be part of the process.

Tips for Enhancing Teamwork

- Be direct in explaining the teamwork approach and what it will mean for the patient.

- Wherever possible, use "we" instead of "us" and "you."

- In terms the patient will understand, clarify the concerns that members of the health-care team have regarding treatment options.

- Emphasize that information is being shared and that the patient's opinions and questions are important.

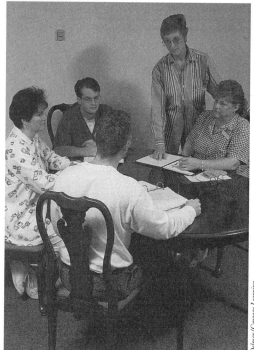

Delmar/Cengage Learning

ENCOURAGING SELF-EFFICACY

Advising patients and educating them are subtly different. When patients feel advised, they assume that the health-care professionals are telling them what to do. While patients may appreciate the offer of advice, they may distrust its content based on the assumption that it reflects the health-care professional's personal **biases**. Furthermore, patients who perceive that they are being directed toward certain treatments will be less likely to feel in control of their health care and less likely to take responsibility for it.

Health-care providers enhance **self-efficacy** by encouraging patients to be independent and self-directed while making medical decisions. Guiding patients toward their own information-gathering can start those patients building a sense of control. Allowing patients to make simple choices whenever possible, such as where to report for tests or what kinds of exercises to perform, can begin to instill the idea that patients can, and should, be active in their treatments. While patients have limited power over their treatment destinies, encouraging as much self-efficacy as possible helps to provide feelings of involvement and influence, which can help to counter the sense of helplessness that all newly diagnosed patients experience at some point.

Sample Dialogue

HEALTH-CARE PROFESSIONAL: We talked about getting another MRI before we decide on treatment. Do you remember that?

PATIENT: Yes, I do. I remember you wanted to see if I had done any additional damage when I fell last week.

HEALTH-CARE PROFESSIONAL: Exactly. When I explained what was going on with your back, you had mentioned that you were going to look up your condition on the American Association of Orthopedic Surgeons Web site. Anything you learned that you found useful?

PATIENT: Actually, I printed out a few pages to go over with you.

HEALTH-CARE PROFESSIONAL: Great idea. But before we do that, I want to schedule the MRI. Your insurance company will allow you to have it done at the hospital or at a private lab that might be closer to you. Do have a preference?

PATIENT: Yes, I work near the hospital, so I'd like to try to do it there.

HEALTH-CARE PROFESSIONAL: It's your choice. Let me make a quick call, and then we'll talk about what you found on the Web site.

Tips for Building Self-Efficacy

- Use "You can" statements.
- Provide options for newly diagnosed patients whenever possible.
- Encourage self-directed exploration of information regarding the condition and its treatment.
- As a means of building confidence, when evaluating treatment options allow the patients to express their preferences and concerns before health-care professionals express theirs.

BEING SENSITIVE TO THE READINESS FACTOR

The importance of readiness to listen to information and to make decisions has been implied throughout this book, but patients progress at their own levels. Some patients can, immediately after diagnosis, begin to listen to information and consider their options, while others cannot. Emotions, experiences, intellectual ability, and knowledge level all play a role. Unresolved fear can cause concerns of readiness to linger. Unfortunately, situations may sometimes dictate that patients make decisions before they have achieved emotional readiness. For health-care professionals, there are no clear guidelines. They must weigh patients' readiness against the urgency of beginning treatment.

Sample Dialogue

HEALTH-CARE PROFESSIONAL: The doctor has asked me to talk to you about scheduling your first treatment. We'll sit down together and talk about potential dates, and then I'll call the hospital and see what they have available.

PATIENT: Do we have to do this right now?

HEALTH-CARE PROFESSIONAL: Sounds like you're feeling some hesitance about getting started.

PATIENT: It's happening too fast. It's like I'm being railroaded into something I might not want to do.

HEALTH-CARE PROFESSIONAL: That certainly isn't our intention. Maybe we need to take a couple of steps back and talk about your treatment.

PATIENT: I'm just not sure I'm ready to do this. I'm not sure if I've really considered the options.

HEALTH-CARE PROFESSIONAL: Okay. Let's go through them again, and I'll clear up any questions you might have.

Tips for Gauging Patient Readiness

- Watch for patients to demonstrate hesitancy, verbally and through body language.

- To avoid stressing patients or building their resistance, avoid pushing too hard for further actions around treatment, such as scheduling.

- Encourage patients to talk about any hesitancy they might feel.

- Listen to their concerns, and encourage patients to ask any questions.

Aiding Health-Care Professionals Who Feel Helpless

Because health-care professionals have partnered with patients throughout their journeys, from diagnosis onward, and have committed to those patients' recoveries, they may become frustrated or alarmed when patients appear to hesitate moving forward. Health-care professionals may even start to feel helpless. The danger is that the health-care professionals may act out of their helplessness and cross professional boundaries by imposing their will on patients. Patients will, in turn, become afraid or alienated. It is important, therefore, to establish boundaries between what health-care professionals want for their patients and what the patients are ready, willing, and able to process.

When professional boundaries are at risk, health-care professionals should bring other health-care professionals into the relationship. Remember that when you make a decision for someone else, what feels like helping is actually taking power away.

Getting Family Members Involved in Decision Making

Newly diagnosed patients do not make treatment decisions in a vacuum. Family members, for one, are directly affected. They experience their own fears as they consider not only how the treatment will affect the patient but also themselves and other loved ones. Providing emotional support during the decision-making process can be stressful; family members may be even more aware of the risks than the patient. Treatment that requires a lengthy recovery time, or a chronic illness, presents issues that include finances, assignment of caregiving duties, and changes in daily routine.

As discussed previously in this chapter, patients' treatment decisions are not always complicated. Depending on the condition, the treatment options may be relatively limited, or treatment may be based on established best practices. Treatment for other conditions may be less clear cut. Regardless of the treatment route chosen, household routines will be impacted, and the potential for change presents the need for numerous decisions. Questions arise, such as, "How will we get by with a reduced income during the recovery?" "What will our meal routines be like when one family member is on a different diet?" "How will help watch over compliance with medication regimens?"

Following are considerations for working with family members to make medical decisions. To gain more perspective of communicating with family members once patients are diagnosed, refer to Chapter 11, in which family communications are discussed in depth.

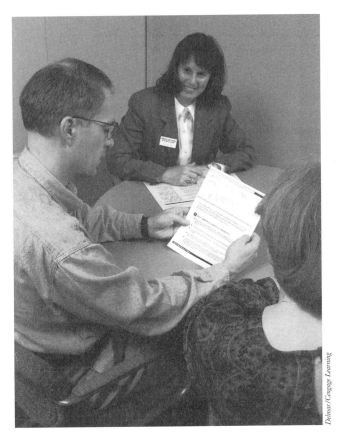

Delmar/Cengage Learning

- Provide the same information to patients and their family members so that they are making decisions based on the same set of facts. This reduces the suspicion that patients often feel they are not being given the complete picture.

- If possible, outline the treatment options, including the treatment itself and ongoing lifestyle management considerations in a joint discussion with patients and family members.

- Family members often feel overwhelmed by the potential responsibilities of caring for an ill family member. They may hesitate to voice their concerns out of a sense of guilt, though these concerns may influence the advice that they give to the patient. It can be helpful to provide family members with an opportunity to discuss their concerns separately with a health-care professional who can answer their concerns honestly but also inform them of available resources.

- As needed, make referrals to other allied professionals, like home care services and social workers, who can offer services to family members.

- Emphasize that the patient is the ultimate decision maker when discussing treatment options with patients as well as with family members.

When working with patients in freeze reaction, it may be necessary for family members to step in and make all treatment decisions. For patients like this, family involvement may be the only option. Patients in flight reaction may also require family involvement. Fighters can inspire confidence in family members as they face their conditions and take responsibility for their destinies, but they may also be perceived as stubborn when their independence clashes with a family member's need for involvement in the process.

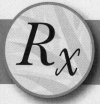 Coming to a Treatment Decision with a Patient

Walter, the patient at the beginning of the chapter diagnosed with prostate cancer, sat down with Toni, one of the nurses in the hospital oncology clinic. Toni will be responsible for overseeing Walter's care, pre- and post-treatment. Dr. Shapiro has gone over Walter's file with Toni, and she knows that Walter is struggling with making a decision about his treatment.

WALTER: I feel like this whole decision is being dropped in my lap. I don't want to be told what to do, mind you, but I'm also not sure if I trust myself to make the right choice.

TONI: You're really feeling scared about this decision and what it's going to mean to you.

WALTER: You're darned right I am.

TONI: We're here to help you decide, Walter. You're not alone.

WALTER: That's good to know.

TONI: You've probably heard that knowledge is power. For you to be as comfortable as possible with the direction your treatment takes, we want to make sure you're fully aware of the treatment options and what each option will mean to you. I know you're aware what the doctor is recommending at this point.

WALTER: Yes, but I'm the guy who has to live with this decision, so I know I need to have my part in making it.

TONI: Exactly. Now let's talk about where you are right now with this decision. What's on your mind?

WALTER: I listened to the doctor, and I did some research on my own. I printed a lot of stuff from the Internet. Some of it's pretty scary.

TONI: We can go through the options together. I've been through this with a lot of patients dealing with the same thing as you. But before we do that, let's take a step way into the future, and then work backward from there.

WALTER: What do you mean?

TONI: Well, you have a prostate cancer diagnosis. Looking into the future, what would you say is your treatment goal?

WALTER: Easy. I want to be alive. I want to be at my job. And I want to have sex with my wife on some kind of a regular basis.

TONI: Okay. So that's how you want to end up. You're certainly clear on that one. As the doctor told you, these are all possibilities, though the return to your sex life may be somewhat gradual, and we can't guarantee that things will be exactly like they were before your treatment. Can you work with that?

WALTER: I guess I'll have to.

TONI: Here's my suggestion. Let's take a look at your goals, and then consider each treatment option based on these goals. Does that sound good?

WALTER: Why not?

TONI: I'll start by making a chart on this sheet of paper. At the top, I'm going to list your goals based on what you told me: alive, working, having sex. And then I'm going to list the potential treatments along the side. Are you with me so far?

WALTER: I think so.

TONI: Good. And then as we go through each of the options, we're going to evaluate it according to your goals. As we do this, I'm going to show you the statistics about each treatment. And I'm going to go over the advantages and disadvantages and tell you about my experiences with other patients. Okay?

WALTER: Let's do it.

Following is the discussion after Toni and Walter discuss treatment options:

TONI: What are you thinking, Walter?

WALTER: Well, I at least have a better idea of the direction I don't want to go in, so I guess we're doing a process of elimination. I'm not there yet, but I guess since there used to be three options and now there are two, I'm 33 percent closer. And I'm leaning toward the doctor's recommendation, so maybe I am even closer. Not too shabby.

TONI: That's a good way to look at it. What would you say are your biggest questions now?

WALTER: I'm not sure if I know what my questions are. I'm kind of loaded with information right now. Maybe I need to sit with this for a while.

TONI: I could offer you some additional help, if you would like me to.

WALTER: Help is a good thing.

TONI: You'd mentioned wanting to get an opinion from another practitioner. I could give you the name of a Web site with a few local doctors to follow up with. I could also give you the names of a support group you could attend where you could meet other men who have also been treated for prostate cancer. You might learn something from them as well.

WALTER: I'm not sure if I'm a support group kind of guy, but I'll think about it. But I'll take the name of that Web site. I'd like to get another opinion before I jump into anything.

TONI: Great. I'll write it down for you. And I'm standing by whenever you want to talk more. But I'll also be following up with you in a few days.

Guidelines for Coming to a Treatment Decision

Following are guidelines to consider when working with patients during the treatment decision-making process:

1. ***Help the patient articulate a realistic goal for treatment.*** The starting place for a treatment decision may actually be the end point. Patients and health-care teams may be talking around treatment but not have actually taken the time to discuss specifics in terms of treatment expectations. Questions to ask include: Is it full recovery or partial? Will the condition require ongoing medication management and lifestyle modifications? If the treatment will result in changes, what kind of changes?

   The health-care team may want to meet first and determine what is realistic for the patient and what is not so that the determination can be presented during the conversation and discussed with the patient. The team's perspective also must be reflected in the **goals**. It can be difficult to discuss treatment goals, because patients may need to adjust their expectations. Notice that, in the preceding example, Toni reminded Walter that he might have to modify his expectations regarding his sex life. If discussions like these did not occur, patients may enter treatment less than fully informed.

2. ***Work backward from the goal, determining what to do to reach it.*** Once patients define their goals, they will most likely be in better positions to understand treatment options, short and long term, because the options will

be grounded in reality. The patients will be clearer on what is possible and can begin to understand what it will take to reach the treatment goals. Any ambiguity—over- or underexpectations—will be resolved. All diagnosis aspects—treatments, recovery, outcome probabilities, lifestyle modifications—can be discussed in terms of the goal. In the example, Toni took the time to write Walter's goals on a sheet of paper to ensure that the discussion remained focused on goals.

3. *Educate the patient about the treatment options.*   With predetermined goals to work from, patients are likely to be more receptive to information about each treatment option. As discussed previously, patient education begins with assessing what patients know, and at what levels they can comprehend information. In the example, Toni's approach was to describe each treatment option in terms of Walter's key goals. During this process, it is important to ensure that patients understand each option and the implications for recovery, relationships, and day-to-day lifestyle.

4. *Help the patient narrow options.*   During the process of reviewing the options with Walter, Toni helped him narrow the options. She was able to do this because, in discussing the options in the context of Walter's goals, it became clear that at least one option would be unacceptable. Of course, the options are more straightforward with some conditions than they are for others, depending on the condition itself, and whether it is life-threatening, acute, or chronic. Therefore, the level of guidance health-care professionals may need to offer will vary. Also, the physician may have one or more recommended courses of treatment, with minimal flexibility for patient choice. This may cause skepticism on the part of the patient, as well as resistance. In the

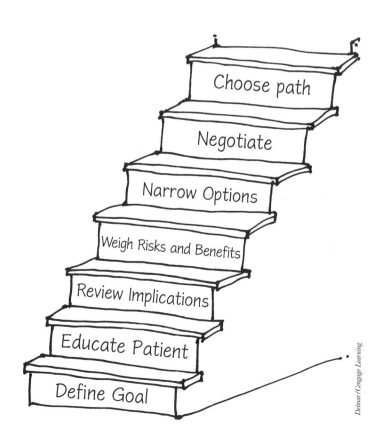

Delmar/Cengage Learning

example, Toni offered Walter referrals for a second opinion and the opportunity to talk with other patients facing the same condition.

Health-care professionals will want to use their judgment in terms of how the patient is guided is weighing options and how the physician's recommendation is reflected in the discussion. Professional ethics, as well as the guidelines established by the individual clinic or physician's office, will guide this discussion.

5. *Some negotiation may be needed.*   Clearly, some aspects of treatment are not negotiable. Patients need to feel some control over their destinies, however, and they are more likely to participate in—and subsequently embrace—treatment decisions when they feel they have some input. While some aspects of treatment are determined based on best practices and are nonnegotiable, there is often at least a small amount of flexibility in areas like start dates, morning versus afternoon schedules, and, in some cases, the venue in which the treatment is delivered. Patients are more likely to comply with lifestyle-management decisions when they are allowed some control. Diet and exercise requirements, for example, may be flexible depending on patient preferences. Consequently, the health-care professional and the patient may go through some negotiations as they come to an agreement regarding direction of the treatment.

6. *Patients may simply decide not to decide.*   Some patients may decide that they do not want a role in decision making but instead prefer to leave decisions to their health-care providers or families. Patients who are not fighters may choose this route. While not optimal, the physician may be left to make this decision for the patient, with the other members of the health-care team charged with carrying out the physician's directions. Some physicians prefer to take this role with their patients. The risk is that patients may later resist these decisions, which can affect compliance and ultimate satisfaction. When patients are unwilling to be involved, however, this may be the only option.

KEEP IN MIND

Patients may respond poorly to feeling like their health-care professionals are forcing decisions on them or that they are being pressed into making decisions prematurely. Have you ever resisted when you felt someone in authority was trying to dictate your actions? What approach would have worked with you?

SUMMARY

Making treatment and other health-care-related decisions is daunting to patients who, after all, generally have no medical backgrounds and minimal experience in decisions of these kinds. The emotional impact of a medical diagnosis further affects the ability to make these decisions, beginning with the ability to process the information required to make informed choices. By understanding the challenges patients face as they contemplate their choices, health-care professionals can effectively facilitate the decision-making process.

Chapter REVIEW

Multiple-Choice Questions

1. When faced with the need to make a treatment decision, a newly diagnosed patient, likely in _____ reaction, immediately goes on the Internet to evaluate treatment options.
   - a. Flight
   - b. Freeze
   - c. Fight
   - d. Any of the above

2. When lacking real information, it is human nature to:
   - a. Create a story based on experiences
   - b. Craft a story based on worst fears
   - c. Assume that positive thinking will make everything better
   - d. Any of the above

3. When newly diagnosed patients are repeatedly presented with the same information from a family member, they tend to respond by:
   - a. Becoming stubborn and ignoring it
   - b. Assuming the information is not to be believed
   - c. Lending the information more credence
   - d. Immediately asking if the information is true

4. When making treatment decisions, what is the relationship of a patient's emotional and cognitive sides?
   - a. The two sides must be kept separate so that the patient thinks clearly.
   - b. The patient should focus on emotions so decisions can be intuitive.
   - c. Acknowledging and experiencing emotions can cause the patient to focus more clearly.
   - d. A patient who is rational and avoids feelings will make better decisions.

5. Newly diagnosed patients may push themselves to make decisions when emotionally unprepared because they:
   - a. Have a sense of urgency about getting treatment under way
   - b. Feel overloaded with information and are trying to avoid stress
   - c. Want to please the health-care professionals advising them
   - d. Any of the above

Fill-in-the-Blank Questions

1. Newly diagnosed patients who fear that asking too many questions about their treatments will render the treatments less effective demonstrate _____ thinking.

2. _____ overload occurs when newly diagnosed patients feel overwhelmed by information about their conditions and recommended treatments and feel they can take in no additional information.

3. The fears and hopes a patient may be experiencing but is denying are called _____ in the room.

4. Newly diagnosed patients, especially fighters, may respond better to health-care professionals who try to

_____ as opposed to lecture.

5. Health-care professionals who help patients be as independent and self-directed as possible when making a

treatment decision promote _____.

Short-Answer Questions

1. Newly diagnosed patients sometimes face major, life-changing treatment decisions. Health-care professionals can sometimes experience a feeling of helplessness as the patients struggle with these decisions. What is the best action for a health-care professional feeling this way? Why?

_____

_____

_____

2. What is the best action to take when a newly diagnosed patient "decides not to decide" on a treatment option?

_____

_____

_____

3. What is the best way to approach a newly diagnosed patient who is clearly having an emotional reaction to the diagnosis but is suppressing emotions?

_____

_____

_____

4. The starting place for health-care professionals in facilitating the treatment decision-making process is to build trust. What can a health-care professional do to establish this trust?

_____

_____

_____

5. In what ways can health-care professionals educate newly diagnosed patients about their diagnoses?

_____

_____

_____

Critical-Thinking Questions

1. Realistically, family members may need to be brought into the treatment decision-making process. What benefits and challenges does family involvement present for health-care professionals?

_____

_____

_____

_____

_____

_____

2. It may help to define a treatment goal for a patient and then to work backward in terms of evaluating treatment options that will best facilitate reaching that goal. If you were using this method, what would you do to ensure that you and the patient had a realistic treatment goal in mind?

_____

_____

_____

_____

_____

_____

3. Making a treatment decision invariably leads to the question of the role of a second opinion. Newly diagnosed patients may or may not be open to seeking second opinions, whether or not they are recommended or required by managed care. What is the role of a health-care professional in discussions around obtaining a second opinion? Are there times when recommending a second opinion may be advisable but might present a conflict of interest for the health-care professional, who is employed by a practice or treatment center?

_____

_____

_____

_____

_____

_____

Internet Exercise

A number of Web sites focus on decision making, including making decisions regarding medical treatments. Some of this information is provided by health-oriented Web sites, others by nonprofit organizations. Company-sponsored Web sites, including pharmaceutical companies and treatment centers, also offer guidance on making decisions.

Using a search engine as a starting place, explore the topic of treatment decision making. Conduct a general search, as well as one linked to specific medical conditions. This will help you become more aware of the many approaches to making treatment decisions, as well as how this information may be biased in some way. You may also find guidelines for making treatment decisions that will be helpful to you and the patients you work with.

CHAPTER 6

Helping Newly Diagnosed Patients Communicate with Health-Care Professionals

OVERVIEW

After reading this chapter, you should be able to:

- Define and use the keywords of helping newly diagnosed patients communicate with health-care professionals.

- Create a baseline for effectively communicating with newly diagnosed patients, including rapport, open dialogue, and boundaries.

- Identify and optimize the teachable moments that strengthen a patient's communication skills.

- Be sensitive to the experience of helplessness and explain how it impacts newly diagnosed patients' ability to communicate effectively.

- Outline the role of the nonphysician health-care professional in relating with the patient when patient-physician issues arise.

- Understand how to discuss compliance issues with patients.

Accepting attitude

Aggressive manner

Alienation

Assertiveness

Baggage

Boundaries

Compassion

Face time

Generalize

High maintenance

Hot buttons

Open dialogue

Parameters

Passive-aggressively

Patient empowerment

Personality conflict

Rapport

Selective listening

Shorthand

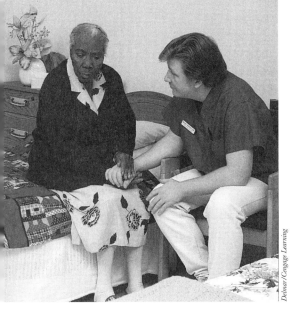

Delmar/Cengage Learning

Case Study

Rhonda calmly told her family that she was ready to face her breast cancer surgery and the treatment that would follow. She had taken pride in being an empowered patient. She had done extensive research on the Internet, had contacted support groups to network with former patients, and had asked acquaintances in the health-care field to give her advice on treatment options and providers. Rhonda had finally decided on a treatment center less than an hour from her home, where she was told that she would be working with one of the best surgeons in the country.

Once Rhonda met her surgeon, Dr. Braghieri, she felt somewhat less empowered, however. While she knew the physician's credentials were impressive, his bedside manner was not what she had hoped for. When she first met him, he quickly shook her hand and then sat down to go over her chart, barely making eye contact with her. He asked her a few questions, but often cut her off mid-sentence to ask her another one. After their first conversation, he reviewed what he called her "presenting symptoms," repeated her diagnosis, and reviewed his recommended course of treatment.

"Let me know what you decide, and we'll get started right away," Dr. Braghieri had said as he stood and prepared to leave the room. He shook her hand again and was gone.

After Rhonda completed her surgery, which was successful, she talked with Monie, one of the oncology nurses at her treatment center, to begin planning her upcoming chemotherapy.

KEEP IN MIND

Patients may vary in terms of how they prefer to communicate with health-care professionals, and these expectations impact their satisfaction with ongoing communications. Have you experienced a health-care provider or professional with an uncomfortable bedside manner? What about the behavior was off-putting? Did you talk to other patients about your impressions? Were their impressions similar to yours?

"Let me start by telling you one thing right now," Rhonda said to Monie. "I didn't expect much of a bedside manner from Dr. Braghieri, and that's what I got: Not much of a bedside manner. I felt like he was a robot and I was some kind of machine he was repairing. I had really checked him out beforehand, and I had decided he was the best. And I still think he is. I wouldn't have chosen anyone else. But I have to say that I'm going to seeing more of my oncologist than I am the surgeon, and I am hoping Dr. Mitchell is a whole lot more patient-friendly than Dr. Braghieri was. Even with all the research I've done on my condition, I feel like I'm in another country, and I don't have a tour guide. I'm going to be around here a lot while I go through chemo, and I'm going to need to work with people I can talk to."

> **KEEP IN MIND**
>
> As a health-care professional, you might be asked to comment on a physician or to indicate whether you agree or disagree with a patient's assessment. What discomforts might arise? How would you address them?

Monie had heard complaints about Dr. Braghieri before, but like Rhonda, she considered him an excellent surgeon and had recommended him to friends who had been diagnosed with breast cancer. She listened as Rhonda talked but offered no comments.

Rhonda was determined to have a different experience with chemotherapy. She had read and heard positive comments about all the oncologists on the staff, but she intended to demand someone with whom she could communicate.

"Can you tell me anything about the oncologist who has been assigned to my case?" Rhonda asked.

Monie was accustomed to this question, so she gave Rhonda the answer she gave to other patients with similar concerns. "We work as a team here, Rhonda," Monie replied. "You'll have one oncologist assigned to your case, but you'll also work closely with the nurses and other professionals on our health-care team. I'll be working with you throughout your treatment and will be overseeing your treatment plan. You can think of me as the go-to person. But let me reassure you that all the oncologists on staff communicate well with patients."

Rhonda considered Monie's words and replied, "We'll see how it goes. I'll let you know if I'm unhappy."

> **KEEP IN MIND**
>
> Patients sometimes have unique, persisting needs when interacting with health-care professionals. How would you respond to Rhonda's concerns and establish communications with her? As a health-care professional, how would you help ensure that Rhonda's needs are met and that her experiences promote healing?

Introduction

"I don't know what to expect."

Hand in hand with the emotions that the newly diagnosed experience are the expectations that they have for their relationships with their health-care providers. Often, these expectations are rooted in misperceptions, unrealistic expectations, and memories of bad experiences. While communication may seem secondary to the role of competent and thorough medical care, the primary concern of the health-care team, health-care professionals should address communications with patients by developing a professional relationship that encourages patients to ask questions, report symptoms, and express concerns. In so doing, health-care professionals will help ensure they are aware of patients' concerns and that their time is used as efficiently as possible.

KEEP IN MIND

Unlike health-care professionals, most newly diagnosed patients have had little experience navigating the medical system. What was your initial exposure to the health-care
establishment like? In what ways were you comfortable adjusting to hospital/clinic pro-
tocol? Working with physicians and other health-care professionals? In what ways have
you had to venture outside your comfort zone? What do you think the major challenges
are for new patients?

Newly diagnosed patients are learning to read their bodies, to know how they
should and should not be feeling, when to report symptoms or problems, and what
language to use in talking about their conditions. Their health-care teams can help
them to do these things effectively by using "teachable moments," opportunities to
guide and instruct.

Starting to Help Patients Express Their Needs and Concerns

For most newly diagnosed patients, the experience of communicating with health-care
professionals beyond addressing occasional illnesses or conducting routine medical
examinations is new. As a result, they do not know how to communicate to ensure that
their needs are met. In general, they are unsure as to what they can reasonably expect
in the medical arena—what they need to express and how they should express it.

While established patients may have developed relationships with their health-
care teams, new diagnoses may introduce new challenges. For example, patients who
have been treated before but by other teams may bring
expectations to their new teams that are unrealistic
given their diagnoses, or they may bring **baggage** from
negative experiences. The relationships between patients
and health-care providers will change as needs and expectations change.

Health-care professionals can greatly enhance communication with their newly diagnosed patients by
taking the first step toward relationship building. The
following sections outline the necessary steps.

CREATING RAPPORT

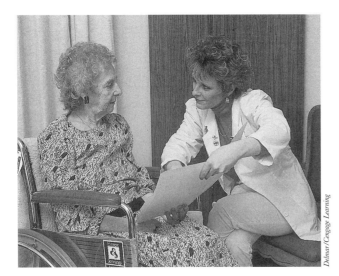

Delmar/Cengage Learning

Health-care professionals begin developing **rapport**
with newly diagnosed patients before speaking any
words. To do so, however, health-care professionals
must first be mindful of patients' emotions and watch for the emotional cues that can
guide initial interactions. As Chapter 2 describes, body language can reveal what
patients are feeling, as well as how open they are to interacting with health-care
professionals.

In addition to being aware of patients' body language, health-care professionals
must be conscious of their own body language if they are to establish rapport with

patients. Smiles, eye contact, and an open posture demonstrate a caring and welcoming attitude, but the gestures must be genuine. Patients sense immediately when health-care professionals are not genuinely caring people, and a hurried, distracted attitude can confirm patients' fears that the health-care professionals view them as cases, not individuals.

CONDUCTING AN OPEN DIALOGUE

From the initial contact onward, health-care professionals can promote communication by encouraging their patients to be open. This means doing things like encouraging patients to express any thoughts or feelings they may have and to ask any questions they might have. Other things include the following:

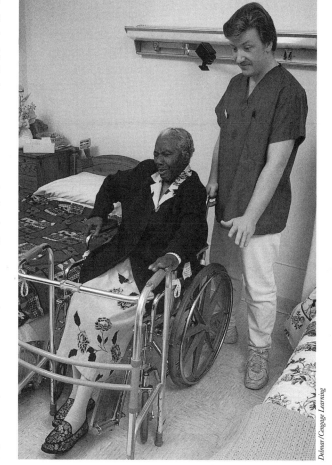

- Listening without interrupting, unless additional detail is needed

- Showing no alarm at symptoms a patient expresses

- Using no negative body language (e.g., eye rolling)

- Avoiding judging or scolding when a patient demonstrates a lack of understanding or compliance

Especially initially, newly diagnosed patients watch the reactions of their health-care professionals both to evaluate their own reactions and to determine how to proceed. When patients perceive that their health-care professionals are open to anything and everything they choose to bring up—within the **boundaries** of the professional relationship—both sides benefit. Patients benefit from having professionals who are focused on their well-being and needs, and health-care professionals benefit from receiving honest information that they can use to make informed decisions and recommendations.

ESTABLISHING BOUNDARIES

Establishing boundaries is always a complicated task for health-care professionals, but without boundaries professional ethics are at risk and professionals are at risk for burnout. Boundaries can be a sensitive issue for newly diagnosed patients. They may be unable to talk to their families or friends about their diagnoses and how they are affecting them, and they may look to their health-care professionals not only as medical resources but sounding boards and support systems.

Because patients rely on them for this kind of support, professionals may feel an additional sense of commitment, if not obligation, that may gradually extend beyond the generally accepted **parameters** of relationships between health-care professional and patient. As caring individuals, health-care professionals want to be there for their patients, and this may include being available during office hours and beyond. Sometimes, the emotional support health-care professionals provide feels more like psychotherapy, which can both drain emotions and present ethical and liability issues.

KEEP IN MIND

When established at the beginnings of relationships, clearly defined communication boundaries can help avoid uncomfortable issues. Have you ever been in a relationship in which you allowed communication to move in a certain direction and then decided that boundaries were crossed? What did you do? What would you do if this occurred in the health-care setting?

KEEP IN MIND

Whatever the relationship, boundaries can inspire strong emotions on both sides—**hot buttons**—and both sides are vulnerable in certain respects. As a health-care professional, in what areas do you most need to establish boundaries with newly diagnosed patients? For example, do you see yourself getting too involved in problem solving? Or do you see yourself at risk for being too available to patients and taking too little time to recharge? What are your plans for fortifying these weaknesses?

None of this is acceptable professional behavior. In fact, it is detrimental to the patient.

When health-care professionals take on too much responsibility and cross boundaries, patients are less likely to develop coping skills or create the support systems of family and friends that are necessary in moving forward beyond treatment. In addition, if health-care professionals offer suboptimal emotional support and advice and patients have complicated emotional reactions, such as extreme depression, those patients are at risk for failing to receive the treatment they need from mental-health professionals.

Health-care professionals should gently establish boundaries when patient relationships start so that the patients know from the beginning what they can and cannot expect on interpersonal and professional levels. Most practices have formal and informal guidelines for interactions between patients and health-care professionals.

Health-care professionals can use the following positive statements to introduce boundaries:

- "I'm only here on certain days, but there are other nurses in the office who could talk to you after you meet with the doctor."

- "I'm willing to listen and tell you about resources other patients have used when they were dealing with similar concerns, but I'm not qualified to give you that kind of advice."

- "I just can't give you my cell-phone number. You might really need to talk to me, and I'd be worried that I wouldn't be available. Let's talk about some other emergency-support options."

- "I'm not the best person for you to have this conversation with, but I do think it's important for you to talk to a qualified mental-health professional. Can I help you find someone who could help you with this?"

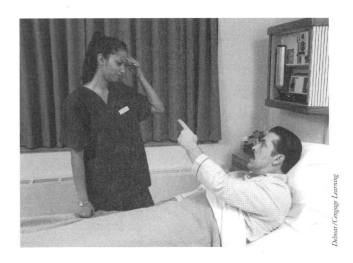

Delmar/Cengage Learning

Educational Moment

Within professional and personal boundaries and any practice guidelines, newly diagnosed patients and health-care professionals have many opportunities to communicate in ways that promote emotional and physical healing. When patients voice concerns or complaints, for example, health-care professionals can offer reassurance and guidance. Further, those professionals can encourage patients' questions and direct patients to the best resources for answers or resolution.

- "I know you have family and friends who would want to be available to you during this time. Is it time to reach out and get them more involved?"

- "Can I suggest that you get connected with a support group in the area? It would be a way for you to meet other patients who could share their experiences."

- "The practice has established guidelines regarding relationships between patients and members of the team. These guidelines protect both of us and help us stay focused on your health. That would be considered a violation. But I can give you a couple of other options."

> **KEEP IN MIND**
>
> Because the health-care environment is often foreign to them, newly diagnosed patients are often unsure how to behave in ways that are appropriate but that get their needs met. Have you ever felt this way? What would you suggest to newly diagnosed patients in this situation?

Seeing How Newly Diagnosed Patients Experience Health Care

When newly diagnosed patients begin to engage the health-care establishment, what they experience is not unlike a visit to a foreign country. The "residents" speak a language that differs from that of the "tourists," and even if they speak the same language, certain words and phrases have different meanings. Similarly, the style of dress and etiquette differ. People behave in ways that are either completely unfamiliar or, most likely, are interpreted differently in the home country.

USING COMMON LANGUAGE

Because they lack the time to articulate every word, health-care professionals must learn to speak "**shorthand**" with each other. Acronyms like SOB for "short of breath," for example, are quick and to the point and help avoid miscommunication. Phrases like "presenting with symptoms" and technical terms like *neutrapenic* and *adjuvant* are perfectly clear in the health-care arena. To outsiders like newly diagnosed patients, however, these examples of "insider talk" are not understandable.

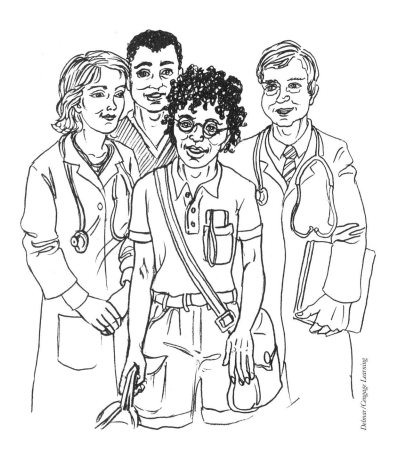

Delmar/Cengage Learning

When health-care professionals use unfamiliar abbreviations, expressions, and technical terms during conversations, newly diagnosed patients can feel confused and intimidated. Quickly, these emotions can give way to fear, because misunderstood words and phrases cause undue alarm, and anger, because medical terminology contributes to a feeling of **alienation**. The result is that patients can feel frustrated and even more out of control. Indeed, learning the language of the health-care establishment is one of the challenges patients confront as they face their conditions and treatments.

Health-care providers can help patients surmount this challenge by watching for signs of misunderstanding or miscommunication and checking to ensure that the terminology is being understood.

What not to say: "Hi, Mrs. Suarez. I'm looking at the physician's orders here, and I see that you came in today presenting some difficulties with Activities of Daily Living. Your complete blood count shows that you are anemic, so she has prescribed growth factors for you."

Encouraging empowered patients: "Hi, Mrs. Suarez. You told the doctor that you were really tired and having some trouble concentrating and getting things done around the house. Your blood test shows that you have some anemia, which would explain why you are feeling this way. We're going to give you a treatment for anemia that should get you feeling better in a few weeks or less. Before we talk about the treatment, though, do you have any questions about your condition? Do you know what anemia means?"

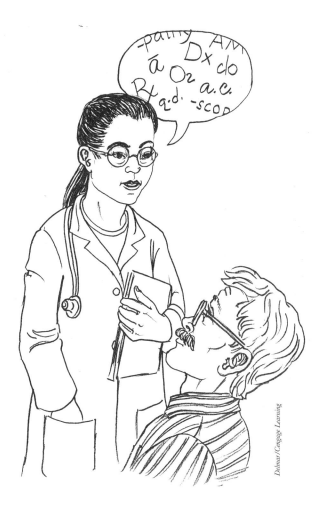

Delmar/Cengage Learning

SHARING POWER IN HEALTH-CARE RELATIONSHIPS

Newly diagnosed patients often struggle to understand who has the power in their health-care relationships: they or their health-care professionals. The concerns patients have about asking questions are one example of this struggle. Generally, patients want to communicate in a way that promotes more communication, but they harbor concerns that their questions will prompt their health-care professionals to avoid them or avoid giving them their full attention. In short, as newly diagnosed patients adjust to their conditions, they want to make sure that they "stay on the right foot" with their health-care providers.

Older patients, who usually have more traditional approaches to health care, are more likely than younger patients to perceive themselves as having less, or no, power, in their health-care relationships. Younger patients, like fighter patients, tend to be more assertive. Superstitious thinking plays a role as well. Newly diagnosed patients often express the concern, directly or indirectly, that they will damage their health-care relationships and, by extension, their treatments and recoveries, if they question their professionals' recommendations. They often fear that they will "jinx" their treatments' effectiveness or somehow alienate their health-care providers.

By encouraging patients to ask questions, health-care providers can ease patients' power concerns and enhance communication. Patients who ask questions are more

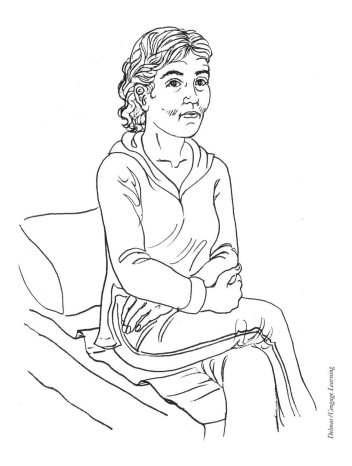

Delmar/Cengage Learning

likely to comply with treatment, because they will understand their conditions and treatments and be more likely to accept their health-care-providers' recommendations. Physicians may have limited time to answer patient questions, however, and patients may feel especially hesitant to question their health-care providers for the reasons described.

What not to do: "I'm going to go through the list of prescriptions with you to review how and when you should take each one. This information is also on the prescription bottle."

Encouraging empowered patients: "I see that you have some different prescriptions to take. This might feel like a lot to keep track of at first, so I'll go through each prescription with you, one at a time. Before I start, though, I want to see if you have any questions. And as we go through the list, feel free to jump in if you have a question."

AVOIDING OFFENSIVE BEHAVIOR

As discussed previously, newly diagnosed patients can find the health-care establishment as alien. Not only is the language foreign, so are the customs. For example, Health Insurance Portability and Accountability Act (HIPAA) rules may require that a patient not approach the reception desk if another patient is already being helped, as a means of protecting patient confidentiality. Therefore, if the receptionist requests that the patient step aside until the first patient is served (and on a busy day this may

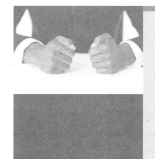

Body Language

Patients experiencing conflicts and other communications issues with members of the health-care team may exhibit body language that includes the following:

- Shoulder shrugging and head shaking
- Arms folded across the chest
- Avoiding eye contact
- Patting/fondling hair
- Standing with the hands on the hips

not be conveyed by the receptionist in the friendliest of terms), the patient being dismissed may feel as if he or she has made an egregious error or feel embarrassed.

Clinics or hospital units that serve a large number of patients often have customs and rules that can further contribute to the confusion that a newly diagnosed patient is feeling. Having to report to the billing office, for example, may leave patients confused if forms and policies are not carefully explained or if they are not treated in a humane manner. This treatment is something that the health-care professionals who subsequently treat them have no control over, yet may have to listen to patient complaints or provide support for patients who feel additional fears and concerns after this interaction. Hospitalized patients who have to rely on the schedules and procedures of this environment feel the culture shock even more acutely.

All newly diagnosed patients are at a disadvantage in the health-care establishment, because trying to identify what is appropriate behavior while learning to navigate the system can be overwhelming. Patients in fight reaction learn to adjust, but those in flight or freeze feel even more overwhelmed and powerless. Out of a desire to "choose their battles," patients will often hold in their frustration, rather than expressing it, and enlist their caregivers to advocate on their behalf.

Health-care professionals can help support their patients by being sensitive to their feelings and encouraging them to be more assertive. Increasing patients' comfort level in the new-to-them health-care environment cultivates openness, which reduces stress and makes communication more effective.

What not to say: "You can't stand here."

Encouraging empowered patients: "We have procedures here that we need to follow. It doesn't always feel like it, but they really protect you and other patients. We have to ask patients to come to the desk one at a time to protect confidentiality. Don't worry. New patients don't know about that."

NAVIGATING INFORMATION SHARING

As part of adjusting to their diagnoses, new patients must learn what symptoms are associated with their conditions and treatments. Out of a need to try to please their health-care providers, patients may try to anticipate the symptoms they should be reporting on. Unfortunately, patients may inadvertently disregard important symptoms,

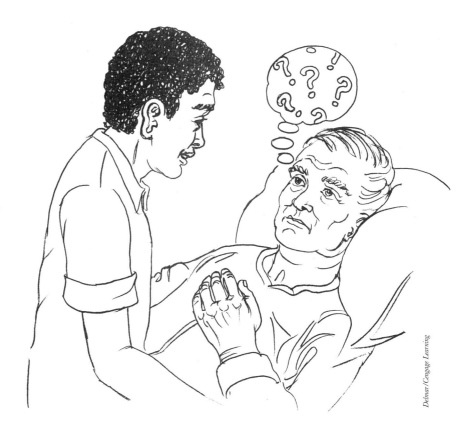

Delmar/Cengage Learning

withhold symptoms to appear well, or overreport symptoms to stay involved with their professionals or secure more treatments, like medication.

Clearly, it is impossible for health-care providers to anticipate how newly diagnosed patients will interpret symptom-related questions, but they can help clarify patient communication by making it clear that, while they are asking specific questions, they are interested in anything that seems out of the ordinary.

What not to say: "How is your appetite? Sleeping okay? How is your energy level? Alright? Sounds like everything is fine."

Encouraging empowered patients: "As you adjust to your condition and its treatment, I'm going to be especially concerned about a few, specific symptoms. But let's start with you telling me how you've been feeling over the past week. Then, I'll ask you some more specific questions."

MANAGING PATIENTS' SELF-PERCEPTIONS

Most newly diagnosed patients want to perceive themselves as "good" patients, and they want their health-care teams to see them as compliant, following treatment guidelines and reporting for checkups or additional treatment as needed. Many pledge secretly to take only the time required of their health-care teams and to raise no unnecessary alarms. They assume that if they are well-behaved, they will receive the best care possible because their health-care professionals will enjoy working with them and will reward them with additional attention and concern. As discussed previously, patients may exhibit superstitious thinking in this area, such as the belief that a positive health-care relationship will lead to a better prognosis as reward for good behavior.

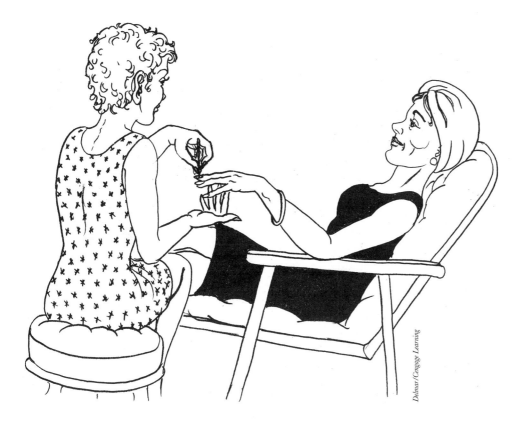

Delmar/Cengage Learning

In busy medical practices, physicians may inadvertently or intentionally convey to patients that their time is highly limited and offer guidelines for deviating from standard appointment schedules. While other health-care professionals on the team, including nursing staff, may be subject to the same guidelines, newly diagnosed patients may assume that they are discouraging physician contact. To avoid appearing overly demanding or "**high maintenance**," some patients may avoid reporting symptoms or discomfort. Others will exaggerate progress so as to appear more attractive.

What not to say: "I see that you're not a complainer. That certainly makes my job a lot easier."

Encouraging empowered patients: "I know this is all new to you and that you're still learning what to expect from your treatment. You can really help us if you let us know what's going on with you as you adjust to your medications."

READING CUES PROPERLY

As discussed in previous chapters, body language is integral to communication. In fact, only 7 percent of communication is based on spoken words and 93 percent is nonverbal. Much of the latter is based on body language (Borg, 2008; Engleberg, 2006). Because body language is so central to communication, an attempt to suppress or over-control it translates as forced or unnatural on conscious and unconscious levels. When health-care professionals attempt to manipulate their body language, they make patients uncomfortable and erode trust.

As newly diagnosed patients form relationships with their health-care professionals, they assess the professionals' body language as well as verbal cues. Patients will watch for signs of concern, such as frowns or arms folded across the chests, and when they see them they will assume that something is going poorly in treatment. In contrast, patients will seek body-language cues that treatment is going well, in this case possibly misinterpreting a smile or a "thumbs up." More subtle body language, such as looking away when speaking, may mean something to a patient even if that patient cannot articulate it.

When they work with newly diagnosed patients, health-care professionals should remember that these patients will likely scrutinize and misinterpret their body language. Professionals with this level of awareness can avoid doing things like appearing overly concerned when in fact they are merely focusing on patients or reacting to unrelated concerns. In return for patients' attention, health-care professionals should observe the patients' reactions to their body language and other verbal cues. When patients appear to be misjudging their messages, the professionals should clarify the patients' perceptions as well as their own intentions.

What not to do: Use body language that fails to reflect the situation (e.g., frown in concentration while discussion a new medication with a patient).

Encouraging empowered patients: "I want to carefully go over how you're feeling with this new medication. I'm going to be very focused while you talk, because I want to learn as much as possible from you." (During the discussion, the health-care professional should listen actively.)

SERVING PATIENTS APPROPRIATELY

We live in an era of assertive patients. While **assertiveness** can strengthen the communication between patient and health-care professional, it can also be less than productive. Patients' questions may, for example, appear demanding or accusatory.

For newly diagnosed patients, inappropriate assertiveness may have more than one cause. Demanding behavior may be an expression of panic or a cry for help. Unrecognized or suppressed fear may manifest as anger. For patients who lack experience with the health-care establishment, assertiveness can translate as distrust. These patients may be operating under the impression that if they do not act in an **aggressive manner**, they will be ignored.

Experience as a caregiver or patient in another health-care setting may influence current patient behavior. Newly diagnosed patients with such experience may **generalize**, assuming they need to be demanding in all health-care settings. Alternatively, they may have simply misinterpreted the current emphasis on **patient empowerment** as having to battle to get their needs met. Media attention has contributed to the misperception that health-care professionals are not trustworthy. Unfortunately, newly diagnosed patients who lack experience with health-care professionals tend to be susceptible to negative imagery and to react accordingly.

When exposed to, or confronted by, aggressive patients, health-care professionals should first recognize their own reactions. It is human nature to respond emotionally, aggressively, or **passive-aggressively** to aggressive or otherwise unpleasant behavior, but such responses tend only to fuel unpleasant behavior on both sides of the conversation.

Instead of responding spontaneously, health-care professionals should pause and evaluate their reactions. Reminders of patients' motivations—fear or stress, perhaps—

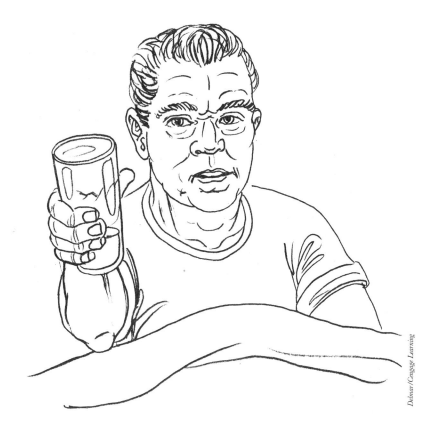

Delmar/Cengage Learning

or relaxation techniques can provide the time and perspective health-care professionals need to help keep patient exchanges productive. Verbal responses that acknowledge patients' needs and concerns can signal to patients that they are being understood, and patients who are understood become less aggressive. Reflective listening, described in Chapter 2, is useful in these situations.

What not to say: "I've got a lot of patients demanding my time. Giving me orders is not going to get you very far around here, so calm down."

Encouraging empowered patients: "I know this is all new to you. You're getting to know us, and we're getting to know you. We're doing everything we can to make sure you get everything you need. Let's try to be patient with each other while we get a routine in place."

Being Sensitive to Helplessness

Helplessness has been an underlying theme of previous chapters. Virtually all newly diagnosed patients experience a sense of helplessness arising from their conditions. For many, diagnosis is the first time they feel no control of their daily lives or destinies. Some patients accept the lack of control and learn to live with their conditions. Others either become overwhelmed by their sense of helplessness or refuse to recognize it.

As Chapter 4 describes, helplessness cannot be denied indefinitely. It finds its way into conversations between patients and health-care professionals, either directly or indirectly. Patients tend to respond poorly when confronted about their helplessness or told that their helplessness is irrational. Patients respond best to health-care

> **KEEP IN MIND**
>
> Newly diagnosed patients enter treatment relationships with experiences that affect their expectations of physician communication. What kinds of experiences have you had dealing with physicians, both as a patient and as a health-care professional? In what ways have you seen physicians be especially helpful? In what ways has communication been less positive?

professionals who show compassion. **Compassion** is an attitude of concern and acceptance of the ways in which patients react to their diagnoses, even when the reactions temporarily complicate interactions with health-care professionals. An **accepting attitude** benefits both patient and health-care professional by neutralizing the stress and frustration difficult patients can inspire and helping to ensure that the health-care professional's reactions do not complicate patient interactions. Compassion can be exhibited through:

- Demonstrating active listening
- Maintaining a calm, patient demeanor when patients express their emotions or are resistant or defensive
- Encouraging patients to express their hesitations or concerns
- Offering referrals for counseling or support groups if patients are open to these options

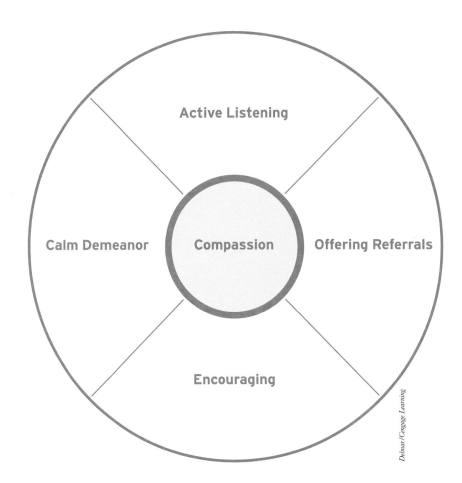

Delmar/Cengage Learning

Handling Problems between Physician and Patient

Situations sometimes arise between newly diagnosed patients and their treating physicians that can result in tension and frustration for both parties. Members of the nursing staff, as well as other members of the health-care team, may find themselves serving as a listening ear or mediator for patient or physician. Most often, health-care staff will be called on to support patients, helping them understand the physician's perspective and coaching them to accept the physician's recommendations and remain compliant. The following sections outline ways to address patient-physician issues that may arise.

ENSURING LISTENING OCCURS

When initially coping with the news of their diagnoses and facing treatment decisions, newly diagnosed patients often need additional support from their health-care teams. While most patients learn what to realistically expect from their physicians and other health-care staff over time, the initial adjustment to the constraints of these relationships can be strained.

Because they are constantly under time pressure, physicians cannot always spend as much time as patients might like answering questions or providing emotional guidance. Whether or not physicians explain the constraints they work under or outline their professional boundaries, patients may perceive their physicians as unwilling to give them the attention they need. As a result, the patients may feel confused or frustrated. Some patients feel their providers are simply not listening. Treating physicians may feel they have answered patients' questions adequately or addressed their complaints, but that does not mean the patients have fully understood, or accepted, the physicians' answers.

Other members of the health-care team—often the receptionists—may hear patients express their frustrations with physicians' perceived unwillingness to listen. The expressions may be direct, through open criticism, or indirect, through subtle hints that their complaints are not being heard. Physicians, for their part, may complain to nursing staff that patients are difficult to work with. They may ask nursing staff to log added **face time** with patients in response.

Practice guidelines that clarify the roles of physicians, nurses, and other health-care staff may help guide patient interactions. Brief explanations of treating physicians' personal styles may also prove helpful. In short, however, patients who feel they are being monitored and treated based on best-practice guidelines are often reassured. Health-care professionals can coach those patients who need additional structure or information. Patients in fight reaction, for example, may request additional information on treatment approaches. Patients of all kinds can help ensure the most efficient use of team resources by learning to record and present symptoms and complaints in ways that most efficiently use their physicians' time. As issues arise, health-care staff must avoid implying that physicians are somehow remiss. Other staff should never volunteer to be the "go-between" of patient and physician.

What not to say: "The doctor is too busy to listen to you again. He's already answered this question." Or "You're right. She's not a very good listener."

Encouraging empowered patients: "You said you don't feel much better yet, and you're beginning to wonder if the medication is working at all. Let's go through some information I have on what to expect when your treatment begins."

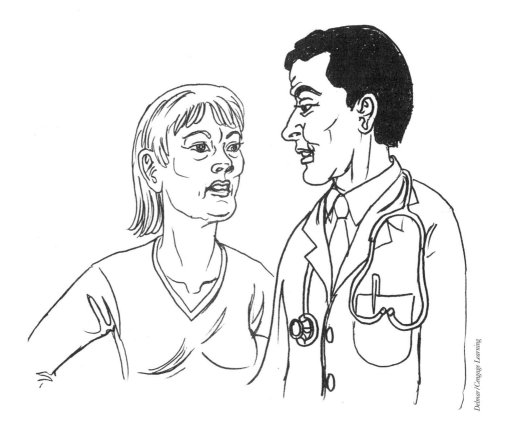

Delmar/Cengage Learning

CHANNELING NEGATIVE EMOTIONS

Newly diagnosed patients tend to expect infinite patience and consideration from their physicians, but physicians are human like everyone else. They may become impatient when patients fail to listen or to comply with treatment. Unfortunately, newly diagnosed patients are often highly sensitive to physicians' negative reactions and may overreact and draw from those reactions irrational conclusions. Patients may fear, for example, that their physicians will fail to deliver optimal services out of frustration. Newly diagnosed patients, because of the impact of their illness on their daily lives, may also feel entitled to what they feel should be infinite patience and consideration on the part of their treating physician, and will consequently overreact to any indications that this is not the case.

When misunderstandings like this arise, other members of the health-care team can help physician and patient alike by asking patients to explain what they believe to have caused their physicians' frustration or anger. With that information, other staff can help provide perspective, both in terms of understanding the physician's perspective and learning how to avoid these conflicts.

What not to say: "The doctor gets in a bad mood. If you aren't doing what she tells you to do, you're going to receive the brunt of it."

Encouraging empowered patients: "From what you described, it sounds like the doctor was hoping you would have your diet in place and be monitoring your blood sugar regularly. As you said, you aren't quite on track with that. Let's talk about helping you put a routine in place that's going to help you get feeling better."

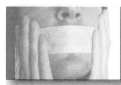

SELF • talk

Patients who have difficulty communicating with health-care professionals may use negative self-talk that includes the following:

Why should I even bother to tell them? They won't listen.

She obviously doesn't like me, so I won't ever get her to help me.

I'm too stupid to understand what he's talking about, and I look like a fool when I ask questions.

They're too busy to spend any time with me. I'll have to figure things out on my own.

They seem to avoid my questions. I think there's a lot they aren't telling me.

Suggested antidotes to negative patient self-talk include the following:

I know the health-care team is busy, but that doesn't mean they don't have time to answer my questions.

No question is stupid. If I need to know something, I can ask someone for the answer.

Health-care professionals may be focused on their work. That doesn't mean they're mad at me.

The health-care team needs to know any symptoms or side effects I might be experiencing so they can help me better.

Just because one health-care professional seems disinterested, it doesn't mean others aren't willing to help. Maybe I need to talk to the right person.

WORKING THROUGH DISAGREEMENTS

Newly diagnosed patients and their treating physicians may sometimes disagree. They may have **personality conflicts**. For example, some newly diagnosed patients resist treatments because they feel the treatments are unwarranted or extreme. Other patients may feel they have information on alternative treatments that their physicians should respect and consider. Patients in fight reaction are most likely to disagree openly with their physicians. Patients in flight reaction, who are emotionally overwhelmed, may overreact to physician suggestions and become argumentative. Patients in freeze reaction, for their part, may use arguments as a means of avoiding important treatment discussions.

Patient-physician disagreements may be so severe as to render patients combative or distrustful of any recommendations. Especially when they feel helpless or afraid, patients at this point may look to other health-care professionals for support or to listen as they ventilate. They may also look to other health-care professionals to intervene with physicians or advocate for them. This situation can be uncomfortable for the health-care professionals. If they handle these conflicts inappropriately, those professionals can contribute to, rather than help resolve, the conflicts.

The key is for health-care professionals to remain objective while being supportive in ways that reduce conflict and enhance patients' trust of their physicians. Often, what patients need most is a listening ear and reassurance that their physicians are experienced and providing the best care possible. Suggestions for presenting concerns

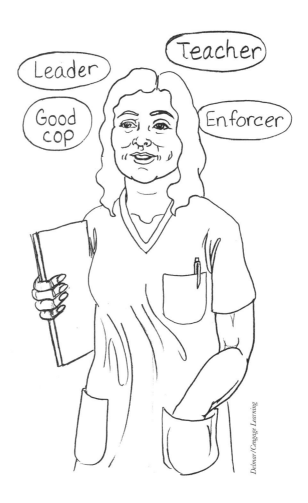

Delmar/Cengage Learning

in collaborative and nonconfrontational ways can really benefit patients, as can reminders that part of the uncomfortable and frustrating diagnosis process is learning to
trust the physician.

What not to say: "The doctor is the expert here, not you. You need to trust her if
you're going to work together." Or "The doctor is not always right. Speak up, and let
him know what you want."

Encouraging empowered patients: "I know it's not easy to begin treatment for
a new condition. A big part of the process is not only learning about your treatment
but learning to trust your doctor. Always feel free to ask us questions. That will help you
to better understand your treatment and the doctor's reasons for recommending it."

Communicating with Newly Diagnosed Patients about Compliance

Health-care professionals share the responsibility of helping patients remain in compliance with physicians' treatment regimens. Asked at times to be teacher, cheerleader,
enforcer, or "good cop" to physicians' "bad cop," health-care staff can be frustrated
by patients who resist compliance, even when those patients do so out of fear or helplessness. When this happens, health-care staff may question their role and responsibil-

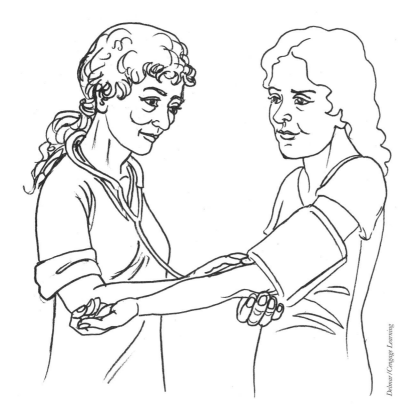

Delmar/Cengage Learning

ities, and boundary issues can occur. Some patients can regress into what can feel like a childlike reliance on their health-care professionals. Effective communication—proactively and in reactions to issues that arise—is crucial to helping patients understand their responsibility in maintaining compliance.

The following sections discuss some common compliance issues.

DEMONSTRATING CARING

The helplessness newly diagnosed patients often experience may manifest as avoidance of responsibility for maintaining compliance. For example, a patient may expect to be reminded to schedule a test the physician has ordered. When the assumption is corrected, the patient may contend, "This was supposed to be the nurse's job," or, "You told me you were going to be watching over me."

While such expectations may feel initially like entitlement on the patient's part, they more accurately reflect the patient's sense of fear and helplessness. Newly diagnosed patients can feel so overwhelmed by their conditions and new responsibilities that they doubt their abilities to handle new demands. Further, the fear factor can interfere with patients' abilities to listen effectively to, process, and then respond to their conditions' demands, which may include things like filling prescriptions, taking medication on schedule, and reporting for labs.

While patients' direct and indirect demands and expectations can frustrate health-care professionals, those professionals, not patients, are responsible for staying nondefensive. Patients may simply need additional guidelines, as well as encouragement to become more responsible and empowered. When patients reassume these responsibilities, they tend to realize they can manage the demands of their conditions.

What not to say: "Scheduling labs are your responsibility, not mine. We can't monitor this for every patient. It has to be your job."

Encouraging empowered patients: "I know there's a lot to keep track of here. Why don't we go over the list together and make sure you know everything you need to do. For the things we don't handle, we'll figure out who to call. If we break this all down into individual pieces, and get them into a schedule, it'll be a lot less overwhelming for you."

WORKING TOWARD COMPREHENSION

A medical condition invariably causes change, and humans resist change by nature. Newly diagnosed patients express their resistance in varied ways, including avoiding treatment compliance by pleading lack of understanding. Through **selective listening**—hearing only that which is palatable and convenient—patients try, consciously and unconsciously, to create their own treatment plans, ones that help them feel their conditions are less serious. When they confront evidence to the contrary, those patients plead ignorance.

The need to deny the unpleasant is, of course, understandable. As discussed previously, newly diagnosed patients may be so overwhelmed by fear and other emotions that they have difficulty processing and acting on health-care recommendations. Health-care professionals can help patients who are listening selectively by being patient and compassionate. Patients who feel their health-care professionals are scolding them, or dictating to them, may become even defensive and resistant. With

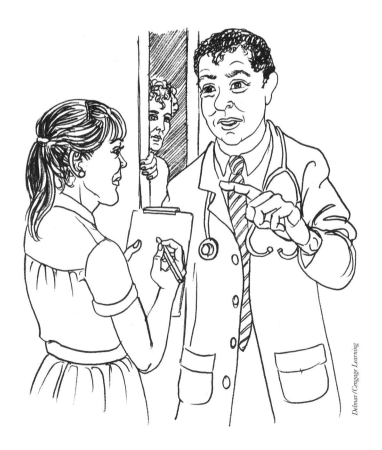

Delmar/Cengage Learning

patients' input, health-care professionals should instead determine patients' understandings of their compliance responsibilities. Offering additional clarification, and compliance assistance, can help reduce patient resistance.

What not to say: "I thought I made it clear to you that you needed to take your medication once in the morning and once in the evening. It's not going to help you if you don't use it correctly."

Encouraging empowered patients: "It's really important to follow the treatment plan your doctor set up. Why don't we go over your treatment plan again? You can ask any questions you might have, and I'll clarify some of the details that slipped through the cracks."

ESTABLISHING ROLES

As they are in any arena, roles in health care are the products of many factors. Constraints of the current health-care system have forced physicians to focus on diagnoses and treatment decisions, while other health-care professionals manage day-to-day treatment planning and patient communication.

Traditionally, physicians have played authoritarian roles, while other health-care professionals have played roles that are secondary and nurturing. In loose terms, these roles have often translated as "bad cop" or "father" for physician and "good cop" or "mother" for other staff. Newly diagnosed patients who adopt these traditions tend to view nonphysician members of the health-care team as their go-betweens

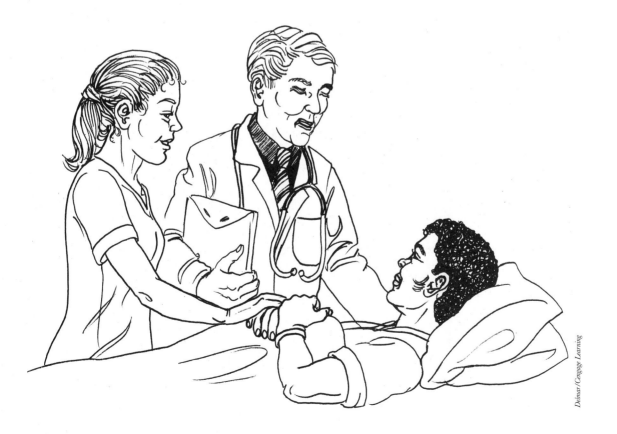

Delmar/Cengage Learning

with physicians. As a result, such patients may do things like ask that members of the health-care team report side effects because they fear physicians do not want to discuss them or will think less of them if they complain. Patients may also approach other members of the health-care team to request changes to their treatment regimens.

Because they have adopted traditional health-care dynamics, newly diagnosed patients can unknowingly infantilize themselves—behave more as children than adults. For their part, health-care professionals may participate in the dynamic but not realize it. While health-care professionals who are serving as physician go-betweens can be temporarily gratified, they often find themselves overextended trying to convey information and honor requests that should be directed to physicians. Further, they can unintentionally cause friction with physicians, who may prefer to develop trusting relationships with their newly diagnosed patients.

Health-care professionals can help avoid physician friction by first being aware that patients may set up this dynamic, albeit unconsciously. For example, professionals should be alert to patients who ask them to communicate with physicians on their behalf, especially when those patients should be addressing the issues directly. Instead of complying with such requests, health-care professionals should encourage patient independence. This might include helping patients clarify what they feel they cannot communicate directly and why. Patients may simply need help defining their needs, such as modifying the treatment regimen or reporting additional symptoms. On some level, whatever the greater office environment, health-care professionals will likely be required to be involved in patient communication.

What not to say: "Sure. I'll put in a good word for you."

Encouraging empowered patients: "Going forward with your treatment, you'll be seeing your physician fairly regularly, and I'm sure she'll want to work closely with you. You mentioned that you heard about a treatment for some of the side effects you're experiencing. Why don't you bring this up with her during your appointment today? I'm sure she'll want to talk with you about this directly."

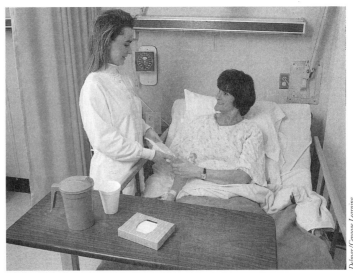

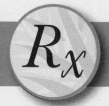 Talking with a Newly Diagnosed Patient with a Communications Issue

In the example at the beginning of the chapter, the nurse, Monie, encountered a patient, Rhonda, who had had a negative experience working with her surgeon. Rhonda had entered the oncology clinic feeling defensive and frustrated from her experience and was both expecting and fearing that her interactions with the health-care professionals in oncology would be the same. Monie knew it was important to reassure Rhonda that patient-professional relationships would be different going forward. She also wanted to set expectations with Rhonda.

MONIE: From what you're telling me, you want to have an open line of communication with the team in oncology and you're worried that you won't find that here. And you're especially worried that the doctors won't be good communicators. Is that right?

RHONDA: Yes. Exactly. I have to say that I'm going to need some hand-holding along the way. I'm hoping you can do that, because this is traumatizing for me. I don't want to come here and be treated like a number.

MONIE: I can understand why you would say that, Rhonda. Chemotherapy is a lot to go through, and I want to reassure you that we don't intend for you to go through it alone. We'll be with you every step of the way. I can also reassure you that our doctors are totally sensitive to the needs of patients. That's what we're all about.

RHONDA: That's really good to know.

MONIE: Now. I'm thinking you must have some questions about how we'll be working together. Why don't I let you start by letting me know what's on your mind, and we'll talk about what you need? Then, I'll fill in any gaps so you have a clear picture of what to expect. Does that sound good?

RHONDA: Sure. One of things I'm wondering about is how I should work with you. Are you the nurse I'll be working with most closely?

MONIE: Yes, I'm the charge nurse on your case. I'm here Monday through Friday, and you can feel free to call if you have questions or want to report anything to me. We also have a general e-mail address for the department, and you can send me e-mail messages, as well.

RHONDA: That sounds good. But I'm worried that something might come up in the evenings or on weekends. What happens if you're off for a day? I was wondering if I could also have your cell phone number and personal e-mail address.

MONIE: We don't use cell phones with patients. Instead, we have an answering service that's always available. If something comes up, you can get assistance right away from whoever is on call. Don't worry. We'll make sure you get the help you need. Our e-mail box is always monitored by someone in the office, so you'll get an answer within a few hours or less during that day, or the next business day.

RHONDA: I'm really worried that I might have an emergency and need you.

MONIE: I understand. That's why we have a system in place to make sure you're covered if anything comes up. It's worked well for other patients when they needed something outside of office hours. It'll also be there for you.

RHONDA: Okay. Now. I'm also concerned about what you want me to report on. If I have a bad day, do you want to know? Are there any kinds of symptoms you're going to be looking for? I have to tell you, this is all new to me. And the only thing I know about chemotherapy is what I've seen in movies and on TV and what I've experienced with a couple of friends. I didn't see anything that made me feel very encouraged.

MONIE: Rhonda, this is something that patients often say to me. I can tell you that the process is unique to each patient. I'm going to go over a list of symptoms that chemotherapy patients sometimes experience. I'll also let you know which ones we are especially concerned about. But I'm going to want to hear anything you have to tell me. Don't worry about whether it's going to be interesting to me or not. If it's on your mind, let us know.

RHONDA: Do I tell you or the doctor?

MONIE: That's a good question. When something comes up, call the office and talk to me or one of the other nurses. We'll enter what you have to say in your chart and pass it on to the doctor. If the doctor has any concerns, you'll get a call from one of us. You can also talk to the doctor about your questions or concerns at your appointment.

RHONDA: This helps a lot. At least I know I'm going to be working with people who are willing to listen to me.

Guidelines for Enhancing Professional Health-Care Communication

Following are some guidelines for helping patients communicate with their health-care professionals:

1. *Look for educational moments.* Newly diagnosed patients can only take in so much information. They tend to tune out when information does not seem immediately relevant or when they feel someone is lecturing them. Health-care professionals can accomplish the most with patients by being sensitive to educational moments that might arise. In the preceding example, Monie listened to Rhonda and, as Rhonda expressed her concerns, corrected misperceptions and provided alternative behaviors. These educational moments present themselves in situations that include when patients express concerns about how they are being treated by health-care professionals, when they make requests that may or may not be reasonable, or when compliance issues arise due to misunderstanding. It is at these moments that the patient is focused on a problem and will be open to a solution.

2. *Maintain a nonjudgmental, nondefensive tone.* Because newly diagnosed patients may expect their health-care professionals to judge them, they may make assumptions about those professionals' body language. Such patients pick up on signs that their providers are judging them in some way, such as expressing annoyance that patients are expressing fear. They may also be sensitive to any sign of provider defensiveness, such as when a health-care professional appears to be caught off guard or becomes argumentative. Because patient communication can be so highly sensitive, health-care professionals should keep an open mind when working with patients and remember that those patients may have perceptions that are rooted in their fear and helplessness, not a desire to criticize health-care professionals. Monie listened to Rhonda's complaints about her surgeon experiences with an open mind and then, rather than defend the surgeon's actions or imply that Rhonda had been needy, steered the conversation toward how she and Rhonda would work together.

3. *Clarify communication processes.*   When communications processes are unclear to newly diagnosed patients, they tend to fill the gaps with assumptions. The result can be discomfort, frustration, and stress for patient and health-care professional alike. The best health-care professionals can do is to guide patients on communications processes as opportunities arise. In the preceding example, Monie explained to Rhonda that she should call the nursing staff if concerns arose, but she also reassured her that the information would be passed on to the doctor who, in turn, would also call, if necessary.

4. *Set expectations, and clarify boundaries.*   Newly diagnosed patients are focused on their own needs, and they often feel overwhelmed. Helplessness, fear, lack of information, and the stress of change all combine to render patients extremely vulnerable. Out of their vulnerability, patients tend to reach out to the health-care professionals with whom they work most closely. Patients in flight reaction are especially likely to want to attach themselves. Rhonda, in the preceding example, exhibited a desire to keep Monie as close as possible. Her fear and helplessness drove her to feel she would need Monie's support to complete her treatment.

Monie used a supportive and empowering approach to help Rhonda realize she would have a team of professionals. She set boundaries in terms of her own availability, being careful to say nothing that might make Rhonda feel unsupported or abandoned. She also helped empower Rhonda but implying that Rhonda would be taking responsibility for making her needs known while working within the patient-professional communication system established by the oncology practice.

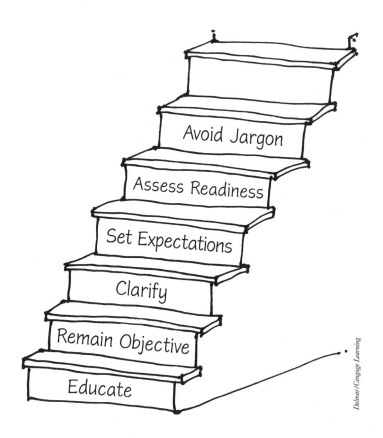

Delmar/Cengage Learning

5. *Begin communicating based on the patient's readiness.* As discussed previously, newly diagnosed patients bring their own levels of readiness to medical treatment, shaped by their unique emotional reactions, experiences and perceptions of their conditions, and expectations of treatment. Instead of reciting a set of guidelines and instructions and expecting patients to respond accordingly, health-care professionals should instead begin by understanding patients' expectations for communication.

   In the example conversation, Monie started by encouraging Rhonda to be open about her concerns and to ask any questions she might have. Then, she addressed Rhonda's issues. This saved Monie time, because she knew what specific concerns to address and could adequately assess Rhonda's expectations.

6. *Avoid jargon.* The requisite vocabulary of medical terms can both overwhelm and confuse newly diagnosed patients. When health-care professionals use terms patients do not understand, the patients can feel as if they are not being acknowledged. They may then become defensive, suspicious, and even irrational. Therefore, it is important for health-care professionals to constantly check that patients understand terminology.

SUMMARY

Newly diagnosed patients take cues from their health-care professionals in terms of the optimal ways to communicate. Team members can guide patients to communicate in ways that will enhance their health-care relationships, thereby ensuring that patients will report their symptoms and side effects and comply with treatment. Effective patient-provider communication supports time management and the honoring of professional boundaries.

Chapter REVIEW

Multiple-Choice Questions

1. Newly diagnosed patients may encounter difficulty communicating with health-care professionals because they:
   a. Learn to read their own bodies and fail to know how they should feel
   b. Cannot identify reportable symptoms
   c. Lack the language to use to discuss symptoms
   d. All of the above

2. The body language that may interfere with patient communication includes which of the following?
   a. Rolling the eyes
   b. Leaning forward
   c. Nodding
   d. Making eye contact

3. When a newly diagnosed patient asks for a health-care professional's mobile phone number, the best response is:
   a. Give the patient the number and be available during this difficult time
   b. Suggest that all members of the health-care team provide the clinic's telephone number
   c. Provide the patient the number and suggest the best times to call
   d. Lecture the patient briefly on self-sufficiency

4. When communicating with patients about their conditions and treatments, it is a good idea to:
   a. Use complicated medical terms so that patients begin to use them on their own
   b. Discourage patients from asking questions that are difficult to answer or unanswerable
   c. Use simple, nontechnical terminology and encourage patients to ask questions as needed
   d. Remind patients that health-care professionals have limited time and direct them to online research

5. When approached by an angry, demanding patient, what should the health-care professional do?
   a. Identify personal emotional reactions and pause before speaking
   b. Inform the patient of the demand's personal impact
   c. State that the behavior will not be tolerated
   d. Inform the patient that such behavior may lead to reduced attention from the health-care team

Fill-in-the-Blank Questions

1. An attitude of concern for patients and acceptance of how they are experiencing their diagnoses demonstrates the concept of _____.

2. _____ includes the terms and abbreviations health-care professionals use.

3. _____ is an expression that refers to negative experiences with health-care providers.

4. Patients who remember only what they most wanted to be told demonstrate _____

listening.

5. Two individuals who have difficulty agreeing or communicating may be experiencing a personality _____

_____.

Short-Answer Questions

1. What are some signs that patient expectations threaten to break patient-professional boundaries?

_____

_____

_____

2. How might a patient interpret a health-care professional's expression of alarm?

_____

_____

_____

3. What can health professionals do to encourage patients who fear they are too demanding or "high mainte-nance"?

_____

_____

_____

4. Health-care professionals can demonstrate a genuine, caring attitude toward patients through what actions?

_____

_____

_____

5. What kinds of statements are disempowering and empowering when patients anger physicians?

_____

_____

_____

Critical-Thinking Questions

1. In today's system, what amount of time is reasonable for health-care providers to spend helping patients address their emotional reactions and gather information? What are key concerns when balancing patient needs with economical constraints?

_____

_____

_____

_____

_____

_____

2. What can health-care professionals do to maintain professional boundaries when patients report that physicians have insensitive bedside manners? What are the options? What are the risks?

_____

_____

_____

_____

_____

_____

3. In the health-care environment, newly diagnosed patients often encounter words and behaviors they fail to understand. What can health-care professionals do to make this environment more welcoming for patients?

_____

_____

_____

_____

_____

_____

Internet Exercise

Search the Web for two or three examples of communication guidelines for patients and health-care professionals. Make sure the guidelines are written from different perspectives. For example, provide an example written from the patient's perspective. Also provide an example from the health-care professional's viewpoint. Guidelines from a clinic's or hospital's perspective might provide a third example. Compare and contrast the communications guidelines, highlighting any similarities and differences.

_____

_____

_____

_____

_____

_____

_____

CHAPTER 7

Encouraging Patients to Gather Information

OVERVIEW

After reading this chapter, you should be able to:

- Define and use the keywords of patient information-gathering.

- Understand the value of information-gathering in helping newly diagnosed patients to become empowered and actively involved in treatment.

- Identify the barriers keeping patients from becoming informed.

- Name the factors that affect information-gathering behaviors.

- Explain how to help patients overcome their barriers to information-gathering.

- Discuss the role of educational moments as opportunities for encouraging patient information-gathering.

- Know the topics that are most useful for newly diagnosed patients.

- Recognize and know how to resolve the situations that challenge information-gathering.

- Describe how to take newly diagnosed patients through the full information-gathering process.

KEYWORDS

Agenda

Avoidance

Barrier

Comfort level

Comprehension

Information-gathering

Socioeconomic status

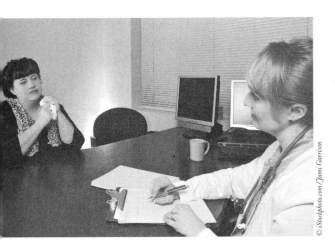

© iStockphoto.com/Jami Garrison

Case Study

Charma had always thought it was normal to feel achy and tired. When she began to feel debilitated, she scheduled an appointment with her physician, Dr. Lopez, who sent her for additional testing. When the test results arrived, Dr. Lopez reviewed them with Charma and then diagnosed her with a condition she had never heard of. Tory, Dr. Lopez's nurse, was also present.

"You have fibromyalgia, Charma," Dr. Lopez said. "It's a chronic condition that causes the joint pain and fatigue you've been experiencing. Do you know anything about it?"

> **KEEP IN MIND**
>
> Diagnoses of unfamiliar conditions can be particularly disconcerting for patients. How would you feel if you were suddenly diagnosed with a condition you had never heard of? What would your main concerns be? How would your concerns affect your willingness to become informed?

Charma did not know what fibromyalgia was. To her, even the name sounded scary. "Am I going to die?" she asked.

"No," Dr. Lopez responded. "Tory and I are going to talk about ways you can adjust your life to live with this condition, but it's going to take some work on our part and yours. We're going to try a medication that's helped other patients with your condition. It may help you, too."

"Okay. I guess," Charma answered hesitantly. She was unsure she wanted to know anything more. After all, at 27, she had a lot of plans that did not include chronic illness.

Continuing the discussion, Dr. Lopez explained fibromyalgia to Charma, what it is and how it developed. Tory described some changes Charma would need to consider to accommodate the limitations caused by her condition. Charma tried to listen, but she was too overcome by shock to understand everything that Dr. Lopez and Tory were telling her.

"Do you have some questions for us?" Dr. Lopez asked.

"I should have a lot of questions," Charma conceded. "But I don't know where to start."

"I know this is a lot for you to hear," Dr. Lopez said. "Right now, I don't expect you to do anything more than listen. But I have to tell you that the best way for you to live with fibromyalgia is to be an educated patient, so you'll understand your symptoms, what to watch out for, and how to adjust to some of the limitations that fibromyalgia patients experience. With fibromyalgia, knowledge is power."

"I understand," Charma answered.

"I'm going to ask you to sit down with Tory to go over some pamphlets we have," the physician continued. "She'll also review the medication schedule with you. Tory is a great resource. In fact, I think she's an expert on helping patients live with fibromyalgia. She'll even suggest some Web sites you might want to visit. Does that sound like a plan?"

"I guess so," Charma shrugged. In truth, however, Charna was unconvinced that more information about fibromyalgia was something that she would want.

Introduction

"I don't know how much information I can handle."

Newly diagnosed patients are inundated with new information at a time when they are not in good positions to process it. The shock of their diagnoses, coupled with the weight of their emotions, makes it difficult to listen to, or process, any information, much less that about newly introduced medical conditions and their treatments. Even if patients were equipped to process their medical information, the sheer volume of that information alone would likely prove a **comprehension** challenge.

Ironically, patients need the medical information they are challenged to process to be able to make informed treatment and lifestyle-management decisions. Patients in fight reaction are likely to educate themselves about their conditions and treatments, while those in flight and freeze reactions are likely to select the information they are willing to learn. Of course, health-care professionals benefit when their patients are educated. In addition to being able to make informed treatment decisions and to understand the implications of their decisions, educated patients are more likely to understand the reasons behind their physicians' recommendations and comply with their treatments as a result. Patients who lack information, in contrast, are more likely to make assumptions that may increase their fear and resistance.

Health-care professionals can help support patients' treatment-compliance efforts by encouraging **information-gathering** behaviors, offering suggestions for relevant information sources, and helping patients understand the information they gather.

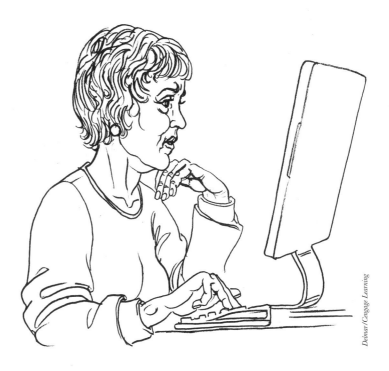

Delmar/Cengage Learning

Identifying Barriers to Information-Gathering

Driven largely by irrational beliefs, ones related to their emotions and concerns, newly diagnosed patients may raise a number of **barriers** to avoid gathering information about their conditions. Patients may feel, for example, that learning more about their conditions may be harmful rather than beneficial.

ADDRESSING INFORMATION AVOIDANCE

Fear is a major barrier to information-gathering. Immediately after diagnosis, patients may want to avoid information out of the fear that what they learn will fuel more uncomfortable emotions. For example, patients may be concerned that they may learn that they could have avoided their conditions, a situation that may lead to guilt. Heredity's role in diagnoses may cause anger, albeit misplaced, at family members. Information about the progression of symptoms or the side effects of treatment may increase patients' sense of helplessness. In short, patients may choose information **avoidance** to avoid more despair.

Among the types of information that newly diagnosed patients want to avoid are the following:

• Evidence that lifestyle choices or heredity played a role in causing the condition

• Treatment options that require decisions patients are unprepared to make

• Treatment side effects that are lengthy, inconvenient, and frightening

• Ongoing compliance requirements that may require major lifestyle changes

Although concerns like these exist, patients must address them at some point to move forward. Some patients are ready sooner than others to progress, driven by their

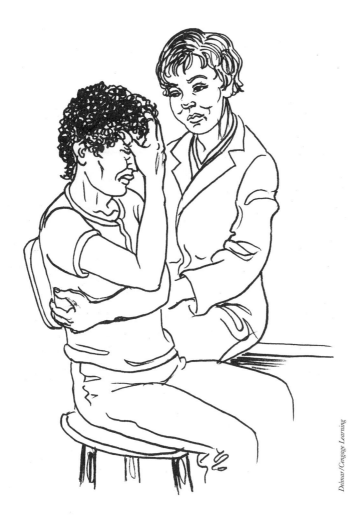

Delmar/Cengage Learning

abilities to address their emotions, gain support from caregivers, and accept the interventions of health-care professionals.

WORKING COUNTER TO FATALISM

Diagnoses can impart on newly diagnosed patients a sense of impending doom, even when their conditions are not considered catastrophic. For example, patients with acute conditions may feel that their treatments will be so disruptive as to rob them of their senses of normalcy.

TAKING POSITIVITY TO THE EXTREME

Newly diagnosed patients, especially those in flight reaction, can carry the need for a positive attitude to an extreme. While positive thinking can help patients cope with the challenges of medical treatment, it can also be a form of denial. By insisting on positivity, newly diagnosed patients can avoid recognizing their emotions, acknowledging the seriousness of their conditions, understanding the urgency of their treatments, and appreciating the need for major lifestyle changes. Some patients may tell themselves that if they stay positive they can avoid addressing their diagnoses and—out of superstitious thinking—will be able to will their diagnoses away. Superstitious

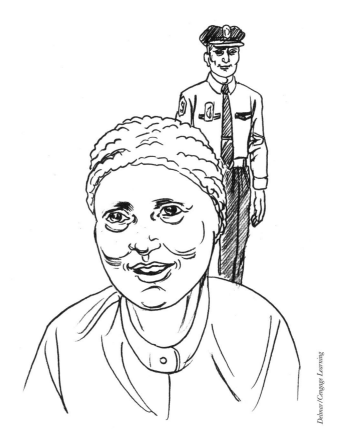

Delmar/Cengage Learning

thinking drives some patients to feel that information-gathering is a sign they distrust in their physicians, one that will somehow interfere with the success of treatment.

Health-care professionals can determine when patients are using a positive attitude as a form of denial by gauging patients' willingness to explore information about their conditions and treatments. Patients in denial express concerns about encountering information that is "negative" and that would place their positive attitudes at risk. They may also express that they are doing their physicians and other health-care providers favors by avoiding information that might erode the team's optimism and trust.

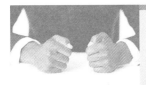

Body Language

Newly diagnosed patients who are starting to gather information about their conditions may demonstrate body language like the following:

- Resting the head in the hands, eyes downcast
- Stroking the chin
- Biting the nails
- Looking away
- Tilting the head forward

FORCING RECOGNITION OF REALITY

Superstitious thinking causes the mainly subconscious belief that not knowing aspects of a medical condition or its treatment can prevent negative events from occurring, particularly as they relate to symptoms and side effects. Newly diagnosed patients with this belief essentially fear that they can cause something to happen by thinking about it too much. They may feel, in essence, that they can "think themselves sick."

KEEPING INFORMATION ATTAINABLE

Physicians and other health-care providers may inadvertently give newly diagnosed patients medical information that is out of their reach because it is too technical, frightening, or confusing. Providers are not solely responsible for the comprehensibility of medical information, however. Patient literature may be confusing in and of itself. Web-based sources can overwhelm patients for a range of reasons. Among other things, Web sites may conflict. Patients cannot easily determine which sites are trustworthy, and patient-generated content may be filled with errors or irrelevant facts. Furthermore, the number of health-related Web sites is vast. Patients seeking information can easily and quickly become overwhelmed with information.

Information overload can especially harm first-time patients. Not knowing where to begin—what basic questions to ask and what sources to target—patients who are exploring medical conditions for the first time are at great risk of becoming lost in a sea of information. After one or two experiences feeling lost, patients may decide against information-gathering altogether.

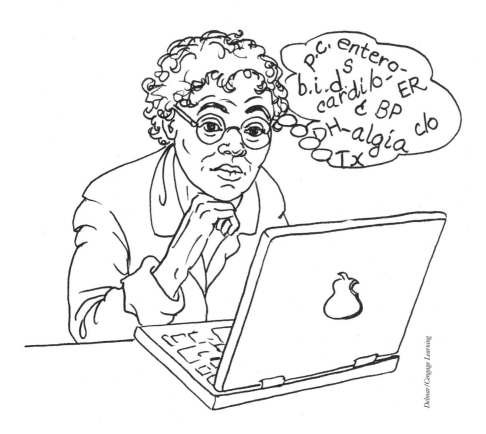

Delmar/Cengage Learning

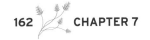

Recognizing Other Factors in Information-Gathering

Beliefs are just one factor that impact the information-gathering behaviors of newly diagnosed patients. The sections following describe some others.

HARNESSING THE FIGHT REACTION

Patients in fight reaction are often enthusiastic information-gatherers, because they want to know as much as possible about their conditions and treatments as a means of making informed decisions. At the start of information-gathering, fighters may need some guidance from health-care professionals. Beyond that, however, such patients are motivated to search on their own.

APPRECIATING GENDER DIFFERENCES

Traditionally, women are more involved medical consumers than men. As an extension, they tend to be more conscientious about information-gathering. Women are often the lead caregivers, and consequently the information-gatherers, for their ill parents, children, and spouses, as well (O'Connor et al., 2003; Pew Internet and American Life Project, 2005).

ASSESSING THE IMPACT OF AGE

Overall, young and middle-aged adult patients are more likely to be active information-gatherers than those who are older. They are more likely to question those in authority, including health-care professionals, and to take responsibility for their health care. In general, they view information-gathering as a means of achieving independence. Older patients, in contrast, come from a generation that unquestioningly trusted physicians and looked to those professionals as sole sources of information and advice. While there are some exceptions—and certainly this is changing with the boomer generation—older patients are also less likely to be active Internet users, so that rich avenue for information-gathering is largely closed off.

CONSIDERING CULTURAL DIFFERENCES

A wide range of multicultural issues impacts the information-gathering of newly diagnosed patients. The first consideration is language. Patients for whom English is not their first language may have difficulty comprehending much of the information they are presented. As a result, they can become confused and uncomfortable. When possible, therefore, medical materials should be in patients' native languages. In addition to grappling with language issues, patients from other cultures may feel uncomfortable asking questions. They may want to avoid appearing not to understand information or to appear disrespectful by questioning someone in authority.

ACCOMMODATING EDUCATION AND SOCIOECONOMIC STATUS

Newly diagnosed patients with low education levels may be uncomfortable reading or have difficulty comprehending what they read. Such patients will most likely benefit from discussions with the health-care professionals who treat them, supplemented by easy-to-understand information and guidelines. Patients from low **socioeconomic status** may share reading issues, as well as discomfort interacting with those they perceive as more educated or in authority.

Facilitating the "Knowledge Is Power" Mentality

Health-care professionals can help newly diagnosed patients become more active information-gathers—and information-users—through a combination of guidance and encouragement. Often, what new patients need are people who are committed to ensuring they are informed and who are willing to take the time, where appropriate, to act as coaches in the information-gathering process.

HELPING PATIENTS OVERCOME INFORMATION AVOIDANCE

Newly diagnosed patients may need help overcoming the fear, denial, or other barriers they have erected against information-gathering. Patients in flight reaction will tend to tune out any information they perceive as frightening or contrary to their chosen treatment paths. Flight patients will also avoid information out of a desire to avoid their conditions. They may even gather information solely to focus on bad news. Patients in fight reaction are generally active information-gatherers, though they may need help identifying which information sources will be most useful.

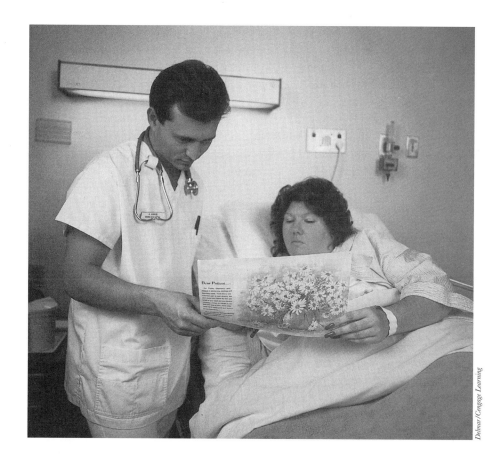

Delmar/Cengage Learning

Sometimes, what patients need most is encouragement to take the first step in getting informed about their conditions. Health-care professionals can help provide this encouragement by taking the time to understand why patients are avoiding information, explaining the benefits of getting informed, and prompting the patients to get started. The following details this step-by-step process:

1. Discuss with patients why they are avoiding information.

    "It seems to me that you don't want to read the pamphlets I gave you. Patients who are diagnosed often want to avoid information at first. Why don't we talk about what's bothering you about getting informed about your condition? I'd like to understand this better so I can see how I can help you."

2. Acknowledge that information avoidance is normal.

    "It's normal to be [scared, confused, overwhelmed] when you first start to learn what's going on with your health. I know you're reading about things you'd rather not know about."

3. Explain the benefits of being an informed patient.

    "If you understand your condition and what to expect from treatment, you benefit in more than one way. First, the things that scare us most are those we don't understand fully. When you understand your condition, you'll know what we can do about it. Also, when you're informed, you can help us by asking questions and by keeping us informed, such as by reporting your side effects. This helps us help you."

MAKING RELEVANT AND APPROPRIATE RESOURCE RECOMMENDATIONS

The health-care information environment is rich and varied. While this means newly diagnosed patients can answer virtually any medical question, and from varied perspectives, it also means that patients may be exposed to information that is biased, irrelevant, or laden with medical terminology. Health-care professionals can help patients start to navigate the sea of medical information by suggesting resources that will meet patients' needs.

Patients may have the best information-gathering intentions while sitting with health-care professionals but lose initiative and focus on their own. As discussed previously, age, education, and cultural background can be barriers, as can be the volume of the information pool. Following are guidelines health-care professionals should consider when helping patients take the first step toward gathering information:

-   Be sensitive to patients' orientations to information.

    "I'm wondering if you'd like to sit down for a few minutes and talk about the best way to take your medication and what you can avoid if you stay on track. If you want, I can write down a few of the most important things for you."

-   Encourage patients to take the first step by suggesting where they might get started.

    "I've listed great Web sites you can visit, as well as a couple of numbers of organizations that specialize in your condition. I'm happy to print this list out for you."

-   Place information in patients' hands.

    "I'm going to give you a handout we put together here at the clinic. A lot of newly diagnosed patients have found that this gave them some useful, basic information, along with a few ideas on where to go for more information. It includes a couple of Web sites we recommend. I'll point out what you might want to pay the most attention to."

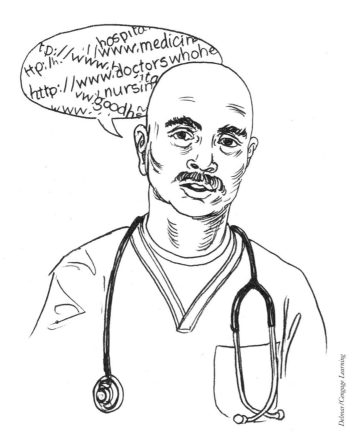

Delmar/Cengage Learning

ENCOURAGING READING AND COMPREHENSION

During the early years of the Internet, only the technologically savvy were active users. Gradually, as more and more people started using the Internet, more and more patients began visiting health-care-related Web sites like WebMD. Visiting a Web site does not guarantee use or comprehension of the site's information, however. Much like the hard-copy materials patients pick up in the office, the information does not necessarily reach its intended audience.

As described previously, newly diagnosed patients may have barriers to reading information about their conditions and treatments. These barriers at once impede patients' willingness to seek and read the information they obtain. Patients may gather information to please their health-care providers but do nothing with it.

Health-care providers can counter patients' resistance to information by gently yet firmly working with the patients to ensure they gain value from it. The following sections outline strategies:

- Time allowing, offer to briefly sit with patients and review information together.

    "Why don't we sit for a couple of minutes and go over the pamphlet I gave you? I can use a highlighter to point out some of the most important points for you to keep in mind."

- Tell patients what they should pay most attention to as they gather information (e.g., treatment duration, side effects, compliance guidelines).

    "I mentioned that you were going to do some searching online. I wrote down a couple of trustworthy sites you might start with. As you read through them, I suggest you pay really close attention to the information on how to get the most from your medication, including the foods to avoid while taking it."

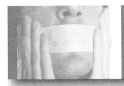

SELF • talk

Negative self-talk around information-gathering includes the following:

I'll never be able to understand all of this. It's all written for doctors and nurses.

I'm only going to read something that makes me feel even more discouraged.

I'll have more questions that nobody will want to answer.

It's better not to know and to let nature take its course.

You can't even believe half of this. Who knows who it's coming from? It's not worth my time.

Antidotes to negative information-gathering self-talk include the following:

A lot of the information on the Web is patient friendly. My health-care professionals can recommend the best sites for patients.

It's better to be informed and to understand what I'm facing than to guess and maybe even think the worst.

I can always ask my health-care team a question if I don't understand something.

Some information is more reliable. I can focus on sites sponsored by reputable organizations.

- Encourage patients to ask questions about what they have read and review key points.

  "I know you looked through some of the materials that were in the new patient packet I gave you. You probably have a few questions about what you read. Do you want to ask me anything now? If not, I can go over a few things with you."

- Gently remind patients of the importance of being informed about their conditions, and ask if they have specific concerns that have prevented them from using information.

  "I know you have a lot to think about, and some of the information can feel overwhelming at first. But it's so important that you have a basic understanding of your condition and the kinds of things you need to be doing for yourself. Do you want to talk about what's keeping you from spending some time getting more informed?"

- Suggest additional information sources when patients appear to be having difficulty understanding what they have been reading.

  "I'm wondering if you didn't find the information I suggested helpful. If you didn't, I have some more ideas about information that could be useful. Would you like a few more suggestions?"

- Offer encouragement in the form of praise when patients discuss things they have read or ask questions.

  "That's a great question. I see you've been doing some information-gathering on your own."

CAPITALIZING ON EDUCATIONAL MOMENTS

While newly diagnosed patients can benefit from conversations about information-gathering, various educational moments arise along the way that health-care professionals can use to convey information and encourage patients to gather information. Take, for example, a patient who has inadvertently been noncompliant with medication, perhaps taking it on an empty stomach instead of with food. The health-care professional might remind the patient of the correct way to take the medication, as well as encourage investigation of information on getting the most from medication. A patient who asks how to maintain an optimal lifestyle gives the health-care professional an opportunity to encourage the patient to gather information around the condition as well as topics like wellness, stress management, and diet/exercise.

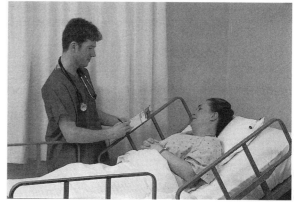

Following are guidelines for taking advantage of educational moments.

- Gently suggest that patients must be informed.

  "It's not uncommon for newly diagnosed patients to run into some glitches when they first start medications. I can give you a couple of rules to follow to make sure you don't run into this kind of problem again. I also have a Web site I can tell you about that really explains what it's like to be treated for your condition and offers a lot of ideas that you might want to keep in mind."

- Suggest related information to help patients maintain healthier lifestyles.

  "You bring up an interesting question about how stress might have been a factor in your recent flare-up. I have some pamphlets here on stress management that you might find helpful. I also know of a couple of great Web sites that explain how stress affects health, and I have some ideas for keeping stress under control."

Highlighting Key Areas of Information

A comprehensive list of information sources, including organizations and Web sites, appears in Appendix A. The following sections discuss some topics to consider when encouraging patients to begin gathering information.

RESEARCHING CONDITIONS AND THEIR TREATMENTS

Patients can benefit from understanding:

- How conditions develop
- Symptoms of treatments
- How conditions may progress when left untreated
- Risks and benefits of each treatment option
- Coping with treatment
- Making lifestyle changes
- Experiences of other patients with the same condition

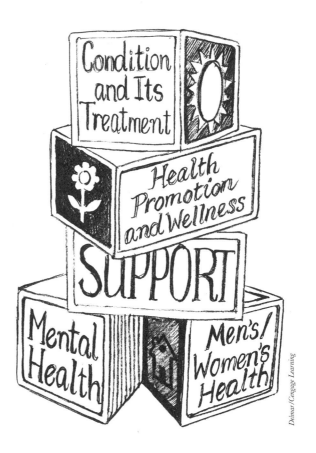

Delmar/Cengage Learning

PROMOTING HEALTH AND WELLNESS

While it is not in the best interest of newly diagnosed patients to research unproven, alternative treatments, they can benefit from the health and wellness practices that support traditional medicine, including the following:

- Biofeedback

- Yoga

- Meditation

- Natural foods

- Vitamins (if physician-approved to not interfere with treatment)

- Appropriate exercise

CULTIVATING PATIENT SUPPORT

For newly diagnosed patients, support groups can be valuable sources of information as well as emotional support. Support options range from traditional support groups; online support, possibly developed by pharmaceutical companies producing patients' medications; or condition-focused organizations. Following are some other support options:

- National associations with local chapters

- Local support groups

- Online chats
- Online behavioral modification programs
- Message boards

DIFFERENTIATING MEN'S AND WOMEN'S HEALTH

By their very natures, some conditions are specific to men or women (e.g., ovarian cancer or prostate cancer). For certain conditions that men and women share, like diabetes, the implications for men and women differ. Patients can benefit from exposure to gender-specific topics like the following:

- Recovering sexually after prostate cancer treatment
- Self-image after breast cancer treatment
- Coping with Type II diabetes

APPRISING MENTAL HEALTH

As mental-health issues arise with patients, health-care professionals should consider the following topics:

- Depression and what to do about it
- Stress management
- Coping with a medical diagnosis
- Local counselors and therapists
- Local support groups
- What to look for when choosing a mental-health professional
- Low-cost options for mental-health treatment

Conducting Information-Gathering Despite Challenges

While medical information can usually be extremely helpful for newly diagnosed patients, at times, it is less than helpful. Information that is based on unsound medical practice or that is misunderstand or misinterpreted qualifies as the latter. The following sections outline challenges that may arise during information-gathering.

ADDRESSING CONTRADICTIONS

Brochures from pharmaceutical companies or even nonprofit organizations may be biased in some way. While the information they carry is not incorrect, it may appear to contradict what patients were told at their health-care clinics or offices. Patients may find other contradictions in sources like the Internet.

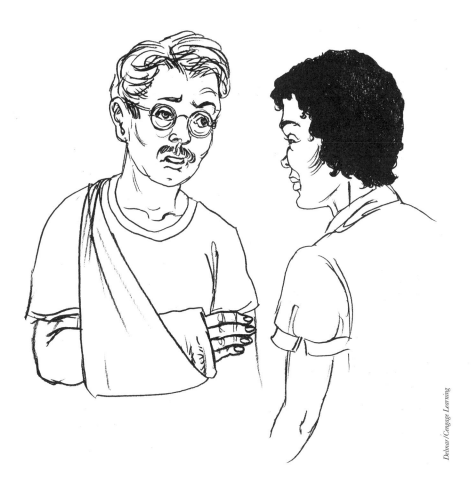

Delmar/Cengage Learning

In the following example, a newly diagnosed patient, Christa, visited a patient blog that discussed the benefits of an arthritis treatment Christa's physician had indicated was not the best treatment for her condition. She discussed her concerns with Tony, her health-care professional.

CHRISTA: I just read that the medication I had originally asked for works much better than the medication I'm using. So now I'm confused. Why aren't I taking it?

TONY: You know the doctor said that arthritis is not a one-size-fits-all condition. Some medications are more appropriate than others.

CHRISTA: Well, I don't know anymore. What I read made a strong case for another approach.

TONY: Can you show me where you read this?

CHRISTA: Sure. (They go on the Internet together.)

TONY: Christa, I just want to point out that this is a blog written by a patient, not a medical professional. The guy who wrote this is talking about his experiences. So this is his perspective and opinion. It doesn't apply to everyone.

CHRISTA: I see. I hadn't thought about that.

TONY: But if you want to talk with the doctor about what you've learned, I'm sure she'd be able to answer your questions.

HARNESSING INFORMATION-INSPIRED FEAR

Inevitably, newly diagnosed patients are going to read things that cause them to be concerned about their conditions or treatments. Most concerned about symptoms, side effects, and disease progression, patients may read something contradictory on a patient blog, as Christa did in the previous example, or they may read biased information on the Web that tries to gain support for a specific treatment.

When health-care professionals and patients have trusting relationships, patients can discuss their concerns with their providers and become both educated and reassured. Health-care professionals are best equipped to help patients determine whether information is credible or not, as well as whether negative outcomes are likely to occur.

Dave, a patient recovering from surgery, visited a Web site that discussed side effects of the pain medication he is taking. He decided to discuss what he read with his health-care professional, Cathy.

> **DAVE:** I'm really worried about this pain medication the doctor prescribed. I read that it causes aplastic anemia. Are you giving me something that's going to cause big problems further down the road?
>
> **CATHY:** Where did you read that?
>
> **DAVE:** Well, I can tell you it was from a reputable source. I read it in the patient information pamphlet from the drug company. I'm sure they know their own product.
>
> **CATHY:** That's a reliable source, Dave, but I'd encourage you to keep in mind that the drug companies have to report any and all potential side effects of their products. The FDA requires it. The package insert will let you know the percentages of patients who've experienced a specific side effect. Most likely, very, very few patients have experienced aplastic anemia. Did you notice the percentage?
>
> **DAVE:** No, I don't think I noticed that.
>
> **CATHY:** Let's take a look and see. Any drug has risks, but when a side effect hardly every occurs, then you don't need to be so worried about that.

KNOWING WHEN INFORMATION-GATHERING IS EXCESSIVE

Patients have their own unique orientations toward information, and so do their physicians. Some physicians encourage information-gathering. They want their patients to explore their conditions, to know as much as possible, so they welcome discussions around what their patients learn. Other physicians have had negative experiences with patients who have been frightened or misinformed through biased information. Still other physicians feel it best that they serve as patients' main sources of information so they can control what patients know about their conditions. These kinds of physicians who have a low **comfort level** for uncontrolled access, want to try to avoid patients who worry too much or ask too many questions.

It is impossible, of course, to control patients' information access completely. Out of concern for how information may affect patient trust, compliance, or decision making,

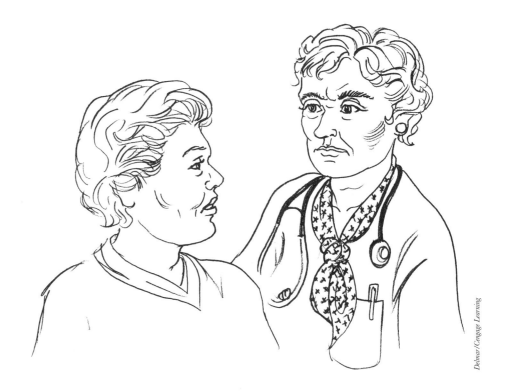

Delmar/Cengage Learning

physicians may express frustration or discomfort with their patients' information-gathering. To keep the lines of communication open, physicians should reassure patients that their questions are welcome despite any controversy.

Rennie, a patient recently diagnosed with a chronic condition, was scolded by her physician recently for reading too much frightening information on the Web. She discussed the incident with her health-care professional, Melissa.

RENNIE: My doctor got kind of mad at me. I thought it was a good idea to understand how I'm being treated, and I have to get informed if I'm going to be able to do that. But I think I asked him a question that made him mad.

MELISSA: What were you talking to him about when you felt he got mad?

RENNIE: I had read an article on a health Web site that said a new injectable drug might be more effective than the pills I'm taking. I asked him if he had heard of it and if he thought it was time for me to try it.

MELISSA: What made you think he was mad at you?

RENNIE: He said that he's comfortable with my treatment at this point and that it's working. He said he's treating me according to best practices for my condition and that I need to trust him and not second-guess him all the time.

MELISSA: I can't speak for the doctor, Rennie, but in this office we encourage patients to be informed about their conditions, and we're all here to answer your questions as they come up. If you have concerns about how your treatment is working, feel free to let one of us know.

Getting Caregivers Involved in Information-Gathering

Caregivers can play varied roles in the process of gathering information for newly diagnosed patients.

As discussed in previous chapters, caregivers feel as much—and sometimes more—fear and helplessness than patients themselves. As they watch their loved ones cope with medical conditions, they may feel the urge to "jump in and make everything better." One of the ways they cope with their own helplessness is to learn as much as possible about the patients' conditions. They are looking for ways to help the patients—to find the best treatments possible and, in the process, feel like they are taking active roles. Family members can play active roles in information-gathering or in encouraging patients to become informed. They can also play roles that are less productive.

The following situations may arise with family members in information-gathering.

KEEPING FAMILY PARTICIPATION EQUITABLE

Family members may become so involved in information-gathering that they discourage the newly diagnosed patients from involvement. They may fear that the patients will learn something that will interfere with the patients' positive attitudes. Caregivers may not trust patients to use information correctly in decision making, so they take charge of the process. They may assume that patients prefer someone else handle the details. Caregivers, especially those from immediate families, may want to avoid their own emotions around their loved ones' medical diagnoses. They fear that patients will express emotions that are uncomfortable for the caregivers, emotions that will stir emotions in the caregivers.

Patients in freeze reaction are so emotional they shut down or deny, so they may welcome caregivers' intervention. Patients in flight may be similarly accommodating, because they are emotionally unprepared to process information. Unfortunately, when caregivers assume control of information-gathering and patients cede control, caregivers disempower patients at a time when they should become empowered.

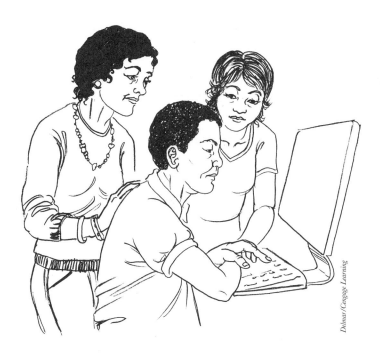

Delmar/Cengage Learning

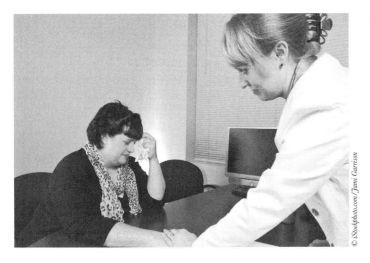

© iStockphoto.com / Jami Garrison

GIVING PATIENTS LEEWAY

Caregivers may expect the newly diagnosed patients to become empowered immediately, to take charge of their information-gathering immediately. Some caregivers are motivated by the recognition that their loved ones must become involved and begin to do whatever is necessary to cope with their diagnoses and get treatments and lifestyle-management activities under way. Other caregivers, however, are motivated by an **agenda** to avoid their own emotions and a desire for patients to put their diagnoses behind them. Patients may sense how their caregivers are feeling and assume that they are on their own with information-gathering. Alternatively, they may resist information-gathering efforts.

Guidelines for Introducing Patients to Information-Gathering

Following are some guidelines to keep in mind when getting newly diagnosed patients started in gathering information about their conditions:

1. *Sell the benefits.* Newly diagnosed patients are often initially hesitant to get involved in information-gathering. For all but the most motivated patients, information-gathering sounds at first like a large undertaking, if not punishment, with a lot of time spent researching topics they have no desire to learn about. Explaining—selling—the process's benefits can help patients to be more open to the idea of learning about their conditions. Patients will feel more in control, know when to be concerned about symptoms, make the best treatment decisions, and choose the lifestyle adjustments that will yield the best results. Tory described information-gathering to Charma as a team effort with the physician and other health-care professionals.

   Success stories of patients who became educated and benefited from reliable information can be powerful motivators for newly diagnosed patients.

2. *Start slowly.* Like Charma did, newly diagnosed patients feel shock initially at diagnosis, then they feel overwhelmed. Information-gathering may feel like yet another mountain to climb. Tory suggested a few areas that Charma might want to research to help her get started, but not many. When she sensed Charma hesitate, she took a step back and asked Charma where she wanted to start. This gave Charma a sense of control and allowed her the option of starting at her own pace.

3. *Consider doing your own research first.* Because health-care professionals cannot be experts on every condition they treat, a list of reliable resources for common conditions can be helpful starting points for information-gathering. Dr. Lopez had had enough fibromyalgia patients that Tory took it upon herself to maintain a resource list. With it, she could more easily start to educate patients.

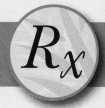

Introducing a Patient to Information-Gathering

Tory sat across from Charma, who looked totally devastated by her diagnosis. She had tears in her eyes, and she slumped forward in her chair. Tory sat for a moment without speaking to give Charma time to gather her thoughts.

TORY: I know this is a lot to hear about. Did you have any expectations about what your symptoms might be caused by?

CHARMA: Not really. I just thought I was tired.

TORY: (Smiles) You are tired. And now we know why. We're going to do everything possible to get you feeling as well as you can. To start that process, I want to go over some information with you. Dr. Lopez already explained some of the basics of fibromyalgia. First, I'm going to review your treatment plan and answer any questions you might have.

Tory explained the schedule for the medication Charma would be receiving, as well as how she might learn to live effectively and as normally as possible with her symptoms.

TORY: Dr. Lopez mentioned that we really want to work with you as a team, and that means that all need to be informed. Can I suggest some information that might be helpful for you to look through?

CHARMA: I guess so.

TORY: Are you an Internet user?

CHARMA: Yes, I am.

TORY: Great. There are a lot of fantastic sites out there that have some excellent information. I'm going to suggest a support site for young women like you who are dealing with chronic conditions. You can get information and find out about support groups that are in the area. I also want to give you the address of a Web site that gives you the basics about fibromyalgia. You might also be interested in information on stress reduction through techniques like meditation and yoga. Does this sound good?

CHARMA: It sounds like too much.

TORY: Okay. Where do you think you could comfortably begin?

CHARMA: I'll just read the pamphlets you gave me. And then maybe I'll check out the site for women with chronic conditions.

TORY: You're married, right, Charma?

CHARMA: Yes, I am.

TORY: I'm wondering if you might talk to your husband about what you learned today and see if he would like to partner with you in learning more about fibromyalgia. Remember, we're going to need him involved in your treatment. Do you think he'd be up for that?

CHARMA: This is going to be hard on him. But I know he's going to want to be by my side.

TORY: That's great. Don't forget that I'm here to answer any questions that come up. We can even go through information together if you want to print it out and bring it in.

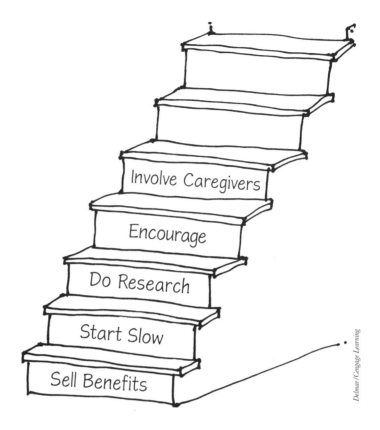

Delmar/Cengage Learning

4. ***Stand by to encourage and interpret.*** Tory made it clear to Charma that she was not sending her into the "forest of information" unaccompanied. She said she was willing to answer questions and to review information Charma might want to print out and bring to the office. In addition to motivating Charma, Tory may have laid the foundation for a productive patient-provider bond.

5. ***When possible, involve caregivers.*** Caregivers can partner with patients who are learning about their conditions. Tory assessed Charma's openness to involving her partner in information-gathering as an option for research and support.

SUMMARY

Information-gathering is a critical step toward patient empowerment. Informed patients are better able to actively participate in their treatments. They understand their conditions and are more likely to comply with treatment because they understand rationales and implications. They also know what they most need to report so their health-care teams are best positioned to help them. Health-care professionals can play an active role in both motivating and guiding patients in this process.

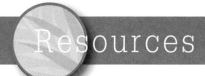
Patient Information-Gathering Worksheet

Patient Name   _____

Condition   _____

Medications Prescribed   _____

_____

Patient was given the following printed information:

_____

_____

_____

_____

Suggested additional resources:

Web sites

_____

_____

_____

_____

_____

_____

Other resources

_____

_____

_____

_____

_____

_____

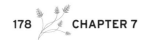
Checklist for Patient Orientation Package

Condition _____

Brochures

_____

_____

_____

_____

Resource list (condition, treatment, mental health)

_____

_____

_____

_____

Self-monitoring checklists

_____

_____

Diet/exercise guidelines

_____

_____

Emergency contacts

_____

_____

Office procedures and policies

_____

_____

Chapter REVIEW

Multiple-Choice Questions

1. Most newly diagnosed patients are motivated to avoid information about their conditions by:
   a. Fear that knowing more will cause more fear
   b. Guilt that they might have contributed to their diagnoses
   c. Concern that they will become angry at their family members
   d. All of the above

2. _____ occurs when newly diagnosed patients express concern that knowing too much about their conditions will be too negative and interfere with their positive attitudes.
   a. Reprisal   c. Reversal
   b. Denial   d. Deconstruction

3. Patients are justified in complaining that information from their health-care professionals or the Internet is:
   a. Too technical   c. Too accurate
   b. Not positive enough   d. Not negative enough

4. Health-care professionals who assure patients it is normal to fear information about their conditions at initial diagnosis are:
   a. Inappropriate, because they encourage patient resistance
   b. Appropriate, because patients should avoid information for as long as possible
   c. Appropriate, because they accept patient responses
   d. Inappropriate, because patients benefit most from direct confrontation about their resistant attitudes

5. In information-gathering, patients' family members or caregivers should do which of the following?
   a. Complete all information-gathering with patients
   b. Avoid information-gathering because it disempowers the patients
   c. Work with patients to help the patients become more informed
   d. Interpret information for the patients

Fill-in-the-Blank Questions

1. A patient who has recently received a cancer diagnosis at first refuses to learn anything about her condition and then, after getting some help coping with her emotions, is willing to read an informational pamphlet. This is an example of _____.

2. A patient who is provided with information that is written for health-care professionals, and not patients, will most likely have difficulty with _____.

3. Patients from low _____ _____ may have had less opportunity to use technology and, consequently, have difficulty looking up information on the Internet.

4. Patients who avoid learning about their conditions out of a belief that knowing too much will worsen their conditions demonstrate _____ thinking.

5. Health-care professionals who take time to understand their patients' customs around illness are sensitive to _____ issues.

Short-Answer Questions

1. What impact does a patient's age have on willingness to gather information on a diagnosis and ask questions?

_____

_____

_____

2. In your opinion, what information is most important for newly diagnosed patients to be aware of?

_____

_____

_____

3. When patients encounter information that seems to contradict what they have heard from health-care professionals, what should other health-care professionals say?

_____

_____

_____

4. Why may family members discourage newly diagnosed patients from gathering information about their conditions?

_____

_____

_____

5. What is an example of an educational moment for patient information-gathering?

_____

_____

_____

Critical-Thinking Questions

1. A patient's cultural background affects willingness to get informed about a medical diagnosis. In the United States, information-gathering approaches may be unique to different regions of the country, as well as to socioeconomic status and educational background. Individuals who grew up in other countries may also have unique approaches to getting informed. What are some of the cultural differences that you have encountered or would expect?

_____

_____

_____

_____

_____

2. Health-care professionals sometimes become concerned about the information newly diagnosed patients encounter online, as well as frustrated by the misperceptions this information may lead to. How would you describe the benefits and potential dangers of Web-based information to a newly diagnosed patient? What would you recommend to a patient who is unfamiliar with the Web and who you are concerned may be unable to distinguish between valid and invalid information?

_____

_____

_____

_____

_____

3. Sometimes, physicians and other health-care professionals question whether there is any value to independent information-gathering, given that patients may become overwhelmed with information, which may lead them to assumptions or misperceptions. Is there a point at which patients become too informed? What is the best balance between being independently informed and trusting in the recommendations of the treatment team?

_____

_____

_____

_____

_____

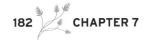

Internet Exercise

Choose three medical conditions. For each condition, conduct a search for information about:

- The condition and its treatment
- Complementary treatments
- Psychosocial support options
- Online patient information exchange

What was your impression of the information you encountered? Its depth? Patient friendliness? Who sponsored the information: nonprofit organizations, bloggers, treatment centers, pharmaceutical companies? How would you compare the sponsors' approaches? What concerns would you have for a newly diagnosed patient searching for information on one of the conditions you chose?

_____

_____

_____

_____

_____

_____

_____

_____

CHAPTER 8

Developing a Support Plan with Patients

OVERVIEW

After reading this chapter, you should be able to:

- Define and use the keywords of developing a support plan with patients.

- Define the range of support needs newly diagnosed patients may have.

- Understand barriers newly diagnosed patients may have to receiving support and how they express them.

- Recognize the signs that patients may feel disempowered.

- Explain how to assess readiness for the support conversation and how to focus this conversation on patient needs and solutions.

- Tell where to look for patient support resources.

- Discuss how to initiate collaboration on the patient support plan.

- Understand the role of family members and other caregivers in providing patient support and making support decisions.

KEYWORDS

Activities of daily living	Disempowered	Psychosocial
Brainstorming	Lifestyle	Resources
Burden	Medical regimen	Self-talk
Case manager	Open posture	Social work department
Collaborate	Openness	Support
Compliance		

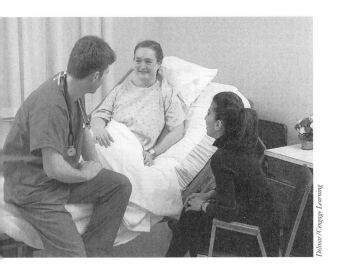

Delmar/Cengage Learning

Case Study

Karina had been warned that her smoking might lead to a diagnosis of Chronic Obstructive Pulmonary Disease (COPD), so when she received the news she was not surprised. She was, however, sad and guilty. Still, she described herself as "somebody who doesn't give up," so she set out to become informed about her condition and do whatever she had to live a full life.

When Karina's respiratory therapist, Josh, and her medical assistant, Sophia, opened the discussion about the kinds of support Karina might need going forward, her resolution to be a fighter began to waver.

> **KEEP IN MIND**
>
> Medical diagnoses often come with a host of medical challenges, particularly when the conditions are chronic. As a health-care professional, what would you be thinking and feeling if you were going to discuss support options with a newly diagnosed patient who is facing many medical challenges as a result of a progressively debilitating medical condition?

"I was prepared for *some* changes in my life," Karina said to Josh and Sophia. "I've been having breathing problems for a long time, and I had already started to feel myself slowing down. Let's say I haven't been hitting the treadmill in the gym any time in recent memory."

Because he had already reviewed the results of Karina's lung-capacity tests, Josh had been administering Karina's breathing treatments. He had shown her how to use the inhaler she would be relying on daily, as well as demonstrated how to use the oxygen she would need at home.

"You've responded well to the breathing treatments," Josh said encouragingly. "And the medication your doctor prescribed for you has really benefited other patients."

"But I have to have oxygen at home now," Karina protested, "and that means to me that my breathing may get worse over time."

"We're always available to you," Josh responded. "We'll be monitoring you closely and doing everything we can to help you maintain your health. One of the things I want to talk to you about is what you can do to take care of your lungs and what supports we can put in place to help make that happen. Sophia is going to be helping me put a plan in place for you."

Josh and Sophia had already discussed Karina's at-home support, including activities of daily living. As Karina talked, however, Sophia realized that emotional support would also be an important part of her plan.

KEEP IN MIND

As Sophia pointed out, emotional support is one element of a comprehensive support plan for a newly diagnosed patient. What concerns would you have regarding Karina's emotional state? Ideally, what would you want to be able to offer her at this point in her treatment?

While Josh and Sophia had begun formulating a plan, they knew that Karina is sad and scared. They also knew she wants to be a fighter and remain as independent as possible. Therefore, they wanted to encourage her to be as self-sufficient as possible but also to embrace the support that will help her maintain her physical and emotional health. Her next comment made it clear that Josh and Sophia had their work cut out for them.

"I don't know if I'm supposed to become an invalid," Katrina said. "When I read about what happens to people with COPD, I don't know if I have any choice. I want to stand up to what's happening to me and make the best of it. At least, I do on some days. On other days, this sounds like a lot of work, and I wonder if I shouldn't get all the help I can to lead a life that is as easy as it can be. Maybe I should just let nature take its course."

"We've a lot to talk about," Sophia said.

"That's what we're here for," Josh added.

KEEP IN MIND

If Karina was your patient, how would you be feeling at this point? Thinking about what you have learned about body language, what body language would you be looking for in Karina? What kind of negative self-talk do you think she might be using?

Introduction

"I don't want to burden other people."

Who likes asking for help? Like most human beings, most newly diagnosed patients do not relish having to rely on their family members and friends to care for them in any way. **Support** is associated with images of neediness, perhaps needing help using the bathroom or with other **activities of daily living**, like preparing meals or getting to the doctor. While few patients need this level of care, they may avoid the topic altogether to avoid imagining where needing support could lead. Not surprisingly, patients who have not yet dealt with their fears or are in denial about their conditions tend to resist the idea of support the most.

Whatever their conditions, most patients need support on some level. They might need temporary support while they recover from surgical procedures, undergo lengthy treatment processes like chemotherapy, or modify their activity levels. Some patients need help complying with treatment requirements for medications or diet. As discussed in previous chapters, newly diagnosed patients may need to plan for short- or long-term emotional support.

Patient support comes in varied forms. If you were going to list the kinds of support newly diagnosed patients need the most, what would you include? Consider reviewing previous chapters for ideas.

As they create treatment plans, health-care professionals often talk to newly diagnosed patients about their support needs. To plan effectively, professionals must help patients overcome their resistance and realistically assess their needs.

Identifying Patients' Support Needs

Because newly diagnosed patients cannot know the kinds of support they might need as they progress through treatment, health-care professionals should bring that knowledge to the team. Armed with that information, the professionals can suggest the kinds of support patients might need, as well as begin to explore patients' perceptions of their needs and potential support options.

The following sections briefly describe support areas. Later sections address these areas with **resources** to consider.

EXPLORING PSYCHOSOCIAL SUPPORT

Because they experience complicated emotions, virtually all newly diagnosed patients can benefit from ongoing **psychosocial** support. All previous chapters have discussed the role of psychosocial support in coping with the emotions of a medical diagnosis. Health-care providers, friends and family members, and mental-health professionals can all provide psychosocial support. Simply having access to someone who can provide a nonjudgmental, listening ear is a basic psychosocial support requirement.

DEFINING ACTIVITIES OF DAILY LIVING

Newly diagnosed patients generally resist the idea of needing help with activities of daily living—things like household chores, grocery shopping, meal preparation, and transportation to appointments—because they associate the need with a loss of normal functioning, a fear-inducing possibility. However, support in this area need not be long term. Some patients simply need assistance immediately after surgery and during and after medical treatments.

INSPIRING LIFESTYLE CHANGES

Newly diagnosed patients may need various kinds of support when changing their **lifestyles**. For example, they may need professional guidance when changing their diets or starting exercise regimens. Support "buddies" who offer encouragement and, potentially, the benefit of their own experiences can help patients maintain the motivation and focus they need to succeed in treatment.

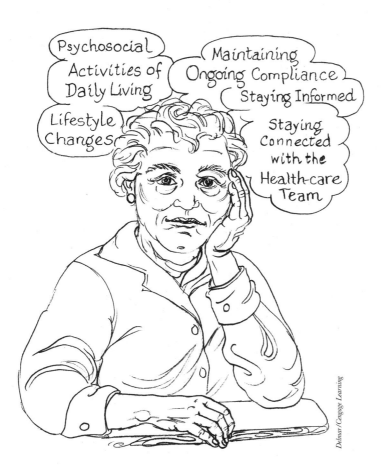

MAINTAINING ONGOING COMPLIANCE

Because some **medical regimens** are more difficult to adjust to and maintain than others, newly diagnosed patients may need support in both the early and later stages of their treatments. Patients may, for example, resist daily injections or medications but with the support of the health-care team assimilate the regimens into their routines.

KEEPING PATIENTS INFORMED

As discussed in Chapter 7, patients are motivated to varying levels to gather information about their conditions and treatments. They are similarly varied in their motivation to continue to stay informed. Patients, especially those in fight reaction, may stay informed on their own, or they may rely on their health-care team to keep them informed and/or suggest relevant information. Patients who want to stay informed may need continuing encouragement and guidance.

STAYING CONNECTED WITH THE HEALTH-CARE TEAM

Once treatment is completed or regimens have been adopted, patients tend to become less vigilant, failing to report for needed checkups or to report any concerns they may have. Depending on where they are in their treatment cycles, patients like these need encouragement from their health-care teams to varying degrees.

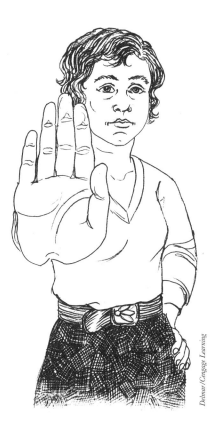

Delmar/Cengage Learning

Overcoming Barriers to Support Acceptance

Newly diagnosed patients may erect barriers to receiving the support they need to adapt to their conditions. The following sections detail those barriers.

EXPLORING DENIAL: SHERRY'S STORY

> *"I'm not going to be sick enough to need any additional help," Sherry insisted when the nurse in charge of her case, Perry, suggested that she consider accepting the services of a home health aide while undergoing chemotherapy. "This isn't going to be a big deal at all," she proclaimed. "As long as I keep my positive attitude, I'll be fine."*
>
> *"The home health aide will only be coming in to help with the more difficult tasks, like cleaning," Perry contended.*
>
> *"These are exactly the kinds of things I need to be doing," Sherry argued. "If I keep active and don't let myself slack off, I'll get through this with no problems."*

Denial can be a powerful barrier to accepting help during a time of need. Newly diagnosed patients often express their denial by insisting that they have to "think positive," which often means avoiding anything counter to the view of the world they want to see. In this example, Sherry does not want to accept that her chemotherapy treatments may take a temporary toll and that this toll may prevent her from being able to function at her normal level. For Sherry, discussing the possibility that she needs help is admitting to the possibility. In her mind, as long as she stays positive, the scary possibilities will go away. Unfortunately, denial can be so strong that newly diagnosed patients will listen selectively to their health-care providers, hearing only what they want to hear.

How denial is expressed:

"All this talk about people helping is just negative thinking."

"Don't try to tell me I'm sick. You're treating me like I'm going to be an invalid."

"This will all be over before I know it."

"I want to keep living my life as if nothing bad is happening to me."

"What you're telling me doesn't make any sense."

WORKING WITH LACK OF INFORMATION: LATOYA'S STORY

"I heard that most people go on doing what they usually do with this thing. The medicine takes care of it," LaToya said to Jana, her health-care professional, when Jana suggested that she may want to talk to a dietician and join a patient group to help her to change her eating habits. "These medications do what your body can't, and you go on living your life."

"Have you been reading the information we gave you that describes your condition and how to best protect your kidneys from further damage?" Jana asked.

"I glanced through it," LaToya answered. "But I talked to a couple of people who have something like what I have, and they haven't had any problems."

Lack of information can be a powerful barrier to proper support. Newly diagnosed patients may listen to people they only assume are informed but are not, or they may listen to only those who tell them what they want to hear. They may also read unreliable literature. Even when information is valid, comprehension is not guaranteed. Valid information is of little help if patients fail to understand it or skip over important facts.

Patients who are uninformed are more likely to make assumptions about their support needs. As they do when in denial, patients are more likely to embrace, or avoid, or distort, information when doing so is consistent with their desire to avoid thinking about anything unpleasant.

How lack of information is expressed:

"I heard from some other people. . . ."

"I know what I'm talking about. I did a little research on my own."

"I can't believe this could be any different than _____ [another, possibly unrelated condition]"

"I trust my judgment on this."

"I was reading something on the Web. . . ."

FEARING LACK OF FINANCIAL RESOURCES: TYLER'S STORY

Tyler realized that, after his heart surgery, he was no longer going to be able to maintain his life's hectic pace. He was going to have to start conserving his energy, which would mean relaxing more at home, spending time with friends, and cutting back on overtime. He was also going to have to get some help maintaining his home.

"You're telling me to cut back on my hours, and that means less money," Tyler protested to Javier, his cardiologist's medical assistant. "And you're telling me I have to hire people to help me with my household chores. That doesn't make any sense."

"Have you looked into the options that might be available to you?" Javier asked.
"A little bit," Tyler answered. "And they're all expensive."

Finances are always top of mind with newly diagnosed patients. They see the statements from their health-care providers and, even if they are not responsible for these costs, they become aware of how much medical care is costing. If they are responsible for co-pays and deductibles, they feel the costs even more directly. If they have to take time away from work for treatment, concerns about job security may arise. And if, like Tyler, they are forced to reduce their work hours, finance-related concerns are increased.

Patients may express their financial concerns directly, as Tyler did, or they may express them indirectly, by doing things like insisting they need no additional help or can return to their former routines once they have recovered. Patients who are financially responsible for others will feel, if not express, additional concerns about how the costs of their medical care may impact others in their households.

How fears about lack of financial resources are expressed:

"I have to keep costs under control, so I'm going to handle things myself. I just need to pace myself."

"My family depends on me. I'll scare them if I start acting like an invalid."

"I'll recover faster if I stay active."

"There are so many people out there looking to rip off someone like me. I'm better off without them."

"I'm already feeling stronger. I'll be back to normal in no time."

WANTING TO AVOID BEING A BURDEN: VIVIAN'S STORY

Vivian took care of her mother as her mother grew older and could no longer care for herself. During the last 2 years of her life, she lived in Vivian's home. When Vivian was diagnosed with chronic fatigue, her medical assistant, Edina, talked with her about the kind of assistance she herself might need going forward.

"I know I don't need that much care right now, but I have to be honest about what I went through caring for my mother," Vivian started. "She needed constant emotional support, and that was hard on me emotionally. She needed me to be an expert on her illnesses so I could help her keep the doctor informed. And then there was all the day-to-day care as she got weaker. I loved her, but she became my life. My kids tell me they're ready to step up to the plate, but I don't know if I want to put them through that."

"So it sounds like see yourself as becoming a burden to your family," Edina reflected.

"That's exactly right," Vivian responded. "I can't let that happen, even if they're telling me I can. I wouldn't do that to anyone."

Fear of being a **burden** to others is common among newly diagnosed patients, especially those with conditions that will require extensive treatment and/or that might be debilitating over time. Patients most often express this fear as a concern that loved ones will be inconvenienced by the responsibility of their care, but they may also fear that family members will become resentful and either continue to care for them begrudgingly or simply walk away. Some even fear that their family members will refuse this responsibility altogether, leaving the patients to face lack of care and their loved ones' lack of concern at once. When family relationships are tense or strained, patients may fear that the relationships will not withstand any additional pressure. Self-image plays a role in these dynamics as well. Human beings have a sense of pride that is based on self-reliance, so asking for help from loved ones can erode self-esteem, especially for those who have previously viewed themselves as the "strong ones" in the family.

How fear of being a burden is expressed:

"This is going to be too much for everyone to handle."

"My family is going to resent me if I start making all these demands."

"I want my family to have their own lives, not to have to take care of me."

"I don't need that much help now, but what about farther down the road?"

"I don't think they'll know what to do. I better take care of this on my own."

EXPRESSING THE DESIRE TO BE (TOO) INDEPENDENT: DAVE'S STORY

Dave was initially angry and fearful when his physician informed him that he had an intestinal blockage and would need surgery followed by a lengthy recovery. His friends, however, have always described Dave as having a "take charge" attitude. Not surprisingly, then, within a few days, Dave had completed extensive research online, networked to find the best surgeon in his area, and, once he was satisfied he had made the right decisions, scheduled his surgery. It was only then that he told his family about his diagnosis.

> *"I'm not a typical needy patient," Dave informed Brian, his nurse. "So don't start telling me what I'm going to need. I've already told my wife that she doesn't need to take any time off from work, and I've told my kids I won't need any help from them. I plan to be back to work within a few days."*
>
> *"The doctor has indicated that you're going to need a lot of bed rest, for a couple of weeks or more," Brian responded. "From there, your strength is going to come back gradually. We think you're going to need to build yourself up over a couple of months or more. We need to talk about having a nurse's aide available a few hours a day while you do that."*
>
> *"That's nonsense," Dave argued. "I don't need anyone getting in my way and holding me back."*

Dave's health-care professionals might call him a classic example of a newly diagnosed patient in fight reaction. He took charge of his health care almost from the moment he received his diagnosis. Like other fighters, though, Dave's insistence on independence could become extreme, to the point that he develops an unrealistic attitude toward the potential effects of his condition and its treatment. Ultimately, if Dave fails to accept the support he needs, his independent attitude will harm him. The health-care team, for its part, will be challenged trying to treat him, because they will have no assurance that he is complying to the level he needs to support his ongoing recovery. Dave's independence may be a way of expressing denial of the seriousness of his condition and the effect his treatment will have on his life.

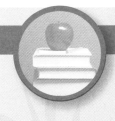

KEEP IN MIND

Newly diagnosed patients tend to struggle with help-lessness throughout their treatments and recoveries. The helplessness patients feel at initial diagnosis may be resolved but return when the patients face the challenges of treatment, medication regimens, side effects, and routine changes. As a health-care professional, how can you support patients facing these challenges?

How a desire for independence is expressed:

"I'll let you know if I need any help."

"Don't try to take charge of my life. I know what I'm doing here."

"If you baby me, you'll turn me into an invalid."

"Just let me make the decisions here."

"The sooner I get back on my feet, the sooner I'll have this behind me."

Accommodating Patients Who Want Unneeded Support

While some newly diagnosed patients reject support, others opt for as much support as possible, much more than they need. These patients have adopted a **disempowered**, victim role. Patients in flight reaction may seek as much support as possible, due primarily to being so overwhelmed by emotions that they are unable—or at least perceive themselves as unable—to care for themselves. Like patients in flight reaction, patients in freeze reaction may insist on more support than they need, but they do so because they have resigned themselves that ongoing decline and dependency are all they have to look forward to.

Patients who see themselves as needing more support than they actually need tend to express their perception in terms of activities of daily living, although it extends to other areas of support as well. Patients who feel this way will insist that family members and health-care professionals perform their household chores and such tasks as meal preparation and even self-care. Patients in flight reaction may ask for extensive emotional support, while patients in freeze reaction may seek additional support in communication with health-care professionals, sometimes insisting that their team members assume responsibility for ongoing tasks like scheduling appointments and updates.

IDENTIFYING OTHER EMOTIONS AT WORK

While helplessness is a rather obvious factor helping create patients' perception that they need unnecessary support, other factors are also at work. Newly diagnosed patients may demand support out of a sense of loneliness. Whether it preceded diagnosis or not, health-care-related support becomes a way patients can gain the nurturing and socialization they crave. Patients who continue to be overwhelmed by the fear factor, or helplessness, may fear that they will somehow "fall through the cracks" if

Educational Moment

Much like newly diagnosed patients benefit from discussions about their support needs, as opportunities arise they benefit from brief reminders of areas in which they will need support and resources. For example, when patients express concern about administering medications at home, health-care professionals could reassure the patients that they will not be expected to do this themselves and that support resources are available.

someone is not constantly watching over them. Anger is yet another emotional factor. Demanding unnecessary support may be a passive-aggressive means of retaliating at whatever, or whomever, the patients have decided are responsible for their situations. Under the surface, complicated psychological issues, rooted in unresolved issues with family members, may be at play.

ENCOURAGING SELF-EFFICACY

Inadvertently, health-care professionals who help newly diagnosed patients make support decisions imply that they need help to choose the appropriate support. Instead of ceding complete responsibility for their care, patients need to be encouraged to accept the support they need yet still use their own emotional, intellectual, and physical resources to avoid becoming victims. In this dynamic, health-care professionals are key to helping patients gain realistic perspectives of the support that they do and do not need.

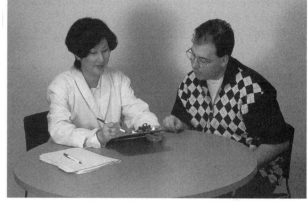

Going forward, the discussion of support in this chapter is intended to help health-care professionals help newly diagnosed patients assess their support needs accurately so those patients can enjoy the support that is consistent with their needs, preferences, and available resources. Consequently, the information and guidelines that follow use situations in which patients resist support as well as demand more support than is necessary.

Assessing Patient Openness to Support

Health-care professionals begin assessing newly diagnosed patients' **openness** to receiving support by listening to patients' perspectives on their health situations and how those situations are impacting their lives. Generally, discussions revolve around activities of daily living, because such activities are heavily tied in with patients' routines, which patients want to maintain as much as possible. With professionals' prompting, discussions also often touch on patients' perceptions of their abilities to cope emotionally, stay informed, and remain compliant.

The success of discussions like these hinges on the ability of health-care professionals to listen. Professionals who listen set the tone that they are considering patients' wants and needs when planning support. In return, patients feel a sense of control at a time when feeling in control is important. As the discussions progress, health-care professionals will have opportunities to gauge patients' willingness to consider support, identify any resistance or other barriers to support, and determine if patient helplessness is amplifying patients' support requests.

MEETING PATIENT POTENTIAL

Clearly, decisions about support can be complicated. Realistically, newly diagnosed patients may need support in certain areas, such as activities of daily living and **compliance**. Unfortunately, patients may resist. Health-care professionals often begin support discussions with details, including needs and suggested solutions. While this approach may appear straightforward and efficient, it risks confusing patients.

The desire to be "normal" is a key motivator for newly diagnosed patients. By asking, "What will it take to be the best possible you?" the health-care professional gives the patient the opportunity to collaborate on the means of maintaining the standard routine as much as possible.

Patients may not immediately understand the connection between support goals and the health-care professionals' suggestions. Some patients could assume that their providers are trying to control their lives.

The optimal way to introduce the support discussion is to invite the patient to **collaborate**, to help create the support plan. Ask, "What are you going to need to be the best possible you?" This question subtly implies to patients the following facts:

- Support is directed toward wellness—being as "normal" as possible—and not toward being "sick" or in any way encouraging a victim role.

- Patients are tasked with helping set the ground rules for support, and the health-care professional values their input.

- The discussion will focus on choosing solutions that are most in line with patients' preferences.

In addition to engaging the patient, beginning the support discussion by providing an opportunity for the patient to talk first gives the health-care professional an opportunity to understand how the patient views the prospect of needing support in some form. In answering this question, patients will express their hopes, fears, and any barriers to support. With this information, health-care professionals can best guide the balance of the discussion.

DEFINING THE ROLE OF SELF-TALK

Newly diagnosed patients most likely have images around what it means to be ill and in need of assistance. They may have faced health problems—or are facing other ones now—or they may have observed, or been caregivers for, family members or friends with medical conditions. Media portrayals of health care may also be in the mix.

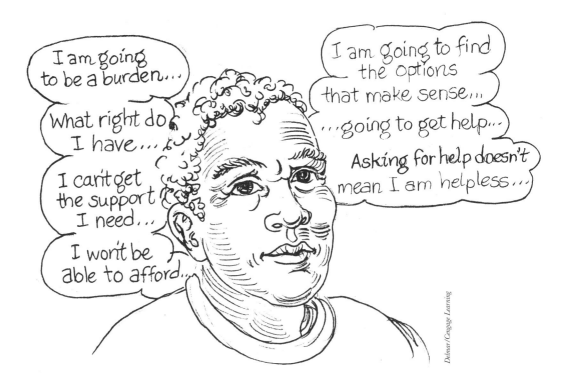

Delmar/Cengage Learning

All these images contribute to patients' **self-talk** about support, which is often accompanied by emotions. Patients may be angry about past responsibilities, disappointed in those who did not come through, or guilty about having failed someone in the past. Patients also worry about contributing to their loved ones' fears about them.

Patients who identify with their negative support self-talk can be hard to reach. Health-care professionals should encourage patients to express their support concerns, and then help the patients identify when they use negative self-talk. As Chapter 2 describes, one contributor to negative self-talk is lack of information, which results in either-or thinking. Health-care professionals can help dispel patients' fear, and counter their negative self-talk, by educating them on the kinds of support options that are available.

Locating Resources for Key Support Areas

Earlier sections of this chapter described the key areas of support that newly diagnosed patients may need. Following are some suggestions for finding resources to meet those needs.

TAPPING INTO HOSPITAL AND CLINIC RESOURCES

Newly diagnosed patients who have required hospitalization most likely have access to the social work departments of the hospitals where they were treated. Social work departments are staffed by individuals who are well-versed in local community resources and provide guidance on assistance with finances, nursing and personal care, support groups, and other emotional support. In **social work departments**, employees are trained to evaluate patients' needs and to make connections with appropriate resources in the community. Department **case managers**

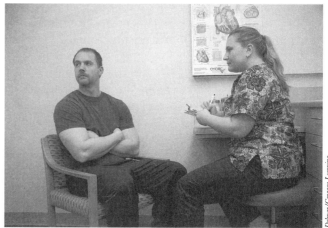

Delmar/Cengage Learning

may also be available to lend support. Hospitals have their own systems for making referrals with the social work department, whether it is initiated by the patient, physician, or other health-care professionals.

HARNESSING THE INTERNET

As Chapter 7 discussed, the World Wide Web has a wealth of health-related information, including sites dedicated to patient support and community resources. Of course, some Web sites are more trustworthy than others. While some provide reliable information, others have agendas that might include selling a product or service or promoting a nonmainstream viewpoint. Regardless, patients benefit greatly from using search engines to locate relevant Web resources.

WORKING WITH COMMUNITY ORGANIZATIONS

Many community organizations exist to help individuals in health-care situations. In large communities, these organizations may be focused on conditions like diabetes,

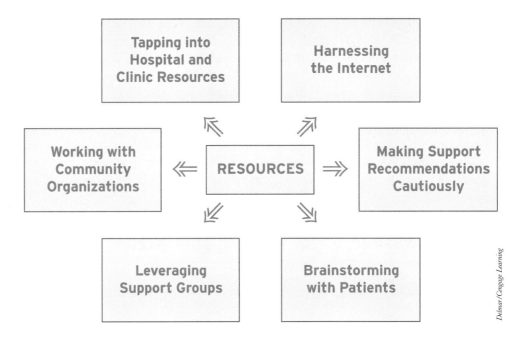

HIV, or cancer. Often, they are local chapters of such large organizations as the American Diabetes Association or the American Cancer Society. These organizations may offer services that include trustworthy information, access to professionals who can answer questions, counseling, support groups, referrals to services like help with chores and meal delivery, and financial grants. A careful search on the Internet will yield the Web sites of these organizations. However, the local yellow pages, the community pages of your local newspaper, and local resource guides all also provide contact information.

It can be helpful for health-care professionals to make the first contacts with these organizations to understand the services they offer and learn the best ways to make referrals. Additionally, professionals can understand any costs that might be involved, clarify eligibility requirements, and obtain the names of patient contacts. In so doing, the health-care staff spare their patients time and frustration when they may have been hesitant to call and/or easily discouraged.

LEVERAGING SUPPORT GROUPS

Support groups are available through hospitals and treatment centers, local organizations, churches and synagogues, and patient advocacy organizations. The Web, the local telephone directory, and your local newspaper are all recommended starting places for locating support groups. These groups not only provide emotional support, they provide information and recommendations for other services. Newly diagnosed patients may embrace support groups, or they may feel exposed in such a setting. Some patients will be frightened or discouraged by other patients' experiences. Given the potential risks, health-care professionals should explain the role and potential benefits of support groups to their patients, keeping in mind that patients may resist the idea, at least initially.

BRAINSTORMING WITH PATIENTS

Newly diagnosed patients often need help tapping into the support options in their communities and networks. For example, a neighbor's child might be interested in making some extra money by mowing the patient's lawn or helping with household chores. A group of friends might be recruited to each make one meal per week. An objective friend or family member might be a good person for the patient to partner with on helping with medication regimens or exercise plans.

Examples and encouragement can lead to the **brainstorming** that often leads to bountiful options. Newly diagnosed patients are often initially reluctant to think of their social circles in terms of support. Consequently, early discussions may be less productive than the discussions that follow. Patients may need time to process the idea of community support, gain perspective in terms of benefits, and acknowledge their needs as well as the willingness of others to step in.

MAKING SUPPORT RECOMMENDATIONS CAUTIOUSLY

For a number of reasons, health-care professionals should make support recommendations cautiously. Of course, choosing appropriate resources, and presenting them in a way that the newly diagnosed patients will understand, is important. More pointedly, newly diagnosed patients may assume that recommendations are endorsements and will likely be disappointed and angry if they have negative experiences. Trust may be eroded as a result. Recommending too many resources may confuse patients. With patients harmed in any way as a result of a professional's referrals, there may be legal implications.

Before making referrals, then, health-care professionals should become well-versed in the policies of their organizations (office, department, hospital, clinic). That way, they will be able to honor any restrictions regarding the kinds of resources they can offer patients. Some organizations maintain official lists of the only support resources staff can recommend to patients. It is also a good idea to clarify with patients that resource recommendations are not endorsements of the health-care professionals or their organizations.

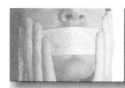

SELF • talk

The prospect of support can trigger a range of negative self-talk messages that include the following:

I'm going to be a burden to my loved ones, and they'll end up resenting me.

I haven't been helpful to other people. What right do I have to ask for help?

Everybody around me wants to turn me into an invalid.

I can't possibly get the kind of support that I'm going to need. If it even exists, I won't be able to afford it.

Antidotes to negative self-talk include the following:

There are a lot of different options for support, so I'm going to find the ones that make the most sense for me.

I don't have to settle for being an invalid. I'm going to get help in maintaining as much of my normal life as possible.

Asking for help doesn't mean I'm helpless.

The people who love me want to see me remain as strong as possible, and they want to participate in making that happen.

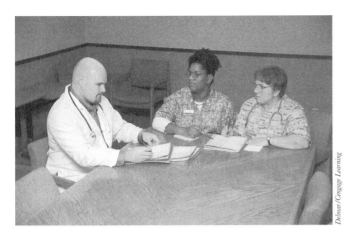

Delmar / Cengage Learning

Networking informally with other health-care professionals can help staff choose appropriate resources. For example, well-established support groups often develop reputations for their approaches and discussion topics. Because support groups can be polarizing for patients, health-care professionals who ask other trusted professionals for recommendations help ensure that the support-group experience is productive for the patient. Networking can be useful in obtaining suggestions and recommendations for other support resources, such as home-health-care agencies.

Initiating Collaboration on the Support Plan

As discussed previously, collaboration is key when working with newly diagnosed patients on support plans. Health-care professionals set the stage by verbally and non-verbally creating environments in which patients feel their feelings, concerns, needs, and preferences are valued.

BEING AWARE OF PERSONAL BODY LANGUAGE

Newly diagnosed patients are highly sensitive to the attitudes of their health-care professionals. Conveying an attitude of openness to collaboration begins with the professionals' body language. Consciously and subconsciously, patients react to even the most subtle cues. While continuously monitoring one's behavior and controlling others' perceptions is impossible, health-care professionals can follow some basic guidelines to effectively portray an attitude of collaboration.

What not to do:

- Avoid eye contact, which may be perceived as a lack of honesty
- Hold a notebook in front of you, which may imply that decisions have already been made
- Stand when the patient is sitting
- Sit with your arms folded across your chest
- Frown or appear distracted

What to do:

- Maintain eye contact
- Smile, convey optimism
- Sit across from the patient with an **open posture**
- Keep paperwork you are holding in plain view
- Nod when the patient speaks to demonstrate active listening

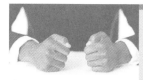

Body Language

Expressing Barriers to Support through Body Language
Newly diagnosed patients may demonstrate resistance to support through body language that includes:

- Looking away
- Stiffness
- Aloofness
- Talking too loudly
- Refusing to communicate
- Frowning

Expressing the Victim Role
Patients may express helplessness through body language like the following:

- Hesitancy
- Talking softly
- Slumping forward
- Speaking haltingly
- Nodding too frequently

REASSURING PATIENTS OF CONTROL

Health-care professionals are often overscheduled and have limited time to spend with each patient, especially on non-direct-care issues that may seem unnecessarily time-consuming. With so little time and so much experience on patient-support issues, it is human nature for health-care staff to start making assumptions about patients' wants and needs. However, those assumptions can easily be inaccurate, and patients tend to respond to a "cookie cutter" approach with the notion that the health-care professionals are trying to control their situations. In response, the patients often resist and withhold cooperation.

What not to say:

- "Here's what we have planned for you."
- "I'll go through the schedule for you."
- "We know exactly what you need."
- "It's all been set up for you."

What to say:

- "We have some suggestions for help with a few things so you can conserve as much of your strength as possible for getting better."
- "I'd like to start with where you think you might need some help."

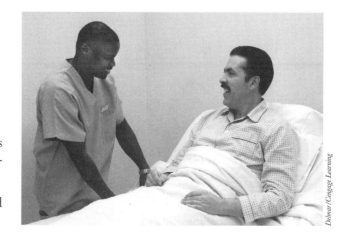

- "Choose the activities that are most important to you, and then let's work together on getting you some help with the other ones."

- "I'm here to help put together a realistic plan for making sure you can do the best you can going forward with your condition. That's my goal."

POSITIONING ASSISTANCE APPROPRIATELY

The support discussion should include an overview of the physician's recommendations, as well as any additional recommendations the health-care professional might have. The patients, possibly already aware of some of the recommendations from talking with their physicians, may try to bargain with their health-care providers regarding the level of support they think they need. Unfortunately, those patients may have based their "deals" on unrealistic expectations. When confronted by patients who are unrealistic about their support needs, health-care professionals may momentarily appear to agree with the patients' assessments as a means of avoiding uncomfortable situations or upsetting the patients. While this approach is understandable, the risk is that the patients will expect their support plans to be based on their unrealistic assessments as well.

Instead of agreeing with unrealistic assessments, health-care professionals should give their patients realistic views of the recommended areas of support, as well as the accompanying rationales. In so doing, the professionals should distinguish between short- and long-term recommendations and review the benefits of receiving the appropriate support. In the spirit of clarity, health-care professionals may find it helpful to review the treating physicians' comments on the patients' charts or to ask physicians to speak with patients. Reminding patients that they will have input into the delivery of their support will likely help soften any disappointment or frustration.

What not to say:

- "Don't worry. You probably won't need much help at all."

- "I'm sure you can have as much home health care as you want."

- "Let's be optimistic. Most patients are on their own in no time at all."

What to say:

- "You'll need this help during your treatment and for a while afterward, until you regain your strength."

- "We'll continue to evaluate how you're doing. We'll leave the support in place only as long as you, and your treatment team, think you need it."

- "Most likely, you'll need this support moving forward with your condition."

- "If you take time to rest and recover, you'll have a better chance of getting back to normal earlier."

STARTING WITH LISTS

Because they are most likely new to the health-care culture, newly diagnosed patients take their cues from health-care professionals as to expected and appropriate behaviors. Health-care professionals who make lists during support discussions can imply to their patients that their meetings are working sessions, that no plans are yet in place, and that the patients' input is desired. It may help to also give patients paper and pens to take notes on. In addition to soliciting participation in the discussion, such an act encourages patients to record any questions or ideas they might have.

As support discussions proceed,, the patients and health-care professionals should compare notes. In additional to providing a sense of control and involvement, this exercise helps patients maintain focus.

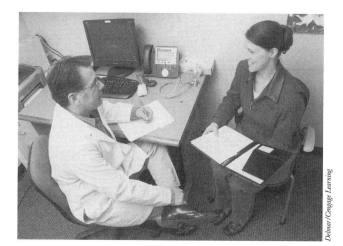

What not to say:

- "I've made some notes for us to go over."

- "I'll go over my ideas. You might want to jot down a few notes."

What to say:

- "I'm going to give you some paper and a pen. If you want to jot down any questions or ideas that you have as we go along, please feel free."

- "Why don't you start by making a list of some of the resources you think might be helpful to you?"

- "I'd like to know what you view as the kinds of support we need to put in place for you while you are in treatment. If you want, go ahead and sketch out what you would see this looking like, and then we can talk."

- "I have some resources I can suggest, but you might want to do some brainstorming on your own, starting with getting some help with household chores."

MAKING SUGGESTIONS BUT ALLOWING CHOICES

Newly diagnosed patients take the recommendations of their health-care teams seriously. While generally this is positive, at times patients might consent when they are uncomfortable in doing so. For example, patients may agree to attend support groups when they have no interest in doing so, or they may agree to checkup schedules they are unsure are realistic. While patients may need suggestions from their health-care team, they will comply more readily with support plans they feel relate to them specifically. To allow their patients choices, health-care professionals should provide suggestions and then discuss the options with the patients to understand any concerns and preferences.

What not to say:

- "Here's what I've got for you."

- "I can tell you what I would do in your situation."

- "I'll tell you what other patients have done."

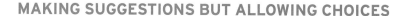

KEEP IN MIND

Health-care professionals may need extreme patience to get newly diagnosed patients to recognize where they may need help and where they can remain self-sufficient. Compassion is key. How would you feel in this situation? What would you like from your health-care provider?

What to say:

- "We're giving you some suggested resources, but it's up to you to decide which ones you want to choose."

- "We want to help you put support in place that meets your needs. I have some ideas for you, but you are the ultimate decision maker in terms of how this all works."

- "I've given you a few ideas, now let's talk about each one."

- "It's important for you to feel comfortable with the support that is put in place. After all, this is all about helping you."

Getting Families Involved in Support

Chapter 11 covers communication with family members and other caregivers. For the purposes of this chapter, it is important to emphasize the critical role that family members play in supporting newly diagnosed patients. Patients do not always want their families involved in support, for reasons that include fear of being a burden and failing to trusting the family members with the task. Family members may also resist this role, for the same reasons.

Realistically, when newly diagnosed patients live with, or near, family members, those family members are involved in patients' health care. Most likely, family members become involved soon after the patients receive their diagnoses by offering emotional support, communicating with the treatment teams, and educating themselves on the patients' conditions. Because they are immobilized to some degree by their emotions, patients in flight or freeze reaction may need their families involved to a greater degree than if they were fighters.

As families become involved in support delivery, the right of the newly diagnosed patients to be in control is an important consideration. Patient and their health-care teams alike may perceive families as "taking over," insisting on being involved in support discussions and dictating how support should be delivered as well as by whom. While family involvement can initially feel overly aggressive and even hostile, it is important for health-care professionals to remember that overinvolvement can arise out of the sense of helplessness that families experience when loved ones receive medical diagnoses. A sense of helplessness may also cause family members to disempower patients by encouraging those patients to do very little.

To offset this possibility, when possible, health-care professionals should gently remind newly diagnosed patients that they are in charge of their support and that others will make decisions only when they allow them to. To keep the families feeling involved and informed, the health-care professionals can offer to answer the questions of family members—with patients' written permission.

While health-care professionals play a key role in helping to organize the patient's ongoing support, they should not become involved in family conflicts. When families make recommendations or choices that are not advisable for the patients, the health-care professionals may need to refer to policy, and enlist physicians, to ensure that the patients' interests are met.

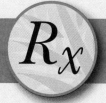

R_x Conducting the Support Discussion

Karina, the recently diagnosed COPD patient from the beginning of the chapter, sat down with Josh, the respiratory therapist, and Sophia, the medical assistant, to begin planning the support she might need moving forward.

SOPHIA: Now that you have a treatment regimen set up, Josh and I want to talk to you about making sure we put in place any support you need. Okay?

KARINA: I don't think I have a lot of choices here. I know I'm sick. But I also know I'm not going to start living like an invalid unless I become one.

JOSH: We don't want to make you weak, Karina. We want to help you to stay as strong as possible.

SOPHIA: Josh is right, Karina. This is about strength, not weakness. Can we think of that as the starting place for what the three of us agree on?

KARINA: Sure, we can start there.

JOSH: Great. So I'd like to ask you to do a lot of the talking while Sophia and I listen. Maybe you could start by answering a question. What will it take to make you the best person possible?

KARINA: That's a big question. Other than making my COPD go away, I'd say making sure I am breathing as well as possible, handling the things I need to do every day at work and at home to keep my life going, being a good wife, and, I guess, just keeping my chin up on the bad days. That's a lot, right?

SOPHIA: It may sound like a lot, but I think this is all doable. I'm going to give you a sheet of paper and a pen. If you don't mind, I'd like to start making a list as we talk. You can jot notes, maybe list any resources you can think of. We'll do the same thing. And then we'll see how we net out. Okay?

KARINA: Yes, I can do that.

JOSH: You mentioned that you want to breathe as well as you can. I certainly want you to do that as well. What kind of help do you need to make that happen?

KARINA: A couple of things come to mind. Making my appointments. Taking my medications. And I guess not pushing myself too hard.

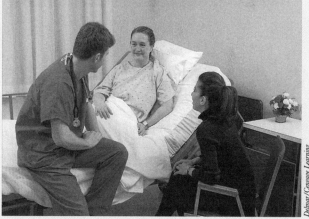

JOSH: Let's start with not pushing yourself too hard. I know Sophia is going to want to have some input here too. So Karina, what will it take to help you with that one?

KARINA: Don't start telling me that I can't go to work or that I have to hire a housekeeper. I take care of my own home. And we don't have money for hired help.

SOPHIA: I wasn't going to make that suggestion, Karina. But I'm wondering if there are some things around the house that you want to keep doing and some things that you can get help with. Remember, you said you wanted to stop pushing yourself so hard. Any ideas?

KARINA: Well, maybe I shouldn't be doing all the heavy cleaning on my own. I have to say it really wears me out. The doctor also told me I shouldn't be doing that anymore.

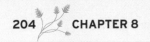

JOSH: What do you mean by "heavy cleaning"?

KARINA: Oh, vacuuming and shampooing the carpet, mopping, washing the windows. Things like that.

SOPHIA: That's a good start. Now. Is there anyone who could help with that?

KARINA: Well, my daughter, Kathy, offered to come home from college once a month and spend a few hours helping me. She probably wouldn't mind. And my husband has offered to do more of this.

JOSH: Fantastic, Karina. We've already got some of your support plan in place. See how easy this is?

KARINA: I guess it wasn't so bad.

SOPHIA: Now. What else can we do to make sure you conserve your energy for what's really important in life?

Josh and Sophia continued to talk with Karina about her activities of daily living and then moved on to discussing areas that included maintaining a healthier lifestyle, staying compliant, and coping with emotions. Together, they formulated a list of key areas and, based on Karina's ideas as well as suggestions from Josh and Sophia, created a support plan.

SOPHIA: Now that Josh and I have discussed your support needs with you, and we've agreed on the best ways to get them met, I'd like to go over them with you. Feel free to ask me any questions you have or let me know if there's anything you aren't sure about. Then, we'll type up the plan so we all have a copy of it. Okay?

KARINA: Sounds good.

JOSH: It's great to know that, at this point, we have a plan for keeping you at your best. Remember that this is a working document. When you stop in for your appointments, one of us will review it with you, and if anything isn't working, we'll find another solution together. Don't forget that we're a team.

Guidelines for Conducting Support Discussions

1. ***Find a common ground.*** At the beginning of resource discussions, newly diagnosed patients may indicate some resistance, or helplessness, or otherwise indicate that they are not going to readily embrace the recommendations of the health-care team or even be willing to have the discussion. When health-care professionals are perceived as forcing their will on patients, either indirectly or directly, the discussions will likely be unproductive. To avoid this situation, the health-care team should focus on a shared goal and use that goal as the starting place for further discussion. In this way, the support discussion is similar to a negotiation, with each party expressing potentially different opinions while staying focused on a common goal. In the preceding example, Sophia and Josh sensed that Karina was resistant and, rather than attempting to sway her opinion in their favor, they took a step back and found a common ground.

2. ***List key needs.*** Given the many issues newly diagnosed patients confront, it is no surprise that the result is often overwhelming. The future may seem so uncertain that discussing it feels like a waste of time, if not frightening. With Karina, Josh and Sophia used a list as a focal point for discussion and thereby helped Karina feel like an equal partner in her care. Psychologically, breaking a large, undefined task into smaller ones, and attaching a solution to each task,

makes the large, undefined task feel less overwhelming and more attainable. In the health-care setting, it might help to organize the list in sections, with each section dedicated to alternatives for each area of support, like household responsibilities, reducing stress, and compliance maintenance.

3. *Ask for patient input.* One of the best ways to help newly diagnosed patients feel in control is to consistently solicit their input. Josh and Sophia made it clear from the beginning that they wanted to know Karina's thoughts and that her input was both needed and valued. One aspect of Karina's fear about the future with her condition was that other people would be dictating how she would be living her life day to day. Therefore, soliciting her input helped to put some of those fears to rest. Furthermore, Karina offered valuable ideas, and, because she was involved in the decision process, she will most likely be more inclined to be compliant.

4. *Make suggestions.* Despite any disagreements, newly diagnosed patients tend to respect the opinions of their health-care professionals. Patients understand that the professionals' training and experience make them uniquely qualified to offer ideas that they would not have or would have considered. The key to acceptance is for health-care professionals to offer their ideas as suggestions to consider and not as dictates that patients must follow. While many aspects of medical care are nonnegotiable, when planning support, there are often numerous options that may all help to solve the problem.

5. *Formulate the best possible approaches.* Much of the support planning process involves patients and the health-care professionals brainstorming, offering alternatives. Once needs and potential solutions have been identified, the next step is to narrow the list of options to the best alternatives. Some further negotiation might be needed to agree on the approach that will meet medical objectives but that is realistic and comfortable for the patient.

6. *Don't let patients leave until committed and they have made initial arrangements.* Once patients have agreed to support plans, the team should encourage them to act immediately. For example, it can be helpful to set dates with the patients, such as when caregivers will begin helping with certain tasks, when the patients will meet with their personal exercise trainer, or when they will schedule appointments with counselors. It may be useful to set a date to review progress so that, if correction is needed, the team can help the patients identify new alternatives. The patients then have incentive to take action as well as stay encouraged.

SUMMARY

Newly diagnosed patients often have a range of support needs as they begin treatment. Those needs may change as they learn to live with their conditions. The right support is an important aspect of ensuring patients successfully complete their treatments. By partnering on the shared initiative of patient support, health-care professionals and patients can help each other choose the options that best meet the patients' needs and enhance ongoing compliance.

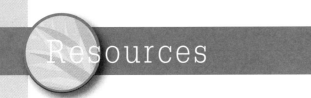

Resources

Support Needs and Resources Worksheet

Task

**Support Resource Available
(name of resource)**

Physical

[ ] Cooking _____

[ ] Cleaning _____

[ ] Shopping _____

[ ] Getting to the doctor _____

[ ] Walking _____

[ ] Taking medications _____

[ ] Self-care _____

[ ] Childcare _____

[ ] Following a diet _____

[ ] Following an exercise plan _____

[ ] Changing bandage _____

[ ] Giving injections _____

[ ] Other: _____ _____

Financial

[ ] Writing checks _____

[ ] Managing finances _____

[ ] Insurance _____

[ ] Making household decisions _____

[ ] Job issues _____

[ ] Other: _____ _____

Psychosocial

[ ] Daily companionship _____

[ ] Listening ear _____

[ ] Occasional check-in _____

[ ] Other: _____ _____

Spiritual

[ ] Group to attend _____

[ ] Someone to call _____

[ ] Someone to visit me _____

[ ] Other: _____ _____

Multiple-Choice Questions

1. In a conversation about support needs with a newly diagnosed patient, which of the following is the optimal starting place?
   a. Support needs the health-care professional has prepared in advance
   b. Support resources the health-care professional has prepared in advance
   c. Patient's perceptions of support needs
   d. Patient's perceptions of support resources

2. The areas of potential support for newly diagnosed patients include:
   a. Psychosocial support
   b. Support in activities of daily living
   c. Support in lifestyle changes
   d. All of the above

3. A newly diagnosed patient responds to an offer of support with the statement, "All this talk about needing people to help me is just negative thinking." This is an example of:
   a. Denial
   b. Lack of information
   c. Positive thinking
   d. Superstitious thinking

4. Health-care professionals should present potential support options for patients cautiously primarily because the patients assume that the:
   a. Health-care professionals are offering to be paid, part-time caregivers
   b. Health-care professionals own the support resources being considered
   c. Recommended resources are endorsed by the health-care professionals
   d. Recommended resources are part of a special program

5. A newly diagnosed patient in fight mode is most likely to:
   a. Resist support that is not comprehensive enough
   b. Resist support to maintain independence
   c. Accept support out of a desire to be as independent as possible
   d. Proactively bring in support before it is actually needed

Fill-in-the-Blank Questions

1. Newly diagnosed patients may refuse to accept support from their families out of a concern that they will become _____.

2. Support for emotional and relationship issues is called _____ support.

3. When the patient, family members, and health-care team work together to develop a support strategy, they demonstrate the concept of _____.

4. The _____ member of the health-care team is tasked with making recommendations and arrangements for such services as home care.

5. Newly diagnosed patients who are allowed no input into their care decisions can be left feeling

_____.

Short-Answer Questions

1. What fears do newly diagnosed patients commonly express in regard to support?

_____

_____

_____

2. A patient who is faced with a range of lifestyle changes might benefit from what types of support?

_____

_____

_____

3. What may motivate newly diagnosed patients to request more support than their situations warrant?

_____

_____

_____

4. Newly diagnosed patients may need to be reassured that being offered suggestions for support does not mean that their control is being taken away. What can health-care professionals do to help reassure patients that this is not the case?

_____

_____

_____

5. What is the value of sitting with patients and creating lists of potential support needs and options?

_____

_____

_____

Critical-Thinking Questions

1. What is the ideal role of health-care professionals in regard to helping newly diagnosed patients assess their support needs and connect with resources? What is realistic? Can health-care professionals become too involved?

_____

_____

_____

_____

_____

_____

2. While health-care professionals are likely to be aware of community resources, making suggestions can be risky if patients or their families assume that suggestions are recommendations or endorsements. What can health-care professionals do to make sure that their intentions are not misunderstood? Should health-care professionals avoid this activity altogether?

_____

_____

_____

_____

_____

_____

3. When patients and family members disagree about support, they may try to involve health-care providers in their conflicts. What role should health-care professionals play when newly diagnosed patients and their family members experience conflict? Should this role change when health-care professionals are asked to intervene in patient-family disagreements? Is it possible for health-care professionals to advocate for patients while avoiding involvement in conflicts?

_____

_____

_____

_____

_____

_____

Internet Exercise

Using resources found entirely on the Internet and a fictitious patient with a medical condition requiring extensive treatment and home confinement for a time, write a support plan. While you can include both local and national resources, keep them realistic and accessible to the patient. As you develop your resource plan, consider the following:

- Psychosocial needs
- Spiritual needs
- Support for activities of daily living
- Lifestyle changes
- Ongoing compliance

Be sure to also consider the availability of local resources in your community, eligibility, cost, and fit with the patient's cultural background.

_____

_____

_____

_____

_____

_____

_____

_____

_____

CHAPTER 9

Coping with Effects on Self-Image

OVERVIEW

After reading this chapter, you should be able to:

- Define and use the keywords of coping with the effects on self-image.

- Understand the potential effects of a medical diagnosis on self-image.

- Identify the causes of low self-image in newly diagnosed patients.

- Know the signs of low self-image and how to use educational moments as opportunities for patient interventions.

- Explain how to intervene when a patient is experiencing low self-image.

Appearance

Assessment

Attributes

Body image

False promise

Judge

Lifestyle management

Low self-image

Normalizing

Personality

Self-esteem

Self-image

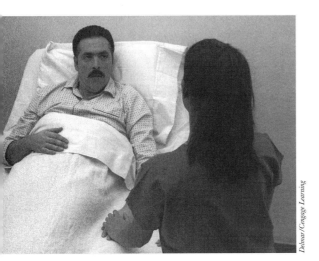

Delmar/Cengage Learning

Case Study

Angel had recently been diagnosed with a tumor in his neck that would require surgical removal. Dr. Rau had been gentle but honest when Angel had asked him how his surgery might affect him. At age 35, the news was not easy for Angel to hear.

"I'll do everything I can to change your appearance as little as possible," Dr. Rau had said. "But with the location of your tumor, I have to be honest with you. You'll have a scar and some disfiguration on that side of your face. You may also experience minimal nerve damage. This will affect your speech, at least for a few months."

Dr. Rau had gone on to explain what he meant when he said that Angel's face would be disfigured. But after hearing that word, and learning that his speech would be affected, Angel had stopped listening. He had lowered his head and looked downward, holding his face in his hands.

> **KEEP IN MIND**
>
> Because we live in a society that is very conscious of physical attractiveness, the changes to patients' appearances that result from their medical conditions can be devastating. Further, in addition to looking one's best, one must be able to speak clearly. How would you be feeling if you had just received Angel's news? If you had learned that you would experience changes in the way you look or speak, what would you be most concerned about? Why?

After meeting with Dr. Rau, Angel went into the lab to see Ava, Dr. Rau's medical assistant, and have a blood sample taken. Ava knew that Dr. Rau would have spoken with Angel about his surgery, and she noticed that Angel was quiet, not smiling or asking about her children like he had on previous visits. This time, Angel seemed to avoid even making eye contact with her.

"Angel," Ava started, "It looks like you're having a rough time today."

"You're right," Angel answered. "I am. And I guess you know why."

Angel liked Ava, so he wanted to say nothing that might seem like he was angry at her, because he was not. Instead, he *was* getting mad at life. He had always been proud of his appearance, and he was often told that he was a good-looking guy. His wife certainly told him he was. Beyond that, as a teacher, how could he be effective in his classroom if he had trouble talking? And what about hanging out with his buddies? Would they even want to be around him?

Shortly after Angel had gotten his diagnosis, he had accepted it. He knew that he needed the surgery to get rid of the tumor and that, even though the tumor was relatively small, the surgery would be complicated.

He just did not expect news like he had received today. He felt even worse than the day he received his diagnosis.

KEEP IN MIND

Newly diagnosed patients who are facing changes that may impact their self-image experience reasonable fears and doubts about their futures. Would you identify with patients' feelings of helplessness in a way that might help you to understand their feelings, or would your feelings of helplessness make the conversation more difficult for you?

Ava placed a chair directly across from Angel, sat in it, and leaned toward him.

"Dr. Rau went over your case with me," Ava said. "So I know your surgery is most likely going to have some long-term effects. I know this is hard for you to have to deal with right now, so soon after learning about your condition."

"It *is* very hard," Angel answered. "I'm a person who takes a lot of pride in how he presents himself to others. I work hard to feel good about myself inside, to feel like a strong person, and to have others think of me the same way. This is who I've always been and who I intended to be in the future."

Angel stopped and looked away. He was afraid that if he kept talking, he would start crying. The last thing he wanted to do was to show any more weakness. He felt that he looked weak enough already.

"We've had a lot of patients go through what you're experiencing," Ava counseled. "I could talk with you about how they have coped."

Ava wanted to at least open the door for Angel to talk with her more. She was unsure if he was talking with anyone else about how his surgery would impact his self-image, so she wanted to be a resource for him. Also, she wanted to help make sure that he was as emotionally prepared as possible for his surgery, both because he had a long recovery period ahead and because it would be important for Angel to be compliant and optimistic during his recovery period.

Angel did not respond to Ava's offer to talk more, but she took no offense. She knew he needed some time on his own to process what Dr. Rau had told him.

Introduction

"I'm not ever going to be the same."

Newly diagnosed patients live with fear and uncertainty regarding how their diagnoses will affect their daily lives. One concern is that they will no longer feel, function, or look like themselves, that their condition or treatments will make them unrecognizable to themselves and others. They may be experiencing cognitive symptoms, such as forgetting or losing concentration, which affect their abilities to interact with others or do their jobs effectively. The emotional impact of diagnoses, as well as the challenges

---

KEEP IN MIND

Ava knows that she has to approach the discussion of Angel's self-image carefully. She wants to neither offer **false promises** nor discourage him. If a patient in this situation wanted to talk to you about self-image issues, what would your goal be? Where would you have the conversation? What body language would you want to adopt?

of going through treatment, can cause mood changes, which can further impact how patients present themselves.

Any of the changes new patients experience can erode self-image. Patients may feel that they have changed in ways that make them "less than" others: needy, unattractive, uninteresting, or ineffective. They may feel that their conditions or treatments have left them so damaged that some or all aspects of themselves—the ones they and others value most—are disappearing. With those aspects gone, they may wonder, "What will remain?"

Patients with **low self-image** present a number of challenges for their health-care teams. When their self-image suffers, newly diagnosed patients are less likely to have the optimism and determination to cope effectively with their conditions and treatments. They are less likely to comply with their treatment regimens and lifestyle-management requirements, and they may fail to communicate symptoms and other changes that their health-care teams must know about to support them properly. Most compellingly, patients' negative outlooks can negatively affect their treatment outcomes (Table 9.1).

Health-care professionals can help patients with low self-image by recognizing the signs so they can encourage patients to do things like focus on strengths and get support.

TABLE 9.1   Signs of Low Self-Image

Following are some signs that patients may be experiencing low-self image:

- Talking mainly about the past

- Apologizing for feelings

- Having difficulty discussing the future

- Feeling anxious, angry, or depressed

- Experiencing low energy

- Speaking bitterly about the future

- Avoiding eye contact

- Hesitating to express opinions

Delmar/Cengage Learning

Understanding How Medical Diagnoses Affect Self-Image

Self-image, a person's personal mental picture, includes a person's **assessment** of **appearance**, success level, and abilities. Some aspects of self-image, like appearance, are observable by others. Others are more personal, such as a person's self-perception of intelligence or success level.

A person's self-image may or may not match others' image of that person. For example, a person may feel he or she is a great singer, but others might have a very different opinion.

Self-image develops over time, shaped by personal experiences and others' opinions and reactions. The process starts when children learn how others view them and respond. Children may learn, for example, that others respond most positively to such **attributes** as an outgoing personality, good looks, or musical or athletic talent.

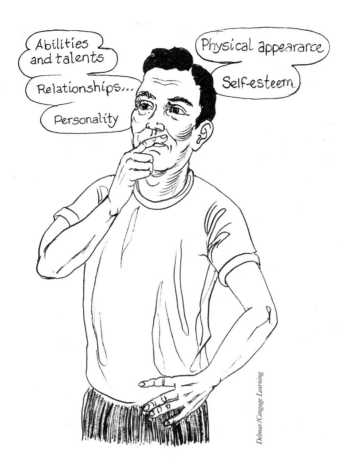

When they have these attributes, their self-image soars. In reverse, when children have attributes to which others react negatively, self-image falters. Self-image continues to develop during adolescence and into adulthood, based on experiences at home and in the workplace. From the perspective of self-image, the diagnosis of a medical condition can be extremely impactful.

KEEP IN MIND

It is human nature to quickly, and often unfairly, **judge** others based on aspects of physical appearance: hair color, weight, age. Imagine how newly diagnosed patients must feel upon learning that their conditions will affect their appearances, temporarily or permanently. Much of patients' resulting concern is based on fear of judgment from others. As a health-care professional, how can you be sensitive to this reality?

APPRECIATING THE IMPORTANCE OF PHYSICAL APPEARANCE

Fairly or unfairly, people judge each other based on appearance. Using physical attributes, we decide whether someone is friendly, a potential romantic partner, or trustworthy. It follows, therefore, that being told one is attractive, and feeling attractive, boosts self-image, while feeling unattractive erodes it.

For those experiencing changes in appearance, no matter how minor, self-image can drop dramatically if they begin to see themselves as unattractive, unusual, or damaged. When the physical appearances of newly diagnosed patients change, the patients experience the changes as losses of important aspects of their identities. They wonder if they are the same people if they look different. They fear that, now that their conditions are obvious, others will single them out for criticism and different treatment, likely negative. They may also fear that others will withdraw from or avoid them or they will embarrass their families.

Newly diagnosed patients often experience anticipatory anxiety as a result of their physical appearances. In short, they fear changes to their appearances before the changes actually occur. Worse, they often base their fears on erroneous information or on assumptions of the worst possible outcomes.

GETTING A SENSE OF ABILITIES AND TALENTS

A sense of being competent is an important aspect of self-image. Competency includes having abilities and talents that others recognize and reward. Examples might include being able to play a musical instrument and performing at church or community events; having a highly technical skill that leads to job security and a good salary; or being a good problem solver and relied on by others to address issues. In American society, individuals often define themselves through what they do for a living and through their abilities and accomplishments.

Unfortunately, newly diagnosed patients may lose certain abilities, at least temporarily. As part of **lifestyle management**, new patients often must change or even discontinue work routines and previously enjoyed activities. Chemotherapy, for example, often dictates the discontinuation of certain life activities as well as work. Post-diagnosis, opportunities to enjoy talents in areas like sports or the arts may become limited.

Because what Americans do is so tightly entwined with their identities, newly diagnosed patients may feel that they have lost much of who they are in losing the ability to perform their regular activities. When they feel they have lost who they are, patients tend to devalue themselves and lose their sense of self-worth. Many end up feeling inept and useless.

PRESERVING THE VALUE OF RELATIONSHIPS

Human beings need to feel that they are parts of social networks, ones made of family members, friends, neighbors, and coworkers. They need to feel wanted and needed, to have their thoughts and opinions valued, to care for others and to be cared for. Relationships with other people are one way in which people define themselves. As a result, productive relationships can boost self-image.

For new patients, diagnoses may change personal relationships. For one, the roles of family members may change. For example, a mother may need care when she was the one who did all the caring. When patients need to rely on family or friends for support for the first time, medical conditions may create new dependencies, ones that may change the overall balance of the patients' relationships.

Relationship changes can cause discomfort and, sometimes, tension. Patients may resent their increased dependency on family or friends, and family and friends, in turn, may become controlling in their desire to care for the patients. Most patients experience as much, or more, anticipatory anxiety regarding potential changes in personal relationships than they experience in reality. In other words, they unnecessarily fear that their conditions will change the ways in which their families and friends relate to them.

As relationships change, and fear and other negative emotions emerge, patients' self-images tend to suffer. Patients struggle with concerns about being burdens to others, somehow falling short of the expectations of friends and family members, and failing to perform fully as members of their social groups.

MAKING THE MOST OF PERSONALITY

Individuals have their own unique qualities—seriousness, humor, positivity, stubbornness, warmth, assertiveness, shyness. Each individual expresses a combination of qualities like these to form their **personalities**. In addition to making human beings interesting to each other, personality is an important part of self-image. People appreciate other people for their personalities.

Fueled by their personalities, people establish patterns of interaction with the people around them, playing roles like "listener," "advisor," "joker," and "leader." When these patterns are interrupted, such as happens when medical diagnoses are delivered, relationships change. When patients, especially, are unable to play their social roles—joker or leader—they naturally fear that they are losing their relationships.

Patients experience other personality changes arising from their medical conditions. The side effects of medication, for example, may include depression. Medical conditions can also affect patients' energy levels and abilities to concentrate, which affects how those patients relate to those around them. Emotions about diagnoses, like sadness or anger, will arise, as will a sense of helplessness and fear. Because patients may not understand what is causing their personality changes, they can also become confused and afraid. Further confusion and fear arise when personality changes cause others to behave differently toward the patients. By the end, patients may not even recognize themselves.

KEEP IN MIND

People share the need to feel valued and cared for. What role do you play with the people you care about? If circumstances prevented you from playing your role, at least temporarily, how would your relationships change?

DEFINING THE ROLE OF SELF-ESTEEM

The term *self-esteem* is often used interchangeably with *self-image*, and while the terms are similar, **self-esteem** is how individuals value their self-worth. It includes feeling capable, pride and self-respect, and being able to project confidence. Having a positive self-image is an important ingredient of self-esteem.

Psychologists usually discuss self-esteem as constant, meaning that self-esteem is a human trait that is relatively unchangeable (Coskun, 2010; McKay & Fanning, 2000). However, life events can change self-esteem, at least temporarily, and a medical diagnosis is certainly one of those events. Patients who receive medical diagnoses can feel that they are no longer of value or that they are incompetent or useless. They may also fear that they will lose value over time. Patients who feel responsible in some way for their diagnoses, perhaps through unhealthy living, may criticize themselves, which further lowers self-esteem.

Feeling Special, Feeling Normal

Human beings highly value their own specialness. Everyone likes to feel that there is something interesting or unique that sets them apart from others, whether it is attitude, skill, or personality. This sense of being special in some way adds to self-image and contributes to self-esteem and well-being. While specialness is valuable, humans also highly value normalcy. Interestingly, most people do not want to be "too special." They want to have a day-to-day routine and be able to participate in daily life without requiring additional assistance or consideration by others. In this regard, people want to be able to "blend in."

A medical diagnosis can threaten the balance between feeling special and feeling normal. Newly diagnosed patients may, because of their medical conditions, look different, eat different foods, or act differently. Because they now stand out—in negative ways—newly diagnosed patients can become fearful and confused, and their self-images will suffer.

Knowing What to Do When Self-Image Is at Risk

Stated simply, the impact of low self-image is that patients who feel poorly about themselves fail to care what happens because they lack the desire to go on. They feel they are "broken" or that, if they do improve, they will be left with losses—in appearance, relationships, or valued activities—that render their qualities of life unacceptable. Medical conditions can so damage patients' self-images that they fail to recognize themselves, and they fear others will not either.

Low self-image issues are not always apparent. Low self-image manifests emotionally, but more likely it will be revealed in patients' statements about their prognoses, the potential outcomes of their treatments, or their willingness to consider lifestyle adjustments and ongoing compliance. Most revealing are seemingly offhand comments, such as, 'Life won't be the same again for me," People will think there's something wrong with me," or "I'll never be normal again" (see Table 9.2 on p. 224).

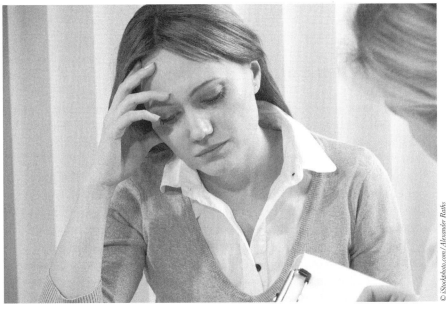

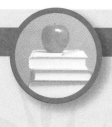

Educational Moment

When newly diagnosed patients express concerns about their self-images or demonstrate body language that indicates they are feeling badly about themselves, health-care professionals should lend listening ears. Most likely, the patients are too embarrassed or ashamed to discuss their self-images with friends or family. The professionals should also encourage patients to focus on their strengths and not their weaknesses.

BEING ALERT FOR EDUCATIONAL MOMENTS

Health-care professionals can help newly diagnosed patients recognize how their diagnoses impact their self-images by being sensitive to the signs and intervening when those signs appear. These are educational moments, a concept that was discussed in Chapter 3. By way of review, an educational moment is essentially an opportunity for a health-care professional to intervene when patients indicate, through spoken words or body language, that they are experiencing destructive thoughts or emotions. Health-care professionals who recognize the signs can use educational moments to help patients demonstrating low self-image understand that there are other ways to think or feel.

The following sections provide examples of potential educational moments related to self-image.

LEARNING ABOUT BODY IMAGE: TONY'S STORY

Tony's hip surgery left him with a number of side effects. While all were inconvenient to various degrees, the one that bothered him the most was the loss of what he called his "Mr. Atlas physique." He had told his physical therapy assistant, Jenn, that, a couple of years ago, at 49, he had had the highest batting average on his company's softball league. He had also been proud of his adherence to his gym routine, and he told Jenn that he "was still keeping up with the young guys" and had intended to maintain that pace.

When Tony's hip pain became increasingly difficult to ignore, however, he had finally had to take his doctor's advice and undergo surgery. That was 6 months ago. Since then, he has been trying to regain his mobility. For someone as active as Tony, the progress has been frustratingly slow. As he struggled to progress, Tony felt his arm and legs muscles had become weaker, and he gained a few pounds.

Looking at Jenn, Tony said, "I look in the mirror, and I don't see the Tony I used to see, the Tony who was at the top of his game. Instead, I see this middle-aged guy who needs to get to the gym! I like the way I used to look. And I don't think people treat me with the same respect anymore. I know there's more to me than the way I look and how much muscle I have, but my body was an important part of who I was, and I worked hard to maintain it. Now what am I?"

What Tony is experiencing: Tony is a person who highly values his appearance and has worked hard to maintain it. He associates his **body image** with respect and envy. Most likely, Tony assumes that others value his appearance more than his other personal attributes. Therefore, changes in his appearance negatively impacted his self-image. While Tony might be a somewhat extreme example, in Western culture it is common to highly value appearance—attractive face, fit body, and youthfulness. Even minor changes, such as weight gain, can devastate newly diagnosed patients if they are perceived as causing the patients to be "less than" in the eyes of others.

What not to say to Tony: While patients experiencing low self-image resulting from body perceptions may react negatively to comments that they should simply accept the ways they look, they also react negatively to comments that are clearly overly optimistic. Examples of overly optimistic statements include the following:

> "Remember that you're still alive. Isn't that worth not looking the same anymore?"

> "You look great to me. I don't know what you're talking about."

> "You'll be back to normal in no time. I'm sure this won't last."

What to say to Tony: When patients talk about losses like changes in appearance, they are not necessarily expecting their health-care professionals to "make things better." Health-care professionals can help instead by acknowledging patients' feelings about their changed appearances. Simply being heard may be what patients need, especially if their friends and families cannot have these discussions. **Normalizing** this experience by explaining that other patients in the same situation also have concerns about their appearances can also help patients realize that they are not alone. It can also be useful to encourage patients to talk to their physicians about their appearance concerns. Examples of normalizing statements include the following:

> "I know you're really upset about the way you look right now."

> "People recovering from this kind of surgery often experience changes in the ways they look. And this can be disappointing."

> "It's always hard to adjust to change."

KEEP IN MIND

If you have a healthy self-image and someone asked you, "What do other people think about you?" your answer would most likely be positive, a good summary of your self-image. Think about how your answer might differ on a day you are feeling especially good about yourself versus a day you have experienced a disappointment. As a health-care professional, how can you help patients in these types of situations?

FEELING HELPLESS: DENISE'S STORY

Since she began her medication regimen, Denise has been asking for more and more help from her family and the health-care professionals at the clinic where she receives her treatment. She has told them that she is having trouble both to adjusting to "all this medication" in her system and to caring for herself. She has asked for help with household chores her family feels she should be able to do on her own. Denise has been reluctant to learn many of the self-care techniques the nursing team has tried to teach her, complaining that they are too hard and that she might hurt herself if she makes a mistake.

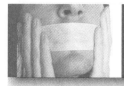

SELF • talk

Negative self-talk can reinforce a low self-image. Following are some examples:

I'm never going to be what I used to be.

People are going to look at me like I'm an invalid or a freak.

Why try when you'll only be reminded of what a failure you've become?

Don't push yourself, or you'll only get sicker.

What good am I if I can't _____ [work long hours, take care of everybody, head up the fund-raiser, etc.] anymore?

Antidotes to the negative self-talk that lowers self-image include:

I haven't lost everything. I still have a lot to offer.

I'm doing the best I can. It doesn't matter what people think when they look at me.

I can take a few steps at a time and regain some of my strength.

I'm dealing with a medical condition, but I'm not a victim or a loser.

I don't have to _____ to be a valuable person.

Last week, one of the nurses, Monica, tried to teach Denise how to give herself an injection. Denise held the syringe in her hand, then laid it on the table and burst into tears.

"I don't think I can do this," Denise cried. "I'm going to need to have someone else do this for me. I don't think I can take care of myself anymore. There's too much to do, with these shots and everything, and I'm afraid I'll make a mistake and make myself even sicker. I wish you had known me a couple of years ago. I didn't need anybody to do anything for me back then. Now I feel like I'm so incompetent I can't do anything for myself. I'm about two steps away from being a total invalid."

What Denise is experiencing: Newly diagnosed patients with low self-images as a result of new and unfamiliar medical regimens may be concerned that their overall competence levels, beginning with the ability to care for themselves, are declining. While new patients may need additional assistance, which signals some change in activity level, they may be reacting in part to a fear about further, more serious decline.

What not to say to Denise: Newly diagnosed patients with self-images characterized by helplessness may resist comments from health-care professionals that make them feel as if they are overexaggerating their inabilities to meet all their challenges. For the health-care professionals, it is risky to encourage patient helplessness by implying that the demands may indeed be too much, because doing so may lower patients' self-images yet more. Examples of inappropriate statements include the following:

"You're only giving yourself an injection. It's no big deal. We give hundreds of them here every day."

"You really need to help us more. There's no reason you can't be taking care of yourself."

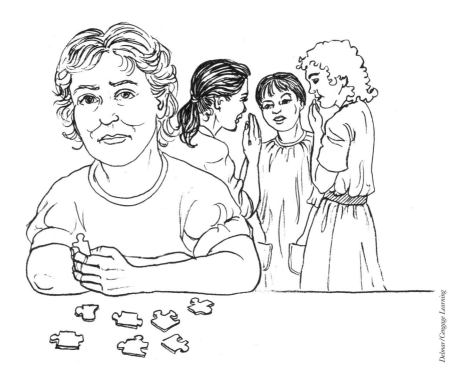

Delmar/Cengage Learning

"This is probably all a lot more than you can handle."

"You're not the strong person you used to be, so now you may need a lot more help than before."

What to say to Denise: The encouragement of health-care professionals can benefit newly diagnosed patients who feel that their diagnoses have jeopardized their competence levels—their abilities to be effective adults and care for themselves appropriately. Providers should listen for self-defeating words and body language and respond with gentle encouragement to focus on strengths. Careful to avoid a patronizing tone, health-care professionals should make sure patients do not feel as if they have done something wrong and are somehow being scolded or that the health-care professionals are implying that life is "a bed of roses" when clearly it is not.

To keep the focus on strengths and positivity, health-care professionals should identify the abilities patients value the most and/or those that help patients feel "normal." Reminding patients of their strong support networks, which include friends and family as well as the health-care team, can also be helpful. The benefit of acknowledging patients' feelings is twofold. First, it can help patients feel understood. Second, it gives patients the chance to discuss the fears that their loved ones may be unable to listen to. Examples of supportive statements include:

"I know it's hard to go through this. It feels like you're different in a lot of ways than you used to be."

"I see that you really enjoy _____ [activity that the health-care professional has observed]. Has that always been important to you?"

"I know you feel disappointed that you've had to cut back on your activities. This doesn't mean, though, that you can't adjust your activity level and stay involved in life. What things can you keep on doing?"

"I've noticed that you have a lot of people around you who are on your side. You seem to have a lot of support."

ACCEPTING CHANGES IN PERSONALITY: SEAN'S STORY

If Sean were to describe himself, he would probably say "the life of the party." He was president of the Lion's Club in his community, often assisted the minister at his church, and, at his job, was known for his sense of humor, which he had a way of using in a way that put his coworkers at ease during times of stress. Sean and his wife, Marion, often hosted barbecues in their backyard, and their friends looked forward to the fun and great food.

When Sean received his diagnosis, his doctor told him he would need to curtail some of his activities and that, at least initially, he might have less energy and enthusiasm while his body adjusted to his prescribed medication. In completing his treatment, Sean developed a relationship with Bennett, the phlebotomist at the lab he visited weekly, and he talked often about what was going on in his life as he adjusted to his condition.

"Everybody looks to me to keep their spirits up," Sean said. "They know I'm going to walk into the room and get the energy going. They know I'm going to find the bright side to whatever's going on, and I'm going to crack a few jokes to break the tension. I'm supposed to be the one that makes everybody happy. If I can't be the Sean that everybody knows and loves, who am I?" After a brief pause, he answered his question himself. "Nobody."

What Sean is experiencing: When newly diagnosed patients fear that their conditions will somehow change their personalities, other related fears emerge. As Sean emphasized, patients may fear that, because others relate to them differently, they are left with no personalities and, therefore, major losses to their identities. Related to this is the fear that, if patients are not themselves, they will lose the recognition and respect of others and, thereby, important relationships. In fact, people may relate differently to new patients after diagnosis. For example, friends of patients may comment that the patients do not seem like themselves.

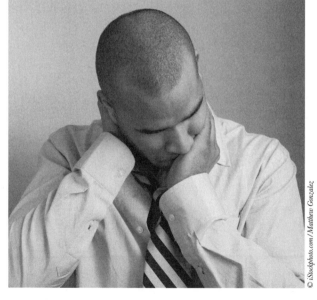

What not to say to Sean: Newly diagnosed patients who are experiencing personality changes are likely to disbelieve suggestions that their personalities have not changed, especially when others have commented that they seem different. Examples of what *not* to say to patients in this situation include:

"You still seem like the same upbeat person to me. I'm sure you're still a lot of fun."

"Even if you aren't feeling well, your friends know that you'll be back to normal soon."

"You told me you've been a steady rock to your family. Do you think it might be time for someone else to do that job while you take a break?"

"Your family and friends will just find a new way to relate to you."

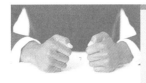

Body Language

When diagnoses impact newly diagnosed patients' self-images, their body language may include the following:

- Shrugging their shoulders
- Smiling sadly
- Shaking the head
- Looking away
- Avoiding eye contact
- Looking downward

What to say to Sean: Health-care professionals can support patients who experience, or fear that they will experience, changes in their personalities by first being supportive listeners when patients express their concerns. They can also help by relating to patients in ways that make them feel they are interesting and valued. Health-care professionals can engage them in conversations, requesting their input and acknowledging their contributions. Examples of supportive statements include the following:

"I know it's hard for you to feel like the take-charge person you've been in the past when you have this treatment ahead of you."

"That was a very funny thing you said. You have a great sense of humor."

"You have an interesting perspective on this. I see you've done some thinking about this."

"It was great to talk to you today."

TABLE 9.2   Determining When a Patient's Self-Image Is in Jeopardy

Newly diagnosed patients often give signs that their diagnoses have in some way impacted their self-images. Among these signs are the following:

- Referring to what life "used to be like" or how things "will never be the same"

- Giving examples of others appearing to relate to them differently

- Avoiding people they care about

- Avoiding activities or responsibilities they once excelled in

- Demonstrating a defeatist attitude (e.g., "I don't even want to try this," or "I know I won't be able to do it anymore")

- Expressing fears about relationships through comments like, "I'm not much good to her anymore," or "I'm sure I won't be any fun to have around"

Delmar/Cengage Learning

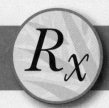

Talking with Newly Diagnosed Patients about Self-Image

Angel entered Dr. Rau's office for his presurgery workup: blood tests and an electrocardiogram test. As part of the visit, Ava was to review the directions for surgery preparation. Angel looked intently into Ava's eyes while she reviewed the directions. He listened intently but said little. After Ava finished, Angel acknowledged that he understood everything and had no questions. However, Ava had a feeling that Angel had not discussed his self-image concerns with anyone, so she wanted to give him an opportunity to talk. She turned from the computer she had been using to update his chart, rested her hands on her lap in an open position, and leaned forward, toward Angel. She paused for a moment before speaking.

AVA: Angel, the last time you were here, you told me how you were feeling about how the surgery might affect you. You told me the surgery was going to cause you to really take a hit to your self-image.

ANGEL: Yes, I did tell you that. I may not look the same and, at least for awhile, I may not talk the same. This is all going to affect my relationships with other people, including my wife and friends, and it may affect my opportunities in my job as a teacher. My self-image is getting kicked pretty hard, I would say. Wouldn't you say the same thing?

AVA: I would agree with you, Angel. As I said before, this is a lot for you to have to deal with at once. I can see that you're having a lot of feelings right now.

ANGEL: Yeah, this is a rough time.

AVA: The team here is standing by to listen and to help you in any way we can.

ANGEL: I appreciate that. But do you have any advice for me?

AVA: I can talk to you about how other patients in similar situations have coped, for one thing. Would you be interested in hearing about them?

ANGEL: I guess I would.

AVA: What I can tell you is that they felt the same way you do. They were scared about how their lives would be if they looked or acted differently after surgery, how their friends and loved ones would treat them. They worried that their coworkers would have different attitudes toward them. And they were afraid that they wouldn't be as useful or as needed by others.

ANGEL: I can relate to all that.

AVA: Most patients going through this, though, have learned how to look at the positive side. They're glad to get back to their lives, even if their lives are going to be different. And they've learned to make accommodations, as have the other people around them.

ANGEL: But they aren't the same anymore.

AVA: No, they aren't, Angel. But they've adjusted by focusing on their strengths and doing as much as possible to maintain the things they value most in life. They tell themselves that they're doing the best they possibly can. Our self-image begins inside, right? And you're still the same person inside that you've always been. That hasn't changed.

ANGEL: I guess that makes some sense.

AVA: A lot has happened in a short time. You got diagnosed, you're going to be treated for your condition, and you're going to experience some challenges. Give yourself some time to adjust to all this, Angel. Be patient with yourself. Can you remind yourself that you're doing the best you can and that you're determined to do what you need to do to get through this?

ANGEL: I can try to do that.

AVA: Great. I recommend to patients that they have strong support groups in place, that they surround themselves with people who care about them. You seem to have quite a support group from what I've seen.

ANGEL: I definitely do. A whole fan club.

AVA: Good. Then that's a strength right there. You should feel good about being cared for that much. They're going to help you get through this.

ANGEL: Yes, I'm sure they will.

AVA: But tell me something, Angel. Do your feelings get overwhelming at times?

ANGEL: I'm handling them okay right now, actually. I'm down, but I'm not out.

AVA: Well, if you do feel overwhelmed, will you give one of us a call?

ANGEL: Yes, I will.

Guidelines for Encouraging Positive Self-Image

Using the conversation between Angel and Ava, following are some guidelines for helping newly diagnosed patients address low self-image:

1. *Show understanding.* When facing a crisis like loss of self-image, newly diagnosed patients need first and foremost to feel like they are being listened to. Friends and family often have difficulty having discussions that involve strong emotions so, to avoid feeling helpless, they may argue there is nothing to worry about or insist that the patients "think positive." The patients, for their part, may want to try to protect their loved ones from discussing potential outcomes and experiencing the patients' raw emotions. Out of a sense of both pride and responsibility, patients may avoid admitting that their conditions have affected their self-images. In the example conversation, Ava began by reminding Angel that she and the other members of the health-care team were available to listen.

2. *Normalize the patient's reaction.* While most newly diagnosed patients think their experiences and emotions are unique to them, they appreciate knowing that others have experienced similar situations and reactions. Health-care professionals who reassure patients that their reactions are normal give patients permission to express themselves fully. They also give them hope that others are coping with similar challenges. Further, relating the experiences of other patients is a way for health-care professionals to offer guidance without specifically telling patients what they should do. Instead, the health-care professionals offer options that patients may decide to exercise or not. Ava let Angel know that she could tell him what other patients in similar situations had experienced, but it was his choice to hear the information. Sometimes, newly diagnosed patients need a little time to be open to hearing information.

3. *Encourage realistic optimism.* Oftentimes, patients newly diagnosed with medical conditions know change is coming. When these patients suspect that their health-care professionals are somehow hiding the truth about the magnitude of that change, or encouraging them to avoid reality, patient-provider trust is at risk. Notice that Ava was honest with Angel in the preceding conversation. She agreed that his treatment was going to cause unwelcome changes. She also spoke about his potential for facing those changes and making adjustments, just as other patients in similar circumstances had been able to do.

4. *Focus on strengths.* Whatever the challenges patients face, they have strengths to meet those challenges. Knowing this can help bolster the patients' low self-images. To support that effort, when health-care professionals know patients' strengths, physical and emotional, they should remind the patients of some of them as needed. Less specific strengths, like determination, a strong support network, and the willingness to be flexible in the face of change, are less readily apparent but no less effective in encouraging patients to look beyond limitations. When identifying strengths is a struggle, health-care professionals should brainstorm with their patients. Ava knew that Angel's fears about surgery were affecting his self-image, so she identified his determined attitude as both a strength and an important aspect of his self-image.

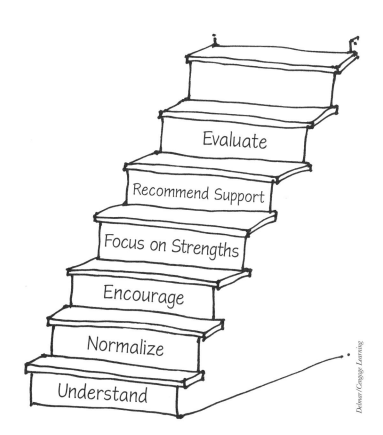

Delmar/Cengage Learning

5. *Recommend support.*   Newly diagnosed patients who are feeling badly about themselves can benefit greatly from the support of friends and family, as well as other patients facing similar challenges. Knowing that others care about them, and are facing their challenges with them, can improve patients' self-images. Ava pointed out to Angel that he appeared to have a good support network, which she also identified as one of his strengths.

6. *Evaluate the need for mental health services.*   Sometimes, newly diagnosed patients with low self-images need the services of mental-health professionals. For example, patients who are helpless or hopeless may be at risk for depression that, if not addressed, will erode the patients' self-images and most likely render the patients despondent to the point they are noncompliant or self-destructive. For guidelines for evaluating patients for depression, review Chapter 3.

SUMMARY

A medical diagnosis, and its accompanying challenges and losses, can impact self-image. Newly diagnosed patients whose diagnoses have impacted their self-images may feel so defeated that they fail to participate actively in their treatments and may be less compliant. Health-care professionals can best help patients with low self-images by listening and offering support and encouragement.

Chapter REVIEW

Multiple-Choice Questions

1. Newly diagnosed patients fear that their diagnoses will affect their self-image in terms of not _____ the same.
   - a. Looking
   - b. Thinking or talking
   - c. Interacting
   - d. Any of the above

2. When a patient expresses concerns about body image, the optimal response is:
   - a. "You won't every look the same again. That's what happens."
   - b. "Aren't you just happy to be alive?"
   - c. "I know you're really upset about the way you look right now."
   - d. "You'll probably be back to normal in no time."

3. When patients feel helpless about their conditions and treatments, the optimal response is:
   - a. "I know this is a hard thing to go through, but I see that you have a lot of support."
   - b. "There's no reason why you can't take care of yourself."
   - c. "This is probably a lot more than you can handle."
   - d. "You're certainly not the person you used to be."

4. The best way to respond to a patient who fears that treatment may result in personality changes is:
   - a. "I'm sure you'll still be the life of the party."
   - b. "I enjoyed talking to you today. You said some interesting things."
   - c. "Your friends must know that you'll be back to normal soon."
   - d. "Your family will just have to find a new way to relate to you."

5. The starting point in talking to a patient who is experiencing self-image concerns is:
   - a. Show understanding
   - b. Challenge faulty information
   - c. Encourage reality checking
   - d. Encourage positive thinking

Fill-in-the-Blank Questions

1. Self-perception of how one looks to others is called _____ _____.

2. Telling patients that the changes they experience are only temporary may be a(n) _____ _____.

3. Worrying that a medication will cause confusion and lethargy without actually knowing whether it will or not is an example of _____ _____.

4. Assuring patients that other patients in their situation experience the same kinds of concerns is attempting to _____ the patients' reaction.

5. Skills, talents, personality characteristics, and physical appearance are considered _____.

Short-Answer Questions

1. What are some of the key signs that a patient's reaction to a diagnosis may be causing low self-image?

   _____

   _____

   _____

2. In what ways might patients' personalities be affected by their medication regimens?

   _____

   _____

   _____

3. What is the value of showing understanding when a newly diagnosed patient has self-image issues?

   _____

   _____

   _____

4. How can health-care professionals involve a patient's support system (i.e., family and friends) as a way of helping bolster the patient's self-image?

   _____

   _____

   _____

5. How can educational moments help patients experiencing self-image issues?

   _____

   _____

   _____

Critical-Thinking Questions

1. Newly diagnosed patients can often benefit from being reassured that their reactions to their diagnoses and treatments are similar to the ways other patients in similar situations react. Is there a point at which helping patients feel "normal" may appear that the health-care professionals are not taking patient concerns seriously or minimizing their reactions? How do health-care professionals avoid this perception?

_____

_____

_____

_____

_____

2. Out of a desire to help patients feel better about themselves, at least temporarily, health-care professionals may be tempted to speak in overly optimistic terms that may, ultimately, cause patients to be disappointed. Being overly direct may leave patients discouraged. What is the best way to discuss the sensitive issues around patient self-image?

_____

_____

_____

_____

_____

_____

3. When newly diagnosed patients suffer blows to their self-images, other issues may emerge (e.g., unresolved experiences that caused low self-image). What are the signs a patient might need additional mental-health intervention? How would you discuss the need for such intervention with the patient?

_____

_____

_____

_____

_____

_____

Internet Exercise

Numerous Internet resources discuss self-image and offer advice and guidelines for individuals experiencing low self-image. Some of these resources focus on self-image as a mental-health issue, while others focus on self-image as it relates to a medical diagnosis. Find at least two resources you think would help a newly diagnosed patient, one from a mental-health perspective and one from a medical perspective.

Why did you choose the two resources you did?

What are the key similarities between these resources? The key differences? Are there any features on either site, such as patient stories, that might be more or less useful to a newly diagnosed patient? Does either resource include services or information at a financial cost to the patient? Which resource would you be most likely to recommend? Why?

_____

_____

_____

_____

_____

_____

_____

_____

CHAPTER 10

Connecting with a Sense of Meaning

OVERVIEW

After reading this chapter, you should be able to:

- Define and use the keywords of connecting with a sense of meaning.

- Relate spirituality to such benefits as wellness, compliance, and communication.

- Be sensitive to patient comments that may be signs of spiritual concerns.

- Define the role of health-care providers in helping patients with spiritual issues.

- Identify the ways in which patients react to self-questioning of spirituality.

- Understand how health-care professionals typically react to patients expressing spiritual concerns.

- Describe how to be a listening ear for patients with spiritual concerns while honoring ethics and effectively setting boundaries.

- Discuss the importance of listening and being supportive without judging.

- Explain how to offer referral sources to patients seeking spiritual guidance.

KEYWORDS

Anxiety

Boundaries

Clergypeople

Despair

Embrace

Ethical

Faith

Higher Power

Interactions

Judgmental

Meaning

Optimism

Organized religion

Peacefulness

Religion

Spiritual community

Spiritual connection

Spiritual counselor

Spiritual direction

Spiritual issues

Spiritual path

Spiritual practices

Spirituality

Urgency

Worship

Yoga

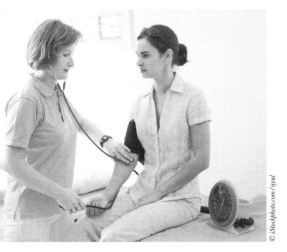

© iStockphoto.com/ryul

Case Study

"I think of my life in two stages," Martina started. "The first was before kidney disease, or at least before I was given the diagnosis of having kidney disease. The second is now, after kidney disease, which started when I was diagnosed last month."

Judy, a dialysis technician in the hospital clinic where Martina is being treated, was used to providing a listening ear to patients as they received their dialysis treatments, so she listened patiently as Martina spoke. Martina told Judy how, even though she had been retaining water and feeling her energy declining, she had been surprised when the nephrologist on the health-care team, Dr. Christoff, had told her she had kidney disease.

"I felt like everything I had worked for and planned for was being snatched out of my hands," Martina said. "Life was dealing me the worst hand possible. I never thought God or whoever is in charge of things would decide that my fate was to have kidney disease. Is this the only meaning that I'm going to have in life?"

Martina continued. "People were always saying to me, 'You don't need to do so much for me. You always do so much.' Thinking back, I'm sure that I was sort of hoping that if I did a lot of good things for other people, like if I really went overboard to be the best person possible, nothing bad would happen to me." Martina stopped and shook her head. "That was kind of stupid on my part, right?"

KEEP IN MIND

Newly diagnosed patients often question what they did or did not do to "deserve" their conditions. If you were working with patients who were beginning to discuss their conditions from spiritual perspectives, what would be your initial concerns?

Judy wanted to be a supportive listener for Martina. While Judy had her own religious beliefs and would have liked to share them, she knew that what Martina needed most at this point was an opportunity to share her feelings, especially the feelings she might feel uncomfortable sharing with family and friends.

From Judy's perspective, Martina's diagnosis appeared to have inspired in her a spiritual crisis. Judy knew that if Martina continued to feel that her life had no **meaning**, she might become easily discouraged with her treatment and not care if she got better or not. Judy also knew that it was important for kidney patients to comply with treatment, so Martina would need to be dedicated to staying as healthy as possible if she were to meet her upcoming challenges of lifestyle changes and dialysis treatment.

KEEP IN MIND

When health-care professionals have patients in spiritual crises, they often recall their own experiences with spirituality and **organized religion**. Some professionals feel helpless and want to fix their patients' problem, while others want to avoid the topics of religion and spirituality entirely. As a health-care professional, would aspects of Martina's spiritual concerns cause you to feel helpless? If so, how would you react?

Judy had long been involved with her church. As a child, she had regularly attended religious services with her parents, and the Sunday routine of rising early to attend church was so ingrained in her as a youth that she maintained the same routine with her own husband and children as an adult. Therefore, when she saw that Martina was questioning life's meaning, she thought her patient could benefit from **spiritual direction**. However, while she would have liked to talk more to Martina about her own religious beliefs, Judy had learned that patients can benefit most from encouragement to seek the **spiritual paths** they are most comfortable with, the ones that fit their backgrounds and views.

"I feel lost," Martina finally said. "I feel like my life is never going to be the same again, and I'm getting no answers about what I should be doing instead. Like I said, it's like life has abandoned me."

Introduction

"I never thought about the meaning of life until this week."

Beginning when they are diagnosed, new patients often have spiritual questions that can take many forms. As they reevaluate their purposes in life—and whether they even have purposes—patients may question the meaning of life. As patients consider what their lives will be like as they face their conditions, they may ask "Why me?" from a spiritual perspective, wondering whether they have been singled out to carry additional burdens, abandoned by God, or even punished for some reason. They may even question whether God, or a **Higher Power**, exists.

A medical diagnosis can lead patients to want to connect, or reconnect, with a greater meaning, God, or their concept of a Higher Power. For many newly diagnosed patients, spirituality offers both meaning beyond the day-to-day experience of illness and a means of coping with illness's stress and discomfort.

For some newly diagnosed patients, **spiritual issues** arise immediately. For others, such issues arise after patients face such difficult emotions as anger, which some patients direct at God or another Higher Power.

KEEP IN MIND

While not a **spiritual counselor**, Judy knew that, as a health-care professional, she had an opportunity to encourage a newly diagnosed patient to enhance her well-being through spirituality. What questions or concerns would you have as you approached this situation?

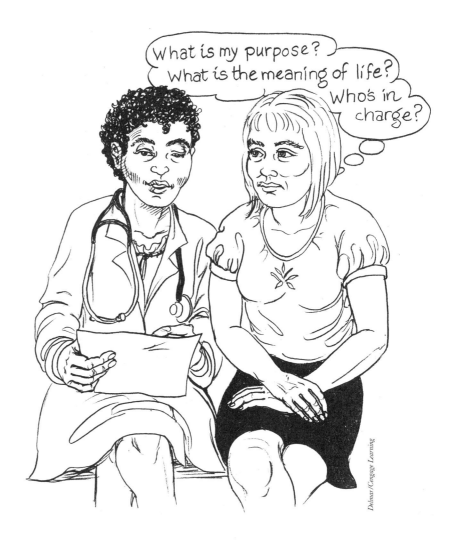

The relationships between health-care professionals and their patients can benefit greatly when patients **embrace** spirituality. For patients, spirituality fosters a sense of peace and overall well-being and can contribute to an attitude of empowerment that can motivate the patients to remain compliant with their treatment and lifestyle regimens.

Health-care professionals can support newly diagnosed patients in their spiritual journeys by first and foremost listening willingly. In many ways, nonjudgmental listening is a spiritual act in and of itself. Newly diagnosed patients may have only their health-care professionals to serve as listening ears, because their friends and family members may be facing their own spiritual crises or are trying to avoid imposing on the patients. In the health-care arena, the goal of spirituality discussions is to encourage patients to make their own **spiritual connections** and, within **ethical** guidelines, explore appropriate resources.

Being Aware of Personal Spirituality

In this chapter, the terms *spirituality* and *religion* are used, but not interchangeably. For the purposes of this chapter, **religion** applies to formal denominations with sets of beliefs and practices, such as the Christian denominations of Catholicism or Methodism or Judaism, Islam, or Buddhism. **Spirituality**, more broadly defined, includes the desire to find meaning in life, have purpose, and connect with one's inner self or to a Higher Power. Spirituality may lead someone to embrace a religious denomination, but it can also lead to practices like meditation, spending time in nature, giving to others, and reading inspirational books.

To serve effectively as a listening ear for newly diagnosed patients, it is important for health-care professionals to be comfortable with their personal spiritualities and to listen to alternate beliefs without being **judgmental** or feeling the need to impose change. For some professionals, these are welcomed and natural tasks. For others, the prospects are uncomfortable.

All health-care professionals can benefit from knowing their comfort levels with spirituality so they can effectively communicate **boundaries** to patients. To that end, health-care professionals should know their institutions' policies and guidelines for discussing religion and spirituality with patients. Guidelines both help health-care professionals avoid any ethical issues that might arise and help professionals be as effective as possible as they help patients through spiritual crises. Some institutions provide additional resources that might also help patients.

> **KEEP IN MIND**
>
> For many, religion and spirituality are unique experiences. How would you define your approach to spirituality? As a health-care professional, what place does it have in your life? In your experience, how do spirituality and religion differ? How are they the same?

Assessing the Spiritual Impact of a Medical Diagnosis

As the following case studies illustrate, newly diagnosed patients can express the spiritual impacts of their diagnoses in many ways.

CONSIDERING THE MEANING OF LIFE: PAULA'S STORY

When Paula received her diagnosis, she described the experience as her "spiritual awakening." The event was important to Paula because, before diagnosis, she had never been involved in any kind of organized religion, nor had she been involved in any informal **spiritual practice**.

> *"After I went through the shock and all the emotions, I started really thinking about my life in a different way. It wasn't what I would call in a religious way, because I wasn't feeling religious. My diagnosis wasn't necessarily life-threatening, but it made me realize I couldn't take my life for granted, that it wasn't guaranteed that I would live forever. And that made me think about what I had accomplished so far in my life and the impact I had made on others. I felt like my diagnosis had given me the opportunity to really take a look at my life in a different way and to think about whether my life was going to have some kind of meaning. And then I started asking what kind of meaning life was supposed to have. I had never asked that question before."*

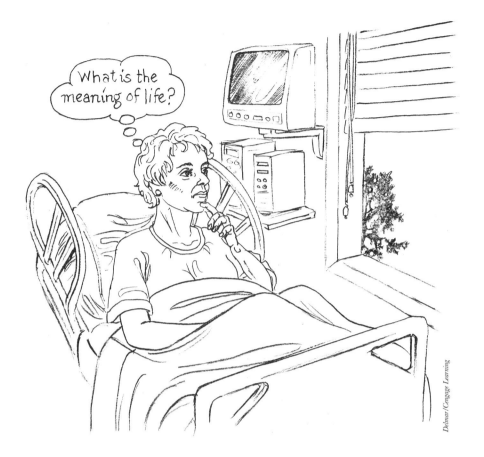

EXPERIENCING LIFE IN THE HERE AND NOW: NATHAN'S STORY

Nathan's diagnosis felt like "someone turned the lights on in my life." Learning that he faced a serious medical condition gave him a new awareness of the world around him, especially of the things he valued most in life.

> "After I met with the doctor and she gave me my diagnosis, I came home to an empty house. My wife was still at work, and my daughter was staying after school for cheerleading practice. So I sat in the living room, thinking about the best way to break the news of my diagnosis. I was glad for the time alone. Sometimes, my favorite classical music helps me relax, so I turned the stereo on and put in a CD. I laid on the couch, and suddenly the music felt so intense. . . . I can't think of any other way to describe it. I could hear the music, and I could feel it. For a second, I wondered if I had a new sound system. It was like my soul woke up to what was important—I mean really important—like enjoying beautiful music. When my wife got home, I held her for a long, long time. Later, she told me that, at that moment, she knew something was wrong, but she also knew something was right. Our relationship has never been better."

FEELING A SENSE OF PEACE: EMILY'S STORY

Emily recounted how, after her diagnosis, she "went through a storm and landed on a peaceful shore," coming to a place of acceptance that, while not religious in the traditional sense, left her with a greater sense of connectedness to the world around her.

"After I received my diagnosis, I learned everything I could about my condition. Some of the information was encouraging, and some not so encouraging. This left me with answers and with questions, many of which my doctor was not able to answer. Mainly, I wanted to know how long I was going to live. I sat with that question, and I kind of went into myself—I guess you could say I did some soul-searching—and thought about whether I wanted to focus on how uncertain life can be or how wonderful it can be. I decided to stop struggling and accept life as it is. This left me feeling a peace I had never experienced before. It was the peace of just accepting life on life's terms and moving on."

ASKING "WHY ME?": PEDRO'S STORY

The "Why me?" question discussed first in Chapter 3 is spiritual in nature. When newly diagnosed patients ask the question, they are basically asking why they were chosen. Was it fate, God, or another Higher Power? Pedro, an active churchgoer, asked the question after his diagnosis.

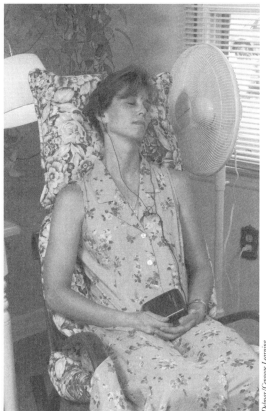

Delmar/Cengage Learning

"I wanted to know why God had either chosen me to face this disease or why He had stood by and allowed it to happen. Either way, He had let me down. I went back and forth in my mind, trying to come up with some kind of answer, and I called out to God to answer it for me. After all, I thought that I'd been faithful all my life, always made it to services, helped out in other ways, treated people decently, and gave as much money as I could. Who deserved to be healthy more than me? Nobody. This went on for a while, me thinking I would punish God back by leaving faith behind. Finally, I talked to my priest, and he helped me get some perspective. I kind of ended up turning the 'Why me?' into 'Why not *me?' In other words, I knew I was going to find the strength to get through this challenge, and I was going to grow from it. That's what helped me get through it."*

FEELING A SENSE OF URGENCY: JULIA'S STORY

Julia experienced her medical diagnosis as a wake-up call to look at what she had accomplished in life and what she still had ahead of her. She described a sense of **urgency** to move forward with her dreams and to contribute more to the world.

"I was what you might call an underachiever most of my life. You know, lots of potential, lots of interests, lots of plans . . . but I never seemed to be able to follow through on any of my goals long enough to see them through. I looked at my life differently after receiving the diagnosis. I felt like I'd been taught a lesson I needed to learn, and the lesson was that I had something to offer the world and if I didn't get busy and start contributing to my own life and the lives of those around me, I might not have much to show for my life. Once my treatment was scheduled, I committed to a plan for what I would do with my life once I had the treatment behind me. I wanted my life to count for something."

WITHDRAWING INTO CONTEMPLATION: LUCIA'S STORY

After receiving the news of her medical diagnosis, Lucia withdrew from her friends and family for long periods of silence. While those around her initially feared she was depressed, Lucia said she simply needed to find her "true self."

"I'd never been into meditation or anything like that. But my diagnosis made me want to find my inner strength. I felt like I'd been so caught up in the rat race of life that I didn't know how to listen to my inner voice anymore. I needed to hear that voice again, and the only way I knew to do that was to be quiet for a while. So I went away to a bed and breakfast for a long weekend and spent a lot of time sitting alone and thinking. When I came home, I found I needed some quiet time every day. Over time, I felt like I finally made contact with my true self and was going to be able to face whatever was going to come my way."

RECONNECTING WITH CHILDHOOD RELIGIOUS PRACTICES: SAUL'S STORY

Saul was an active professional with a busy travel schedule and long work hours. When he was diagnosed, he felt a need for stability and comfort. The need returned him to the religious practices of his childhood.

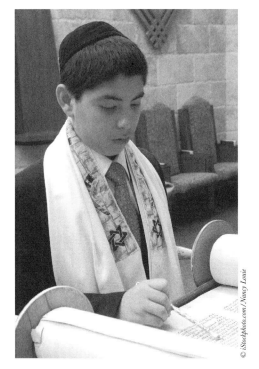

© iStockphoto.com / Nancy Louie

"I was brought up in a religious household, but when I left home, I no longer saw the need for what I thought were a lot of unnecessary laws and rituals that didn't fit into my modern lifestyle. But when I received my medical diagnosis, it was those laws and rituals that brought me back to my faith. My diagnosis was so unexpected that I felt like I had no control over anything in my life. My religious practices gave me a sense of being protected. I felt like as long as I practiced my religion, I would have an anchor, as my parents before me, and the generations before them, had had."

BEING ENCOURAGED TO EMBRACE A SPIRITUAL BEING: GRACE'S STORY

Grace's family reacted to her diagnosis by talking to her about her relationship with God. While understanding their concern, Grace was also alarmed and angry at their insistence that she embrace beliefs that differed from her own.

"I was a little surprised when they all showed up at my house and told me I was in spiritual danger. I didn't think I was at death's door, and I also didn't think I was a bad person. But I also knew that they loved me and that they only wanted to help me in the best way they knew how. I told them I appreciated their concern but that I would make my own decisions about my spiritual life. To be honest, their behavior kind of turned me off from any kind of spirituality for quite a while, until I could think things through and go back to my own spiritual path."

KEEP IN MIND

Patients must often find their own ways to religion and spirituality, if they choose those paths at all. Think about patients you have known who have faced medical diagnoses. Did you witness any of them questioning their spirituality, or seeking greater spiritual connections, as a result of their diagnoses?

Connecting Spirituality to the Patient-Professional Relationship

As discussed in previous chapters, health-care professionals are not expected to function as mental-health professionals, because mental-health services are not within the scope of health-care training. Similarly, health-care professionals are not expected to serve as spiritual counselors. However, when discussed within professional and ethical boundaries, spirituality can benefit newly diagnosed patients and enhance their relationships with health-care providers.

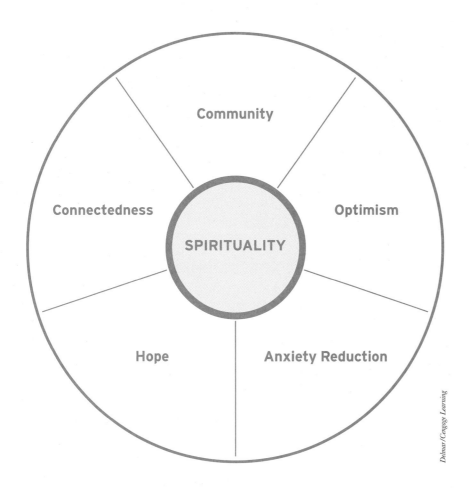

Delmar/Cengage Learning

LISTING THE BENEFITS OF SPIRITUALITY FOR NEWLY DIAGNOSED PATIENTS

The health-care-related benefits of spirituality include the following:

1. *A sense of community.* Whether patients are attending formalized religious services or pursuing spiritual practices on their own, spirituality provides a feeling of community with others holding similar beliefs. Ideally, a **spiritual community** includes people who have experienced their own medical challenges who can reach out to newly diagnosed patients to offer emotional support as well as spiritual guidance. With the aid of spiritual communities, patients can address feelings of isolation and gain support.

2. *A sense of connectedness to something larger.* When facing a diagnosis and treatment, it is human nature to focus on the "small stuff," things like daily fears, frustrations, and discomforts. Single-minded focus on issues like these, however, can quickly become detrimental, causing patients to feel that their days are filled with one crisis after another. Most spiritual practices encourage the belief in a Higher Power that is greater than the challenges of day-to-day life. This belief can help patients maintain a perspective on life and take daily disappointments and challenges in stride.

3. *Hope and optimism.* Each religious denomination offers members a way of maintaining hope and **optimism**. Some encourage followers to focus on

the positive, to view "the cup as half full instead of half empty." Others promote suffering as a means of growing in wisdom and inner strength. Still others offer the possibility of an afterlife that is free of pain and suffering. Whatever the denomination, these beliefs can help patients face whatever daily challenges their medical diagnoses may present.

4. *Anxiety reduction.*   Newly diagnosed patients often feel anxious. They face daily uncertainty in terms of the challenges their diagnoses and treatments might present, as well as concerns regarding their mortality. Spiritual practices like prayer and meditation can reduce the **anxiety** arising from patients' fear and helplessness (Coppola & Spector, 2009; Foley et al., 2010; Sears & Kraus, 2009).

LINKING HEALTH-CARE PROFESSIONALS AND SPIRITUALITY

When newly diagnosed patients embrace spirituality, they can enhance their relationships with health-care professionals. Patients with optimistic attitudes toward treatment, who are hopeful their treatments will succeed, are more likely to comply with treatment regimens (Richards, et al., 2008; Sherr et al., 2008). They are more likely to adhere to medication schedules and to take recommendations for recovery and lifestyle changes. Less anxious and fearful due to spiritual practices like meditation, newly diagnosed patients may communicate more effectively with their health-care professionals, asking more questions, remembering more information, and reporting symptoms and side effects more vigilantly (Bundy, 2001; Hack et al., 2005; Kennedy, 2005). In short, compliant patients make the jobs of health-care professionals easier.

Reacting to Issues with Spiritual Dimensions

Day to day, spiritual issues arise in the **interactions** between newly diagnosed patients and health-care professionals. Patients may, for example, discuss their hopes and fears in terms of their spiritual beliefs, or they may express concern over their lack of spiritual involvement. They may ask their health-care providers for spiritual advice or for referrals to professionals who can offer this advice. Sometimes, patients are simply seeking a listening ear.

In part because they are not trained in this realm, health-care professionals may feel uncomfortable discussing spirituality with patients. Their own beliefs may be

Educational Moment

When speaking with their health-care professionals, newly diagnosed patients often ask questions of purpose and meaning, such as "Why is God allowing this to happen to me?" and "What am I supposed to learn from this?" Questions like these give health-care professionals opportunities to remind patients that spiritual questions are normal. When these questions arise, professionals may suggest that patients with spiritual or religious backgrounds speak with their **clergypeople**.

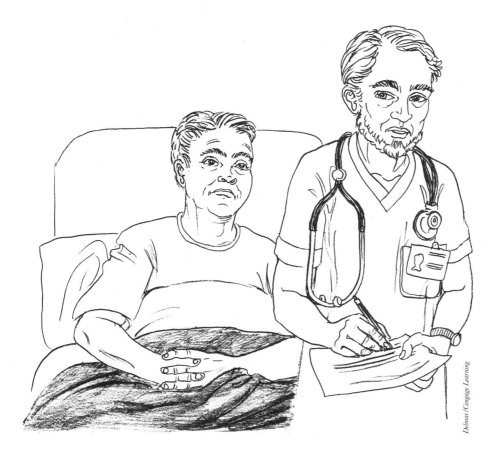

Delmar/Cengage Learning

uncertain, or they may feel spirituality is irrelevant to wellness and effective health-care communication. As mentioned earlier, medical offices and hospitals often have strict guidelines regarding the discussion of spirituality and religion with patients.

To help keep professional boundaries clear and defined, it is important for health-care professionals to be well-versed in their organizations' guidelines for discussing spirituality. They should also clarify their own spiritual beliefs, if they choose to embrace any spiritual beliefs at all. With clear understandings of their spiritual per-spectives, and the latitude they may or may not have in discussing such issues, health-care professionals can more confidently decide whether to have spiritually based conversations with patients. When professionals feel poorly equipped to participate in such discussions, many organizations provide resources to which professionals can refer patients with spiritual issues.

The following sections outline the key issues that arise for health-care profession-als around spirituality and newly diagnosed patients.

KEEP IN MIND

As with all health-care interactions, the personal perspectives of participating parties are factors. How would you describe your initial reaction upon finding yourself in a con-versation about religion or spirituality? How would that reaction play out if you were having the conversation with a patient?

ACCEPTING THE URGE TO AVOID

Ali, a respiratory therapy technician, finished giving a breathing treatment to his patient, Olivia. Noticing that Olivia seemed to be feeling sad, Ali decided to spend a minute to see if he could cheer her up before moving on to his next patient. "How are you doing today?" he asked.

"Not so good," Olivia responded. "I've got a lot of questions."

"Anything I can answer for you?" Ali asked.

Olivia hesitated and then said, "Maybe you can. I know you work with a lot of patients who are sick and don't know why something like this has happened to them. Since you talk to these patients, maybe you have some answers. So let me ask: Do you think God has turned His back on us for some reason?"

Ali did no want to have this conversation with Olivia. First, he was unsure how to answer. He had been raised in a religious household, but he was not currently practicing his **faith**. He was worried that, if he did try to answer Olivia's question, he might say something wrong and harm her. Further, he was unsure if the hospital allowed religious discussions with patients.

"You sure seem to be breathing better today," Ali finally responded. "You're doing a little better every day."

What's going on with the health-care professional: When faced with uncomfortable conversations, it is natural for health-care professionals to want to avoid. Ali avoided Olivia's question by ignoring it and focusing on something he could talk comfortably about, Olivia's physical health. If he had hoped to distract Olivia from her spiritual concerns, Ali more likely succeeded in making his patient feel ignored and, possibly, disrespected. At the same time, if Ali was uncomfortable having a conversation about spirituality, and was unsure of his professional boundaries, he was correct in avoiding.

Health-care professionals who, like Ali, are uncomfortable discussing spiritual issues with patients can avoid these discussions yet honor their patients by doing the following:

- Acknowledging that spiritual questions are normal during times of uncertainty
- Admitting to feeling uncomfortable or unqualified
- Suggesting alternative resources

Following are additional guidelines:

What not to say:
- "I don't want to talk about God with you today."
- "I want to focus on your medical issues."
- "Everything is fine. Let's focus on the positive."
- "I have other things to go over with you."

What to say:
- "It is normal for patients to have spiritual questions when they are diagnosed with medical conditions."
- "I'm not the best person to talk with about spiritual issues, but I can help you to find someone who is more qualified."

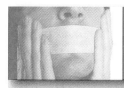

SELF • talk

Self-talk statements like the following can reinforce spiritual confusion:

God has turned His back on me.

If I can't be the way I've always been, then I don't have any purpose in life.

There's never going to be any peace in my life.

I must have done something terrible to deserve this.

I have so much I have to get done, there's never going to be enough time.

Antidotes to negative spirituality self-talk include the following:

I can look to the teachings of my faith to help me to face my illness.

I'm still a worthy human being and can contribute to the world around me.

I'm facing a struggle now, but I'll find peace again in my life.

I have no control over this diagnosis, but I can find the strength to deal with it.

I can be patient with myself and accomplish more in life.

- "Religion is a deep discussion. Do you have someone you can talk to about God?"

- "I can see you have some spiritual issues you want to talk to someone about. Do you need help finding a clergyperson? I have some ideas about how to do that."

AVOIDING ETHICAL CONCERNS

Nicole had been devoutly religious since she was a child. She was born in a home in which daily life revolved around the teachings of her denomination, and she found religion a source of inspiration and peace through high school, nursing school, and into her adult life as a wife, mother, and professional. When patients from similar backgrounds wanted to discuss their faith, Nicole was always eager to share her story.

At the moment, Nicole was worried about Carl, a patient at the hospital clinic where she worked. He had come in complaining about leg pain that was eventually diagnosed as a condition that would require lengthy treatment. Carl had reacted to his diagnosis without emotion, and he came alone to his next appointment. When Nicole asked him if he had support at home to help him during his treatment, Carl had responded, "I don't need anybody but myself."

To Nicole, Carl appeared to have no spiritual foundation. She thought he could benefit from her testimony, so she told him about how her faith had made a difference in her life and asked him if he would like some literature, as well as a visit from the pastor of her church. "You need God during this time in your life, Carl," Nicole counseled. "Don't wait any longer."

"I can't believe you're saying this to me," Carl retorted. "What gives you the right?"

He demanded that another nurse be assigned to his case and indicated he would be sending a letter to his physician and the director of the hospital.

What's going on with the health-care professional: Religious faith can be a source of comfort during a difficult time, and Nicole had benefited from her faith in

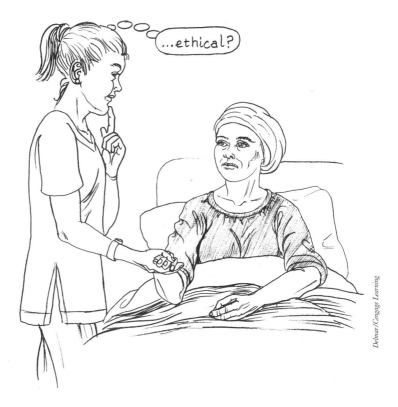

ways she felt would also benefit Carl. As a caring health-care professional, she wanted to help someone who appeared to be in need. Further, Nicole's religious training directed her to reach out when opportunity arises. From the perspective of her denomination, Nicole was fulfilling her obligations. From Carl's perspective, however, and quite possibly the organization that employs her, Nicole crossed ethical and professional boundaries.

While Nicole's intentions were well-meaning, she created harm and may now be reprimanded as a result. In the future, she could avoid situations like these by doing the following:

- Avoiding discussions of spirituality and religion unless patients indicate interest first

- Suggesting spiritual resources with other resources, like mental-health services, and allowing patients to indicate interest

- Adhering to office or clinic guidelines for spiritual discussion

The following provides additional guidelines for handling patients who appear to need spiritual assistance:

What not to say:

- "You need some spiritual direction in your life. I can help."

- "It is going to be easier to get through this if you have faith in God."

- "I'd be happy to arrange for you to receive spiritual guidance."

What to say:

- "Is there any kind of support you need right now? We have some resources that we keep on file here that I can recommend to you."

- "We have resources for mental-health and spiritual counseling. Would any of this be helpful to you right now?"

- "Newly diagnosed patients like you can benefit from spiritual beliefs and practices as they deal with the news of their conditions and start moving forward with treatment. Is this something you'd like me to help connect you with?"

DISCOUNTING SPIRITUALITY

Sara, a medical assistant, describes herself as a rational person who sees life as it is, without trying to pretend that there is some kind of underlying, deeper meaning or Higher Power. Sara thinks that newly diagnosed patients should focus on the realities of their diagnoses and work with their health-care professionals to make informed decisions and comply with treatment recommendations. In her experience, this is the best way for patients to get better. She views positive thinking and prayer as potentially interfering with treatment.

As Sara completed her duties one day, her patient, Carolina, remarked that she was looking for a prayer group to help support her as she began treatment. "Do you have any suggestions for how I might find a good prayer group?" Carolina asked.

"I'd really encourage you to focus on doing what you need to do medically to get back on your feet," Sara answered. "You have a great health-care team in place, you're going to be receiving state-of-the-art treatment, and we have a solid plan of aftercare in place. It doesn't get any better than what you have right here."

"I think prayer would also help me to get through this, though," Carolina responded. "I wasn't asking you to pray with me, just to see if you had any suggestions."

What's going on with the health-care professional: Spiritual disbelief, like spiritual belief, is deeply personal. People who take purely rational approaches to life may be convinced that spirituality is misguided. As a health-care professional, Sara thought that her patient, Carolina, would be better off focusing her time and energy on what she could gain through modern medicine and not be distracted, and possibly disappointed by, beliefs not grounded in science. In her desire to encourage Carolina to stay realistic and focused, she implied a disrespect for Carolina's beliefs and may have offended her.

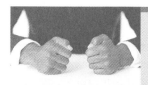

Body Language

Newly diagnosed patients may reflect their struggles with spiritual issues through body language that includes the following:

- Frown or confused expression
- Slumped posture, looking down toward the floor
- Direct eye contact
- Hands held outward in an open position
- Arms crossed over the body

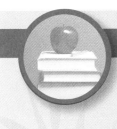

Sara could have accommodated Carolina's beliefs and her own by doing the following:

- Accepting that Carolina has spiritual beliefs she does not share
- Acknowledging Carolina's beliefs without attempting to impose her own
- Offering Carolina any available resources or indicating she has no resources to help

Additional guidelines for handling situations like these follow:

What not to say:

- "I don't believe in any kind of religion. I don't think it has any value."
- "Medical science has everything you need to get you feeling better."
- "You can trust your health-care team to get you through this."
- "We're health-care professionals here, and this is where we all need to be focused."

What to say:

- "I don't know a lot about prayer groups, and we don't really have any resources like that on file here. I'm sorry I can't help you with that."
- "One of the nurses here may have some ideas for you. I'll introduce you to him."
- "You might do some online searching to find a local group. I can give you a couple of ideas about how to get started."
- "Patients sometimes tell me that prayer can be helpful during difficult times like this."

PROVIDING A LISTENING EAR

Franco works in the physical therapy department of a rehabilitation facility that primarily serves patients who are recovering from surgery. He often engages his patients in conversation while working with them, both to distract them from their pain and discomfort and to determine if they want someone to talk to. Franco's patients often raise the topic of spirituality in these conversations. Franco has strong spiritual beliefs of his own, but he knows that his beliefs tend to differ greatly from those of his patients.

One of Franco's patients, Christopher, was recovering from an automobile accident that almost killed him. During his extensive recovery, Christopher became very involved in his religion and talked about it often during Franco's treatment sessions.

Franco did not want to share his differing beliefs with Christopher, but he also did not want to discourage his patient from talking.

"My faith has really made a difference in my life," Christopher told Franco. "I'm striving to get closer and closer to God while I'm here. I would wish the same thing in your life, my friend."

"I can see how important your faith is to you," Franco answered. "Maybe you can tell me more about how your faith is helping you get through your recovery."

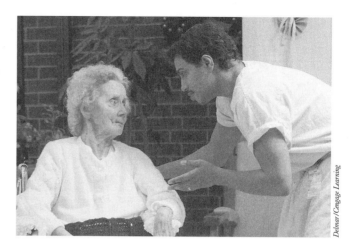

What's going on with the health-care professional: Franco is secure in his religious faith and does not need or, more likely, want to be introduced to Christopher's beliefs. He understands that Christopher's faith has been a major factor in helping him recover from his traumatic accident and that it has helped him comply with a long and difficult recovery process. Franco sees that Christopher's faith has value, and he wants Christopher to feel comfortable and accepted when he chooses to discuss it. In this regard, Franco has chosen to be a listening ear for Christopher and to encourage his patient to do whatever he can to have an optimistic and determined attitude during recovery. If Christopher's newfound religious faith is supporting him in his recovery then, in Franco's mind, this is an important aspect of his treatment. Franco also knows that, by acknowledging and respecting Christopher's religious beliefs, he is enhancing patient-professional trust.

Franco based his approach with Christopher on the following:

- Acceptance that Christopher has chosen his own spiritual path

- Belief that there are multiple spiritual paths available and that what is important is that Christopher is benefitting from his chosen path

- A desire to listen to Christopher in a nonjudgmental, supportive manner

Suggestions for being a listening ear in a spiritual sense follow:

What not to say:

- "Are you sure it's a good idea to be so involved in all this religion?"

- "I think what's really gotten you this far is your hard work and the excellent care you've had."

- "Let's talk about your exercise right now. Maybe we'll have time to talk about religion some other time."

What to say:

- "I'm glad your faith is helping you get through this process."

- "Tell me more about how you rely on God during this time."

- "Sounds like your spirituality is really helping you face the challenges of recovering from your accident."

- "I know physical therapy can be painful at times. How does your faith help you during the rough spots?"

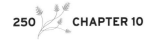

Understanding How Patients Experience Spirituality

Newly diagnosed patients who are seeking, or at least open to, some form of spiritual expression can benefit from the suggestions of their health-care professionals. Organized religious services are not the only ways to experience spirituality. Depending on their interests and abilities, patients can pursue spirituality on an individual basis.

The following sections provide suggestions for pursuing a spiritual existence.

APPRECIATING WORSHIP

Services at a church, a synagogue, or another religious meeting place offer opportunities for **worship** in more formal settings. People who were reared to attend religious services may find this approach most appealing because it is comfortable. For those less mobile patients, radio, television, and Internet broadcasts of religious services are widely available.

GETTING INSPIRATION

Inspirational messages may or may not be based on specific religious denominations. A wide range of books, radio/TV/Internet broadcasts, and Web sites are inspirational but not religious. The stories of individuals who have addressed health-care crises through positive thinking and empowerment can be particularly impactful for newly diagnosed patients.

INTERACTING SOCIALLY

Spending time caring for people, sharing their hopes and fears, can help newly diagnosed patients feel supported and connected to something greater than their day-to-day experiences. Patients can enjoy social support in person with friends and family as well as through online health and spiritual communities.

GIVING BACK

Community involvement, such as tutoring children, can benefit newly diagnosed patients. Volunteer opportunities shift the focus from the patients—their needs, frustrations, and disappointments—to others' challenges. In this way, volunteer work can be a great way for patients to find new meaning in life.

REDUCING STRESS

Practices like meditation, **yoga**, creative visualization, and journaling have been proven to reduce patients' stress levels and promote their wellness. The work of Jon Kabat-Zinn is especially relevant in terms of offering evidence of how these practices can enhance health and spiritual well-being. Kabat-Zinn, a pioneer in using mindfulness meditation with patients coping with illness and pain, founded the Stress Reduction Clinic and the Center for Mindfulness in Medicine, Health Care, and Society at the University of Massachusetts Medical School (Kabat-Zinn, 1990, 2006).

KEEP IN MIND

Spirituality manifests itself in many ways. Each day provides countless opportunities to sense the spiritual. How do you experience spirituality in your own life? How does this translate to your work as a health-care professional?

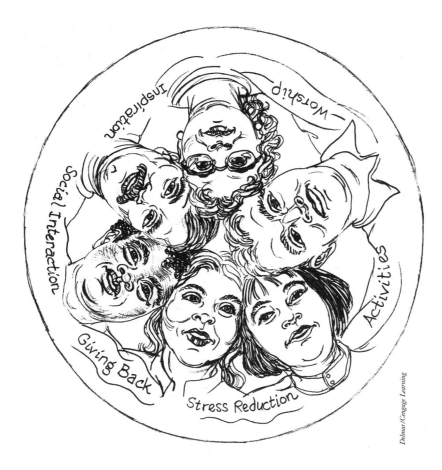

Delmar/Cengage Learning

BEING ACTIVE

Physical activity, which can include vigorous activity but also simply taking walks, promotes patient wellness and empowerment. A walk in nature, for example, can be a spiritual experience, as can a drive in the country, a fishing expedition, or a skiing trip.

Recognizing When Despair Leads to Depression

The feelings of **despair** and helplessness arising from spiritual crises can overwhelm patients, causing depression. To provide the proper level of service, health-care professionals should evaluate patients in spiritual crisis for symptoms of depression and be ready to make referrals to mental-health professionals as needed. Chapter 3 gives guidelines for evaluating depression in patients.

Guidelines for Assisting Newly Diagnosed Patients from a Spiritual Perspective

Following are guidelines to consider when discussing spiritual issues with patients:

1. *Normalize the desire for a spiritual connection.* Newly diagnosed patients often feel like their experiences are unique, that they are the only people in the world who have ever felt the way they feel. As a result, they may

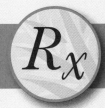

Discussing Spirituality with Patients

Martina, the patient newly diagnosed with kidney disease at the beginning of this chapter, was experiencing a spiritual crisis and questioning if her life was going to have any meaning beyond illness. Her dialysis technician, Judy, wanted to act as a sounding board and give Martina an opportunity to discuss her spiritual concerns. Judy wanted her patient to feel she could at least voice her spiritual issues. She was trained to direct Martina to the hospital's spiritual resources if needed. As she sat with Martina, they talked.

JUDY: Martina, I know your diagnosis has really knocked the wind out of you. Other patients I work with go through the same thing when they first receive their diagnoses.

MARTINA: Yes, that about describes it—wind out of my sails. Add "turned inside out" to the mix and you've pretty much said it all.

JUDY: From what you said, you're not so sure what the meaning of your life is right now. It all seems kind of hopeless to you.

MARTINA: That's the way I feel. Whoever's in charge isn't paying much attention to me right now. Maybe nobody's in charge.

JUDY: Martina, it sounds like you have concerns that are spiritual. I can't give you spiritual advice, but I'm a good listener and I might be able to recommend a couple of resources we have here at the hospital. Would any of that help you?

MARTINA: Sure. No one else wants to listen to me. Right now, my family is so upset by my situation, seeing me so sick and then knowing that I'm going to have to go on dialysis, they can't handle any more. When I start to talk about my disappointment and how helpless I feel, they run for the hills.

JUDY: This is a hard situation for families. They're dealing with their own fears, and sometimes they avoid talking about the hard stuff with their loved ones. Families often wish the patients could just take things in stride and get better.

MARTINA: I can accept that. But I feel like I need something more than what I can get from other people, anyway.

JUDY: Do you have any religious affiliation?

MARTINA: They asked me the same question in the Admissions office. I said I hadn't stepped inside a church in years. I really don't think that's what I need right now.

JUDY: What do you need?

MARTINA: What I need is peace of mind. I want to know that there's something more to life than feeling sick and having to get all this medical treatment, that life has some kind of meaning. If this is all there is to life, then it seems kind of futile to me. Why bother to get better?

JUDY: In my job, I talk to a lot of patients who feel a lot like you do. I've seen some of them adopt spiritual practices that really helped them. Are you interested in knowing what they did?

MARTINA: Sure.

JUDY: Some got involved in practices like yoga and meditation, which helped them feel more calm. Others found inspirational books that helped them get perspective on their lives. I worked with one patient who just started taking walks in nature. She felt like these walks gave her a new outlook on life. I've also seen patients benefit greatly from talking with clergypeople.

MARTINA: Those are some good ideas, Judy.

JUDY: We have a pastoral counselor on staff if you want to talk to her. And we offer all kinds of classes in the Wellness Center. If you're really feeling low, you might talk to the nurses about referring you to a mental-health professional.

MARTINA: I'll give this all some thought.

JUDY: I'd just like to add that, as you know, human beings have an emotional side and a physical side, and they also have a spiritual side. As much as possible, we always encourage our patients to focus on being the best people they can be, from all angles. This contributes to your wellness and helps us all work together better.

feel they should not be having their reactions. Spiritual concerns can be especially difficult for patients to express, because they may feel that, if they are questioning the existence of God and/or feeling hopeless, they may be in some way displeasing God and thereby inviting further difficulties. To protect their self-esteem, patients may hesitate to admit they are challenged spiritually as well as physically.

Health-care professionals can help patients with spiritual concerns by first reassuring them that it is normal to feel uncertain after diagnosis. Judy began her conversation with Martina by telling her that she had worked with other patients with similar reactions.

2. *Clarify boundaries, and offer to be a listening ear.* Particularly when they are not qualified to offer spiritual counseling, health-care professionals should set expectations and boundaries at the start of patient conversations. That way, patients are not confused or disappointed when their providers cannot offer spiritual advice. Institutional guidelines that dictate the role health-care providers give providers additional boundaries in which to operate. Judy informed Martina that, while she was unable to give spiritual advice, she could provide a listening ear if Martina wanted to talk about her spiritual issues.

3. *Avoid judging the patient.* Judy had her own religious beliefs based on her long association with her denomination. She may have liked to have explained her beliefs to Martina and invited her to share in them. She may have also been feeling that Martina was moving in the wrong direction spiritually and should not be questioning the existence of a Higher Power. If Judy was having these thoughts, though, she was careful not to convey them. Instead, she maintained an attitude of listening without judgment. Judy's approach made it easier for Martina to be honest about what was on her mind. She knew Judy was open to whatever she had to say.

4. *Share the experiences of other patients.* Newly diagnosed patients in spiritual crisis often feel alone in their struggle. While health-care professionals cannot generally make direct spiritual recommendations, they can share the experiences of other patients as suggestions for spiritual connection and growth. Learning the experiences of other patients with similar struggles can help patients feel less alone, and it can help normalize their feelings. Judy was able to offer Martina various suggestions based on what she had witnessed other patients do.

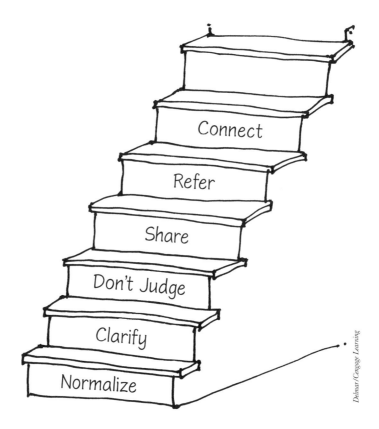

Connect

Refer

Share

Don't Judge

Clarify

Normalize

Delmar/Cengage Learning

5. ***Offer other referral sources.*** In the preceding conversation Judy had noted Martina's general sadness and suggested the services of a mental-health professional. While not able to assist Martina with her spiritual needs directly, Judy knew the value of the referral sources in her hospital, including a pastoral counselor and a Wellness Center, which gave Martina options for moving forward.

6. ***Connect spirituality with general wellness.*** While caution is always advisable with newly diagnosed patients, health-care professionals can gently explain the benefits patients can gain by taking steps to enhance their own wellness. Judy had been trained that newly diagnosed patients who face their diagnoses and treatments with calmness and acceptance are better able to follow treatment recommendations and staying motivated, even when challenges arise along the way. She closed her conversation with Martina with this point for that reason.

SUMMARY

A medical diagnosis can cause new patients to doubt and question their spiritual beliefs. When patients are in spiritual crisis, questioning the existence of a Higher Power, the meaning of life, and their contributions to the world, health-care professionals can serve as listening ears and refer them to resources that might be useful in resolving these issues. Spiritual practices can reduce stress, increase motivation to be compliant, and enhance communication.

Chapter REVIEW

Multiple-Choice Questions

1. Newly diagnosed patients may seek answers to spiritual questions out of a desire to:
   a. Find greater meaning in life
   b. Answer the "Why me?" question
   c. Connect with a higher power
   d. All of the above

2. It is accurate to say that health-care professionals should:
   a. Express their own religious beliefs to get patients on the right path
   b. Use personal religious beliefs to start spiritual discussions with patients
   c. Encourage patients to seek spiritual guidance they are comfortable with
   d. Refer patients to their personal clergypeople

3. For newly diagnosed patients, the benefits of embracing spirituality include all of the following *except*:
   a. Sense of connection to something larger than daily challenges
   b. Fear of the unknown
   c. Hope and optimism
   d. Anxiety reduction

4. A health-care professional who is uncomfortable discussing spiritual issues with patients should say which of the following?
   a. "I don't want to talk about God with you today."
   b. "I'm only here to talk about medical issues."
   c. "Come on. Let's focus on the positive. Let's not talk about this right now."
   d. "Do you need help finding a spiritual counselor? I have some ideas about how to do that."

5. When the religious beliefs of the health-care professional differ from those of the patient, the professional should say:
   a. "I'm glad your faith is helping you through this process."
   b. "Hard work has gotten you this far, not religion."
   c. "Are you sure all this religion is a good idea?"
   d. "I want to talk about your exercise, not your religion."

Fill-in-the-Blank Questions

1. _____ is the process of gaining a sense of spiritual connectedness through silence and thoughtfulness.

2. Being hopeful yet realistic about the future is called _____.

3. Spirituality may include prayer as well as New Age practices like _____ and _____.

4. Because discussions about spirituality and religion can lead to ethical issues, health-care professionals should provide a listening ear but set _____ in terms of what they can discuss and recommend to patients.

5. Spirituality may or may not involve a(n) _____ power.

Short-Answer Questions

1. From a spiritual perspective, why do medical diagnoses sometimes motivate patients to get more involved in life?

   _____

   _____

   _____

2. Why might patients who were actively involved in religious practices as children consider returning to those practices after diagnosis?

   _____

   _____

   _____

3. How do spiritual practices help to reduce patient anxiety?

   _____

   _____

   _____

4. In what ways can newly diagnosed patients experience spirituality?

   _____

   _____

   _____

5. What is the benefit of volunteer work for patients seeking greater spirituality?

   _____

   _____

   _____

Critical-Thinking Questions

1. Spirituality can greatly benefit patients who face medical diagnoses. Are there situations in which patients' religious beliefs may be unbeneficial? How might religious beliefs affect the ways in which patients view their prognoses or willingness to comply with treatment?

_____

_____

_____

_____

_____

2. Health-care professionals are often exposed to interactions between patients and their family members. Are there any aspects of family interactions that might be of concern from the perspective of spirituality and religion? If these interactions distressed the patient, what, if any, is the ideal role of the patients' health-care professionals?

_____

_____

_____

_____

_____

3. What is the ideal role of spirituality or religion in the life of a newly diagnosed patient? Detail your own perspective, as well as two differing ones. How are these perspectives similar? How are they different?

_____

_____

_____

_____

_____

Internet Exercise

A number of Internet resources address spirituality and religion. Consider these resources from the perspective of a newly diagnosed patient who has a background in each of the following:

- New Age spirituality
- Protestantism
- Evangelical Christianity
- Catholicism
- Buddhism
- Judaism
- Islam
- Naturism

Find at least two resources for each of these faiths, one with general information and inspiration and one with local resources. Which of these faiths are in your community? How prominent are they, and why?

_____

_____

_____

_____

_____

_____

_____

_____

_____

CHAPTER 11

Communicating with Family Members and Caregivers

OVERVIEW

After reading this chapter, you should be able to:

- Define and use the keywords of communicating with family members and caregivers.

- Describe how family members experience the news that their loved ones have been diagnosed with medical conditions.

- Identify the emotions of family members postdiagnosis and how they may affect their behaviors toward the patients.

- Understand the role of helplessness and how family members cope with their own helplessness.

- Discuss the communication issues that commonly arise between patients and family members.

- Explain the techniques for encouraging patients and family members to communicate better.

- Outline the ethical and boundary issues to be considered when communicating with family members.

KEYWORDS

Check-in

Communication

Elephant in the room

Normalcy

Sadness

Self-care

Tentative

Withdraw

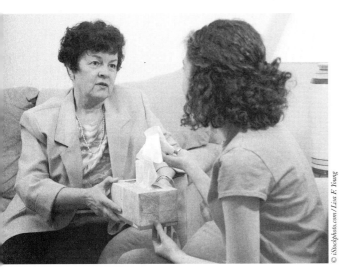

© iStockphoto.com / Lisa F. Young

KEEP IN MIND

Family members feel a great deal of stress when loved ones face medical diagnoses. As a health-care professional, what concerns would you expect a family member in this situation to have?

Case Study

For a month or more, Logan had tried to hide how poorly he was feeling from his wife, Angela. She knew something was wrong, but she could not persuade Logan to see his physician. Finally, Logan's back pain became so excruciating that he was taken from his job to the hospital by ambulance. The emergency room physician, suspecting that Logan was seriously ill, admitted him to the hospital and brought in an oncologist. Within a few days, Logan was diagnosed with lymphoma.

Since Logan had entered the emergency room, Angela had stayed by his side. Distraught, she refused to leave him even to check on their two young children, who were staying with her parents.

Charlotte, a licensed practical nurse (LPN) assigned to care for Logan during the evening shift, chatted often with Angela as she checked Logan's vital signs or administered his medication. Angela was approximately Charlotte's age and, as they learned during one conversation, the two had a few acquaintances in common. Charlotte was concerned about Angela. Charlotte had a child of her own and could identify with Angela's fears about Logan. She could also understand the challenges of trying to watch her children, especially while their father was seriously ill. Charlotte could not help but imagine what she would be going through if her own husband were facing a medical diagnosis.

The second evening Charlotte was on duty, Angela told her she was dissatisfied with the treatment Logan was receiving at the hospital. She disagreed, for example, with the oncologist's medication orders. Angela felt that the oncologist assigned to Logan's case was giving her too little information and that the conversations had occurred while she was home checking on her children. To try to gain the information she was after, she would ask Logan what he and the oncologist had discussed, but she worried that her husband was withholding details.

"Let me give you an example of what I mean, Charlotte," Angela offered. "I spent last night with the kids. When I came to the hospital this morning, Logan was still sound asleep. In fact, he was snoring, he was sleeping so deeply. When he finally woke up, he told me that one of the nurses had awakened him during the night and given him sleep medication. He's only supposed to get that when he can't sleep. So they knocked him out for no reason."

"Gosh, Angela," Charlotte said, thinking how she would feel in Angela's situation. "That doesn't sound good at all."

Family members may feel helpless when their loved ones are diagnosed with medical conditions. They want to help the patients but do not know how to, and they are trying to cope with the added responsibilities they may have to shoulder as a result. Helplessness can lead to stress and may cause family members to become overly critical of patients' health care. As a health-care professional, what is your plan for addressing situations like these?

As soon as she made that comment, Charlotte knew she probably should not have.

"I'm glad you agree," Angela sighed. "So now I know you won't mind helping me with something. I want to persuade Logan to ask for another oncologist to handle his case. As usual, though, he's being stubborn. He insists that he likes his oncologist, and Logan seems to think he knows what he's doing. But since you're a nurse, he might listen to you. Can you help me?"

"Angela," Charlotte started. "I really can't get involved in communication between you and your husband. That's between the two of you."

Angela began to cry. "I can't handle this on my own," she sobbed. "The doctor is on Logan's side, and I need the nurses on mine. And I'm afraid we don't have much time."

Charlotte understood that Angela was extremely upset and unable to have a reasonable discussion at that moment.

"I'd like to bring in Betty, the nursing supervisor, to talk with you," Charlotte said. "Is that okay?"

"If you won't help me," Angela responded, "I guess you'll have to."

While Angela felt her only hope was to bring in a health-care professional to help her persuade her husband to change oncologists, Charlotte knew it would be unethical to get involved in **communication** between Angela and Logan. She was concerned she had already overstepped her boundaries by appearing to agree with Angela's concerns.

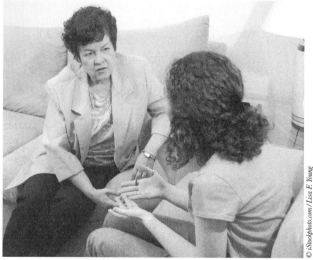
© iStockphoto.com / Lisa F. Young

Introduction

"This has been hard on all of us."

There is no denying it: Patients' medical diagnoses affect the patients' family members and other loved ones. Immediately after learning of the diagnoses, family members, like the patients themselves, may experience flight, freeze, or fight reactions, but they may react differently than the patients. They may also experience many of the same emotions as the patients, including fear, anger, and **sadness**.

As family members experience their emotions, they may hesitate to share them. Family members often fear saying the wrong thing, being unable to maintain patients' positivity, and losing the **normalcy** they once enjoyed. When, conversely, family members feel comfortable sharing their emotions with patients, and offer and receive support, families and patients draw closer.

KEEP IN MIND

Family members feeling stress from the diagnoses of their loved ones may seek allies. Angela asked for Charlotte's help changing oncologists, because the two had formed a relationship. As a health-care professional, what would you do in Charlotte's position?

Unfortunately, the changes required by patients' treatment regimens or lifestyle-management requirements can create stress for friends and family members as well as patients. For example, friends or family may be called on to take over household chores or transport patients to and from their medical treatments. As they worry that the patients, and their own lives, will never be the same, friends and family members allow their fears to amplify their already high stress levels. Further, financial concerns may arise.

Because medical diagnoses can cause such turmoil in patients' lives, patients and their families often have difficulty communicating. When patients and their families cannot communicate, families are challenged to support patients emotionally, help them make treatment decisions, and act as caregivers. Health-care professionals, for their part, may find themselves in the uncomfortable position of having to try to mediate.

Health-care professionals are not required to mediate family disagreements or to provide family mental-health services. When family communication problems are unresolved, health-care professionals can help by being sensitive to the causal issues and offering suggestions and guidance where appropriate.

Asking the Question "Why Us?"

Inevitably, medical diagnoses raise a lot of unanswerable questions, for patients and their families alike. For example, family members may question why their loved ones would develop medical conditions when those loved ones always cared for their health. They may ask why their comfortable home environments would suddenly be threatened. They may even question their own mortality. Their loved ones' diagnoses feel like challenges to their assumptions about how life should progress. In short, whereas the newly diagnosed tend to ask "Why me?" their friends and families tend to ask "Why us?"

Of course, the inevitable, undesirable answer to "Why us?" is "Because bad, unfair things can happen to our loved ones, as senseless and unfair as it may seem." Out of a desire to avoid admitting they have no control over what happens, family members may avoid discussing the answer to this question. They may also avoid such discussions for fear they will appear selfish or negative.

Unfortunately, failing to answer "Why us?" does not make its reality go away. Pervasive in that it is likely on the mind of every member of the patient's family, this question influences the emotions of all involved. As they struggle to surmount these and the other challenges diagnoses bring, patients and their loved ones work to understand how they will interact with each other and their health-care professionals.

KEEP IN MIND

Clearly, medical diagnoses tend to have far-reaching, often negative, impacts on close, personal relationships. How would you react if one of your family members was diagnosed with a serious medical condition? Would you label your reactions as fight, flight, or freeze? Why? How would your diagnosed family member likely react? How would that person's reaction impact the communication you share?

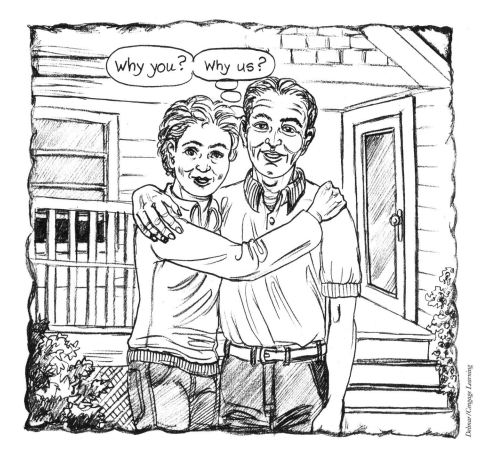

Understanding Family Members' Initial Reactions to Diagnoses

Initially, family members, and others close to the newly diagnosed patient, tend to react to the patient's diagnosis with shock, followed by flight, freeze, or fight, although the latter reactions may manifest differently than they do in the patient.

ASSESSING THE FLIGHT REACTION IN FAMILY MEMBERS

Family members may react to their loved ones' diagnoses with rushes of emotions that, at least temporarily, prevent them from being able to understand the patients' diagnoses and treatments, helping to make treatment decisions, or otherwise thinking rationally.

Fear is the main component of family members' flight reaction, fear for the patients' well-being and fear of how the family members will be impacted. Family members in flight reaction may upset patients. Ironically, patients may feel that they must assist their family members or otherwise reassure them that they can handle their diagnoses. Out of concern for their families, patients may deprive themselves of emotional support at a time they need it most. To avoid making patients emotional with their out-of-control emotions, family members in flight may avoid the patients. To try to feel less helpless, family members in flight may even try to impose less-than-ideal treatments on patients just to do something.

STUDYING FAMILY MEMBERS' FREEZE REACTIONS

Family members in freeze reaction tend to assume two things: (1) that medical conditions are patients' fate and (2) that they as outsiders are powerless to help. It follows, then, that family members in freeze reaction are likely to avoid discussing diagnoses with patients, rationalizing that the patients want to be in control and will reach out to family members if their assistance is needed. In fact, patients who need family support will avoid family members who are in freeze reaction. When the patients are also in freeze reaction, the health-care team may have to motivate patients and family members alike.

EVALUATING FAMILY MEMBERS WHO RESPOND AS FIGHTERS

Even one family member in fight reaction offers a newly diagnosed patient strong support. Particularly when patients are in flight or freeze reaction, family caregivers in fight reaction can make all the difference. When patients are also fighters, however, conflict can result. Patients may feel that their families are trying to control or interfere with their treatments.

Identifying the Emotions Family Members Experience

As the following sections illustrate, as family members and others close to newly diagnosed patients react to the patients' diagnoses, they experience emotions similar to those of the patients.

STARTING WITH FEAR

> *"When I learned about my husband's condition, all I could think about was how scared I was. I was terrified he might get really sick and that I could lose him. I didn't want to be without him. And I was afraid about what this might mean for our children, if he was going to be able to keep working at the same level he had been, and what kinds of responsibilities I might have to be taking on at some point."*

The fear family members may experience should not be underestimated. While some conditions, like cancer and diabetes, raise obvious concerns about disability and even death, virtually any medical diagnosis can cause family members fear. Family members fear loss of emotional support and fear about finances, but, most of all, family members fear for the future of the newly diagnosed patients. Medical diagnoses are confirmation that human beings are not invincible and that the family members they depend on to play certain roles—partners, parents, siblings—may sometimes be unable to fulfill their roles.

Family members often feel pressured to be positive around their newly diagnosed patients, much like the patients do with family members. Fear often stifles the communication between patients and family members. For example, patients and their families may avoid conversations about treatment options out of a desire to avoid both feeling and expressing the fear these conversations inspire. Out of a fear of feeling

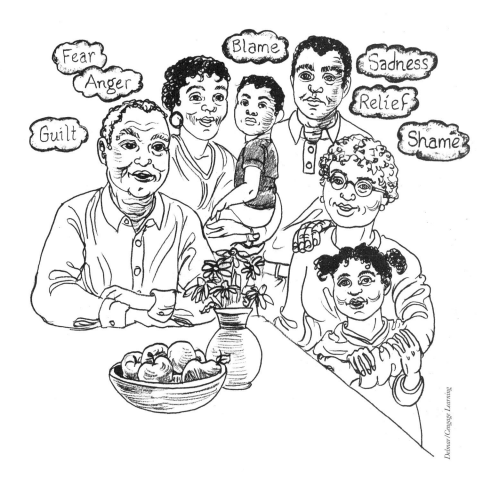

Delmar/Cengage Learning

helpless, family members may become overly controlling, trying to dictate their expectations for the patients' care to the health-care teams. The result is tension and frustration for everyone.

DELVING INTO ANGER

"I was so mad, that's all I could feel. I was mad that my mother was going to have to face all this treatment. What had she done to deserve this? I was mad that she and my father had made so many plans and now they might not be able to enjoy the future they had planned. I walked around feeling angry for a long time."

Family members feel angry for varied reasons. Anger can be a reaction to a sense of unfairness and helplessness that comes from having to watch a loved one suffer in some way and being unable to stop it. Anger also arises from disappointment and fear that life is changing in ways that are unexpected and unwanted and that future plans may not unfold as expected. Anger is both a comfortable and an uncomfortable emotion. In Western culture, anger is an acceptable emotion that, while justified in its own right, also substitutes for emotions that are less comfortable, such as sadness and fear. Some fear that if they allowed themselves to feel as angry as they really are, they might lose control.

Fear of losing control often prevents family members from expressing anger around patients. When angry outbursts occur, family members often feel guilty and remorseful afterward. Most often, families direct anger away from their real sources

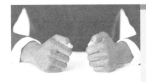

Body Language

The family members of newly diagnosed patients who are experiencing stress may show it through such body language as:

- Angry expressions
- Frightened expressions
- Tears
- Defiant posture (hands on the hips, feet and legs spread)
- Sitting with the arms crossed
- Agitation

and toward targets that are somehow perceived as safer. Unfortunately, family members may direct their anger toward health-care professionals. For example, a family member may make an issue of a task they think a certified nursing assistant (can) should have performed, such as replacing a towel; complain that a nurse did not recommend a test when they thought he should have; or express outrage that health-care professionals were not warm and friendly toward their loved ones. Whether these complaints are justified or not, the anger is disproportionate. Family members may vent their rage at an unmade bed when what is really making them angry is the helplessness they feel in knowing that someone they care about is sick and in treatment.

MAKING TIME FOR SADNESS

"I didn't want to tell my brother how sad I felt, but he must have known. He had been so healthy and strong. I had always looked up to him. I still did, but I couldn't help but think that over time he would likely lose his strength, and he might face other medical conditions related to his diagnosis. I knew his future wasn't looking too bright anymore."

Sadness is a common reaction to learning that a family member has received a medical diagnosis. Sadness comes from a sense of loss, or the fear of potential loss, as family members struggle to accept the patients' conditions and whatever changes may accompany them. Family members may experience sad feelings so intense that they appear to be in grief, at least when the patients are initially diagnosed. As they process the news, their sadness may lessen, but it tends to remain. In fact, family members may find it difficult to let go of their sadness. Some feel that everything they encounter is somehow colored by the sadness they carry.

As with anger and other strong emotions, when family members feel sad, they may be quick to act—and overreact—to events that occur. Their behaviors may even appear irrational. They may break down and cry for no apparent reason, for example, which distresses patients. Family members have difficulty conveying their sadness to patients directly, out of fear that they may upset the patients yet more. Superstitious thinking may play a role here. Family members may feel that if they verbalize their sadness they may make something bad happen. Therefore, they instead often try to hide their sadness from others, if not from themselves. The result is indirect communication—talking around issues, not expressing thoughts and feelings directly.

BEING ABLE TO EXPRESS RELIEF

"I was relieved it wasn't any worse. She had been feeling so badly that I had prepared myself for all kinds of possibilities, most of them pretty bad. As it turned out, she had a lot of medicine in her future, but if she took good care of herself, which I intended to help her do, chances are she would live a full life. I know that everything is going to be just fine now."

As a means of preparation, family members and patients alike often imagine worst-case scenarios so they can celebrate when diagnoses actually come. All parties tend to feel intense relief when the patients' diagnoses are less severe than feared. Feelings are particularly intense for family members who have had experiences with illness, personally or with others, or who knew of conditions the patients could have inherited but did not. Those in denial can feel relief when there is little information about diagnoses and what they might mean for the patients' future.

While relief can be positive, cultivating optimism in family members and patients, it can challenge communication. Family members can feel relieved to the extent that they close off to information that runs contrary to their optimism, and they may try to convince patients to do the same. Health-care professionals may need to help family members modify their expectations so they can cope realistically with the diagnoses, and help patients to do the same.

DEALING WITH GUILT, SHAME, AND BLAME

"I have to say I was embarrassed when my son told me he had been diagnosed with hepatitis C. I always thought of that as a disease that drug addicts and street people get. I felt ashamed. I didn't want to think of him as having been a drug user, though I suspected he might be. If it was related to drugs or sex or something like that, then I thought I must not have done a very good job as a father, like maybe I had let him down, had not taught him how to live a good life. So I felt guilty about being a bad parent, and I felt guilty about being ashamed of my own son. It was terrible."

As emotions, shame and guilt are often closely related. Newly diagnosed patients and their families may share guilt and shame arising from the patients' diagnoses, particularly when the underlying conditions were sexually transmitted, like HIV, or related to illegal drug use, like hepatitis C. Conditions that are lifestyle related, such as lung cancer and Type II diabetes, can cause shame because they may have been avoided with other lifestyle choices. Family members who they could have helped with prevention may feel guilty, or they may feel guilty for things they think or learn upon hearing the diagnoses. Lack of information can compound the guilt and shame some feel. For example, hepatitis C is transmitted in ways other than illegal drug use. To offset negative perceptions, health-care professionals may have to educate family members with patients.

Like ignorance, guilt and shame tend to complicate family dynamics, and family relationship difficulties may be long-standing. Family members may have experienced guilt, shame, and anger for years regarding the patients' behaviors or lifestyles. When diagnoses come, family members may place responsibility and blame on the patients, amplifying any tension. Family members who do not address their feelings of guilt and shame can offer no support to patients. Instead, they **withdraw** or become hostile or judgmental. The patients, in turn, suffer damage to their self-images as they feel yet more guilt and shame.

Health-care professionals can greatly assist families in dealing with patients' diagnoses by offering information about conditions and encouraging family members to do their own information-gathering. Furthermore, encouraging family members to talk with objective people and/or mental-health professionals can greatly benefit patients and family members.

Researching Common Caregiver-Patient Communication Issues

The following sections outline the communication issues that commonly arise between newly diagnosed patients and their family members and friends.

CHOOSING TO IGNORE

Commonly, when family members are diagnosed with medical conditions, both patients and family members may have difficulty discussing many aspects of the conditions and their treatments because they do not want to express, or admit, feelings of helplessness lest they expose weaknesses or discourage one another. Often, helplessness becomes the "**elephant in the room**" that everyone knows about but no one wants to talk about. Avoidance does not achieve eradication, however. Instead, the

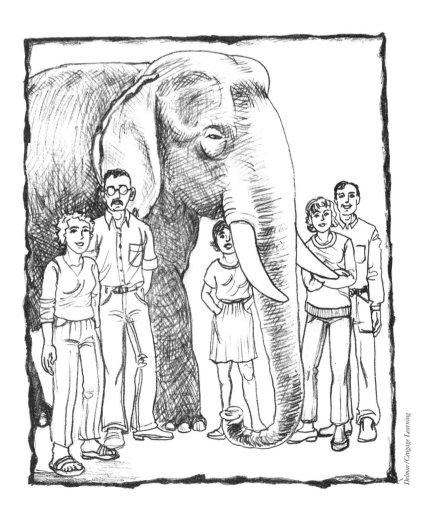

Delmar/Cengage Learning

elephant in the room may become larger and larger and show itself through further avoidance of anything that might cause a sense of helplessness.

Family members may attempt to avoid the feelings of fear and helplessness through "can-do" attitudes and the belief that hard work will conquer any challenge. They may insist on positive attitudes despite any evidence to the contrary, as if ignoring the challenges will make them go away. Family members will often try to influence health-care professionals to join them in ignoring the elephant in the room by avoiding difficult topics, such as potential challenges of treatment and recovery. Ironically, as patients and their family members try to cover their uncomfortable feelings, stress and other negative emotions build.

From the patient's perspective: It was not easy for Connie to deal with the news of her medical diagnosis, but she has learned to accept that she is going to have to watch her diet closely and stay consistent with her medications. Nevertheless, she worries that, even if she is diligent about compliance, she will have additional complications or need changes to her regimen. "We'll watch this closely," Connie's physician had promised her.

> *"I don't know what's going to happen to me. I was symptom free, and now I'm in treatment and have no idea what might or might not be ahead of me. The hardest part is trying to keep a stiff upper lip with Ethan. He must be worried about what's going to happen to me and what that might mean for our family. But it's like he thinks that if I talk about how out of control I feel here, then I'll make more bad things happen. So I keep my mouth shut."*

From the family member's perspective: Connie's husband, Ethan, described himself to a friend as "the walking wounded." Initially shocked at Connie's diagnosis, he quickly mobilized to become an active partner with Connie in facing her condition. He had become educated on her condition and volunteered to meet with her health-care team to learn how he could best help her. In Ethan's mind, the communication he has with Connie about her condition and its treatment is fine. He wants her to "keep her spirits up" and dwell on nothing that might be discouraging.

> *"Connie and I really share information. I know as much as she does about it, if not more, to be honest. Her doctor and I have even talked about potential complications and what we need to do to avoid them. But I don't want to burden her with any of this. Sometimes I can't stop thinking about how worried I am and how I feel like our home life could spin out of control if her condition suddenly worsens. I try not to let it show. If she doesn't talk about things that might upset her, I think she'll have a better chance."*

TRYING TO MAKE EVERTHING BETTER

When something is obviously broken, it is human nature to want to fix it. For better or worse, this is often the guiding principle of family members and other caregivers in their interactions with newly diagnosed patients. Once diagnoses arrive, friends and families tend to jump in to try to fix whatever they can and "make everything better." Unfortunately, family members who take over may benefit neither themselves nor the patients.

When family members step in to help newly diagnosed patients, they often step in uninvited. Patients, especially fighters, most likely want to make their treatment decisions and handle daily life responsibilities. Because initially they know too little to know the best way forward, they perceive the assistance offered by family members

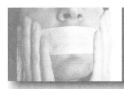

SELF • talk

The family members of patients can reinforce their feelings of fear and hopelessness through self-talk that includes the following:

I can't believe this is happening to our family. We haven't done anything to deserve it.

The medical establishment doesn't care about any of us, and probably won't give us the help we need.

We are surrounded by uncaring and incompetent people.

No matter how hard anyone tries, this isn't going to have a happy ending.

I will never be able to make these doctors and nurses understand me.

Antidotes to family members' negative self-talk include the following:

I'm surrounded by smart and caring professionals. I need to be more patient.

We're all doing the best we can here, despite how we might step on each other's toes at times.

I can take one day at a time and see this through.

The doctors and nurses have been through this with patients and their families before, and they understand what we're going through.

and caregivers as premature and unwelcomed. Ultimately, fighters feel disempowered when their family members offer unwanted advice and assistance. Patients in flight and freeze reactions, in contrast, could benefit from the gentle encouragement and measured assistance of family members.

While well-intentioned, the desire to take over for newly diagnosed patients comes from a sense of helplessness on the part of family members and other caregivers. Family members involve themselves in patients' health care as a means of dealing with their own fear and uncertainty. If they can make the patients' problems go away, they can make their helplessness go away as well. What results, however, is frustration, conflict, and disappointment for both patients and family members.

From the patient's perspective: Jacob has always described himself as a "control freak." He started a successful business and ran it for 30 years and would have continued to run it had he not been diagnosed with a heart condition and ordered by his physician to cut back his workload. Jacob has lived alone since his wife died. His grown children want to be involved in providing any emotional or other support that he might need, including completing work around the house, but, true to form, he has refused.

> *"The kids try to bring up the topic of how they can help poor old dad, but I won't hear of it. I know my daughter, Ellen, is as much of a control freak as I am. She'll want to jump in and take over, thinking that's what I need her to do. First, she'll do the housework, and before you know it, she'll be telling me what I can eat and when I need to go to bed at night. I know she means well, but I'm not going to have them turning me into a guest in my own home. I can handle this on my own. And I don't see any reason to talk about anyone else getting involved."*

From the family member's perspective: Jacob's daughter, Ellen, admits that she has been worried about him since her mother died. She thought her father was eating poorly, getting too little exercise, and working too many hours. Consequently, when he was diagnosed with his heart condition, she was not surprised, although she would never admit that to him. Now that he has been diagnosed, Ellen regrets not having been more outspoken when she was first concerned, and she wonders if her father's heart condition might have been avoided had she been more assertive.

"I feel like I let this happen in some ways. I should have jumped in and made him take better care of himself, even if it might have caused some friction at first. But it's too late. At this point, I feel like I have another chance to make sure he stays as healthy as possible, and that means being compliant with the doctor's office. He doesn't take orders very well, but I'm not trying to order him around. I just want to help out with some of his chores and see where I can give him some encouragement to stay with his program. But if he cuts me off when I bring up the subject, I don't know how far we're going to get."

STAYING POSITIVE

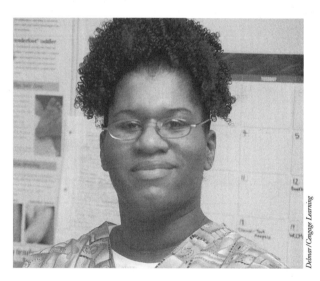

As discussed in previous chapters, denial is a common reaction to a medical diagnosis. After initially denying their conditions, many patients will, over time, come to terms with them and move forward with the decisions they must make. Of course, some continue to struggle with denial.

Like patients, patients' families may follow a pattern of denial postdiagnosis, and some family members are better able to face reality than others. When family members deny patients' conditions, however, communication breaks down. Often, family members in denial are selective in what they will talk about. For example, the denial of family members may manifest as a desire to remain hopeful despite any off-putting evidence. As a result, family members may refuse to listen when patients try to discuss less-than-positive treatment outcomes, side effects, or recurrences. The patients are left feeling unsupported. Family members may even refuse to think about or discuss patients' conditions or treatment at all. For support, patients may look to health-care professionals to have these discussions. Family members, for their part, may ask that the professionals encourage patients not to focus on their concerns.

From the patient's perspective: When Claudia first received her rheumatoid arthritis diagnosis, she refused to believe it. She asked her doctor to order a new set of tests to confirm that the diagnosis was accurate. While Claudia had known that her condition was in her family, and that she and her sisters might be affected, she had hoped that they might all be spared. She and her sisters had occasionally discussed their fears about the condition, but only in general terms because, up until now, none had been diagnosed with it. When Claudia received her diagnosis, she was surprised at the reaction of her sister Carmela.

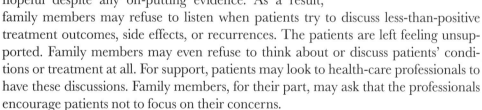

"I said to her, 'Carmela, I have Mom's condition. I might be going through what she went through,' and Carmela might as well have told me to get over myself. She told me to stop worrying, that the medicines were a lot better and that I would be fine. I kind of agreed, but I still

---

KEEP IN MIND

Given the complexity of emotions, and the motivations driving relationships, it can be difficult to always be authentic. Have you ever felt like you needed to think and act positively when you were not necessarily feeling that way? Who benefited more?

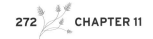
wanted to talk to her about what I might need if things didn't work out so well and to ask her if she would be able to help out with my son if there came a time when I wasn't able to function so well. At that point, she interrupted me and told me to stop being so negative. She told me to think positive and keep smiling and everything would be fine. I feel like she's going to call the positive-thinking police on me if tell her how I'm really feeling."

From the family member's perspective: Carmela had difficulty explaining how she feels about Claudia's diagnosis, because she is uncomfortable with her feelings. She is angry Claudia may experience what their mother did: She does not want to go through that again. She is also concerned about how Claudia will cope with her responsibilities as a mother if she becomes debilitated and what life will be like for her son. Selfishly, Carmela is fearful about her own future. If Claudia got diagnosed, she could too. Although intellectually she knows that Claudia needs to talk about her diagnosis, she has not been able to have that conversation yet.

"I fully intend to be there for my sister in whatever way she needs me. I really do. But I'm not ready now, and I don't know when I will be. And maybe this is selfish, but what I need my sister to do is to be strong and fight this. I need her not to even think about the possibility that she won't beat it and have a normal life. I can't help but believe that if she refuses to give in, and doesn't make any room for it in her life, she'll be fine. That's what I need her to believe too."

MISUSING EMPOWERMENT

In Western society, people are often reared to believe that hard work can overcome virtually any challenge. Patients in fight reaction demonstrate this attitude by becoming educated so they can make informed treatment decisions and feel empowered to comply with their treatments. These patients' families, adopting similar attitudes, tend to partner with the patients and take active roles in the patients' health care. However, families may inadvertently cause tension in their patient relationships. They may, for example, prompt patients to "help themselves" when the patients feel they are doing everything possible. Similarly, family members may leave fighters alone to make decisions and cope with treatment recommendations, when really those patients need the feedback and support of their families.

Like they do fighters, family members with empowerment attitudes impact newly diagnosed patients in flight or freeze reaction. Already on edge, patients in flight reaction may become even more anxious if they perceive that their families are abandoning them. More than some, patients in flight reaction need their family members to help them make more rational, and less emotional, decisions. Patients in freeze reaction also need family support and advocacy, because they are at risk for avoiding

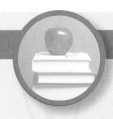

Educational Moment

Most likely, family members have little experience working with medical professionals. By demonstrating direct, compassionate communication, health-care professionals can model desired behaviors for families interacting with patients, each other, and the health-care team.

their diagnoses and consequently becoming passive in making decisions or being compliant.

Family members adopt the "do something for yourself" attitude for reasons other than wanting patients to be as active as possible. Some want to avoid the uncomfortable emotions diagnoses stir up or the seriousness of the situations. From the health-care professionals' perspective, family members in avoidance cannot play key supporting roles for patients.

From the patient's perspective: Daryl's orthopedic surgeon just told him his spinal surgery would be more extensive than expected. Not only, she said, would Daryl require hospitalization for at least a week, it might be a month or more before he could return to work. Even then, he would likely only be able to work part-time until he fully recovered. That was, the surgeon said, all the information she could offer until after the surgery was completed.

Daryl had many concerns, but he was worried most about recovering and how his recuperation would impact his wife, Gale, and their young child. He had tried to voice his concerns to Gale, but she only advised him to return to work as soon as possible and then changed the subject.

> *"I know Gale is worried about me and what this is going to mean for us if I need to delay my return to work. I think she is as scared about it as I am. But instead of being willing to talk about a strategy with me for how we will deal with my recovery if it is slower than expected, she makes me feel like I'm trying to get sympathy or turn my recovery into a vacation. Last night, she told me that if I work extra hard in physical therapy, I can probably shorten my recovery to a week or two and go right back to work. Like it's all under my control. Well, I can tell you that the doctor is not telling me that."*

From the family member's perspective: Gale does not want to admit that she is afraid about the future. She wants Daryl to feel better and to be back to normal, but she also wants to ensure that their income will soon recover, because she is not currently employed. She does not want to imagine the possible outcomes, and she certainly does not want to discuss any of this. While Gale knows Daryl does not control the outcome of his surgery, and that the surgeon cannot make promises, she wants to believe that a determined attitude and hard work on Daryl's part may lead to a miraculous recovery. She is hoping that she can push him hard enough to recover as fast as she needs him to. In short, Gale is in her own flight reaction to Daryl's condition.

> *"Daryl has always been a hard worker and a very determined person, so it scares me when I see he can't live a normal life. I want to do everything I can to encourage him to be the person I know he is and to take charge of this situation. He can do it if he keeps working. If I can keep pushing him, this will all be nothing but a bad memory."*

Encouraging Patient-Family Communication via the Health-Care Team

Through tools like educational moments, health-care professionals can play subtle roles in enhancing patient-family communication. The following sections outline other strategies.

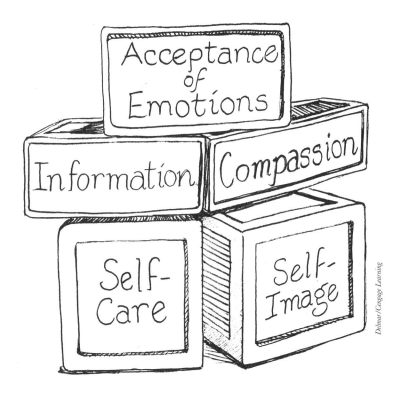

Delmar/Cengage Learning

PROMPTING FAMILIES TO ACCEPT THEIR OWN EMOTIONS

Recall that newly diagnosed patients and their family members together experience the patients' illnesses, sometimes suppressing uncomfortable feelings, like fear or anger. As needed, health-care professionals can serve as sounding boards, encouraging anyone involved in the patients' diagnoses to express their feelings. Health-care professionals should start by reminding patients and family members alike that everyone connected to a diagnosis is affected and that strong reactions around diagnoses are to be expected on both sides. To help ensure that exchanges remain productive, the health-care professionals should be careful to avoid advising either side—patient or family—on how to communicate with the other. Instead, they should keep the focus on expressing emotions, and thereby releasing tension. Patients and family members usually feel great release simply from no longer having to hold their feelings inside, and relaxed participants in communication tend to communicate better. A safe place to discuss emotions adds another layer of comfort.

What not to say:

"You shouldn't be feeling this way."

"You really need to tell _____ [patient's name] how you're feeling."

"You need to focus on how your loved one is feeling, not on how you feel."

"You can't let emotions get in the way of doing what you can to support _____."

Words that enhance communications:

"I can't give you advice about how to talk to _____ [patient's name], but I'm a good listener."

"It's normal to have a lot of fear and other feelings when someone we love is facing a medical diagnosis."

"I can see that you have a lot going on. Anything you want to tell me about?"

"I've worked with a lot of patients facing diagnoses like _____'s. I know it's always hard on family members."

"I know that _____ is going through a lot of emotions from this medical diagnosis, but I can see that you and the other members of the family are too. This is what happens when someone is diagnosed."

FOSTERING SELF-CARE

Family members usually think that the best things they can do for patients is to be totally focused on their care, devoting all their emotional and physical energy to this goal. However, they risk depleting themselves in the process, leaving themselves open to exhaustion, illness, and their own emotional breakdowns. Certainly, family members are less effective when they fail to care for themselves.

Health-care professionals can help family members by encouraging them to get enough rest, eat healthy diets, take breaks to recharge themselves, and lean on their friends/families or mental-health professionals for support. To lend further help, health-care professionals can describe how to delegate caregiving tasks and refer family members to community resources as needed and appropriate. It can be useful for professionals to plan with family members strategies that both meet the family members' physical and emotional needs and meet the needs of the patients. In that way, health-care professionals integrate **self-care** into treatment plans.

Initially, family members may resist the idea of self-care, because they may resist admitting that they may be unable at some point to handle their caregiving responsibilities. Until they experience caregiving firsthand, most family members feel that they are up to the task. To help gain family members' buy-in on self-care strategies, health-care professionals should present the concept as a suggestion, not an order. They may also consider calling patients and families together to discuss ways they can all care for each other. That way, all people involved feel a sense of responsibility.

What not to say:

"Just get through this. You can collapse later."

"You need to be there for _____, regardless of how difficult it may seem."

"If you wear yourself out, you'll be useless."

"Tell your other family members that they have to roll up their sleeves and help you."

"Believe me, it may look easy now, but you probably won't be able to handle all this."

Words that enhance communications:

"Do you think it might help to have some support lined up for yourself, just in case some unanticipated challenges come up?"

"Let's sit down for a minute and talk about how you're doing."

"Would it help if we all got together and put a plan in place, for _____ [patient's name] and all of you, before we start the treatment? I know _____ is concerned about you and will want to be involved in this."

"You have a lot ahead of you once the treatment begins. Can we take a moment and talk about the best way to help you stay strong?"

DELIVERING A MESSAGE OF COMPASSION

Once patients and family members begin to face the patients' conditions daily, uncomfortable emotions like anger are likely to emerge. As dedicated as they may be to maintaining calm, humans sometimes allow their negative feelings—fear and anger—to lead them to words and behaviors they later regret. Feeling guilty, and trying to avoid additional guilt, can only add to the stress that family members are feeling.

Health-care professionals can help ease tensions by gently suggesting that patients and family members be patient with each other and remind each other that everyone involved is doing the best they can under difficult circumstances. In this regard, educational moments are invaluable. Health-care professionals who prompt patients and family members to ventilate with the professionals, and not on each other, generally can help defuse powerful emotions. Professionals who are good listeners and demonstrate empathy as frustration and complaints arise deepen the sense of trust in the health-care team.

What not to say:

"I know how you're feeling. These guys must be driving you crazy."

"Believe me, in your position, I'd tell her to get lost."

"You can take control here. I'll tell you how."

"It must make you nuts when he behaves that way."

Words that enhance communications:

"I know this is really difficult for all of you. It's scary to find out that someone you love is facing serious medical treatment."

"I can see that you're really frustrated. But this is a lot to deal with, and it seems like you're being hard on yourself. Can you give yourself a break here?"

"Anyone would be frustrated in your situation. But it seems to me that you're all doing the best you can under the circumstances."

"It's been my experience in working with patients that everyone is doing the best they can even though it doesn't always seem like it. Can you think of it that way?"

SUPPORTING INFORMATION-GATHERING AND CHECK-INS

Lack of information interferes with effective communication. When newly diagnosed patients or their family members lack information, they tend to provide their own, often making erroneous assumptions. Erroneous assumptions lead to poor conclusions, some more unrealistic than others. The net result is further stress for both patients and their family members.

For the treatment process to be successful, information-gathering must be ongoing. As patients progress, they should continue to gain information that complements their knowledge bases. Patients and family members may gather some of this information on their own, but other information must come from physicians and other health-care professionals. For example, a patient who experiences unfamiliar symptoms can gather some information but should consult with the treating physician before making any assumptions.

Health-care professionals can help patients and family members stay informed by suggesting reliable information resources and ongoing **check-ins** with the physicians and other members of the health-care team. Regular, continued involvement with the right resources—preferably with all parties involved at the same time—helps ensure that all involved are acting on the same information, rather than different interpretations and assumptions.

What not to say:

"You shouldn't be jumping to any conclusions here without talking to the doctor first."

"You seem to know a lot about this, so you're probably right. Let _____ [patient's name] hear what you have to say."

"Stand up for yourself here. You've done your research."

"That sounds really scary. I haven't heard of that, but I'm not up on the latest research."

Words that enhance communications:

"There's a lot of contradictory information on the Internet. Have you all sat down and talked to the doctor about this?"

"It's important to make sure we set up a routine so we can monitor you on an ongoing basis as we move forward with your treatment."

"Let's all sit down and review the treatment plan so we can answer any questions that might have come up. I'll ask the other health-care professionals involved with your case to sit in."

"I'm hearing different opinions from you and your brother about your mother's care. Why don't we go over everything together so we're all in sync?"

"I know the nurse is going to have an opinion about this. Have you talked to him lately?"

DISTINGUISHING PATIENTS FROM THEIR MEDICAL CONDITIONS

With all the emphasis on medical information, symptoms, and treatments, it is easy to begin to view newly diagnosed patients as medical conditions rather than human beings. Family members may become so concerned about patients' health care that they make every issue a medical one and forget that the patients have nonmedical needs. Not infrequently, family members modify their expectations for patients, assuming they cannot participate in certain activities, for example.

> **KEEP IN MIND**
>
> Family members are most likely inexperienced with patients' diagnoses, which means they are unfamiliar with relating to the patients from a medical perspective. Loved ones may require coaching to understand how to help the patients maintain their essential humanity. As a health-care professional, how would you approach this task?

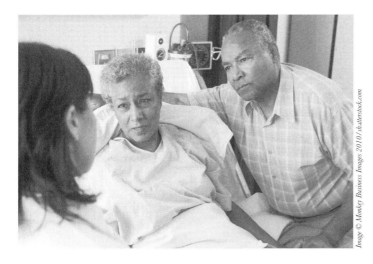

Often, family members shift their behaviors toward patients as a means of adjusting to the patients' diagnoses. By generalizing medical issues, for example, family members may be trying to prepare themselves to live with loved ones with medical conditions. Being hypervigilant to patients may really be family members' ways of coping with their helplessness.

Some patients respond poorly when family members identify them by their medical diagnoses, and interpersonal tension results. For patients with disempowered self-images, such a focus can reinforce dependence.

When family members stop seeing patients as whole people, health-care professionals should gently step in, doing things like subtly reminding loved ones that the patients can choose when medical intervention is and is not needed. Direction as to which activities patients can continue, and which may challenge them, can help family members keep realistic perspectives on patients' abilities. To keep patients engaged, health-care professionals should involve them in all discussions. That way, family members must talk *with* patients and not *around* them.

What not to say:

"She probably can't participate, so just don't bring it up."

"Now that your _____ [sister, brother, spouse, parent, etc.] is a _____ [diabetic, arthritic, cancer patient, etc.]. . . ."

"Stop treating _____ [patient's name] like a sick person."

Words that enhance communications:

"Your _____ [sister, brother, parent, etc.] is still the person [he/she] always was. Medical conditions introduce new challenges, but people stay the same they always were."

"Talk to _____ [patient's name] about how much [he/she] feels like participating."

"Other than some of the restrictions the doctor mentioned, the decision is up to _____."

"Why don't we all get together and talk about what everyone's role is going to be. We'll start with _____ [patient's name] perspective."

"I know you're concerned about how the diagnosis is going to affect what [his/her] life is going to be like, but there's no reason [he/she] can't continue to be a well-rounded person, just like [he/she] has always been."

KEEP IN MIND

As they deal with the impact of medical diagnoses, patients and their family members can benefit from similar guidance and suggestions from health-care professionals. If you were the family member of a newly diagnosed loved one, what could you say that would be most helpful?

Exercising Caution through Ethics and Boundaries

Under any circumstances, family relationships are complicated. Consequently, health-care professionals should always approach involvement in communication issues between patients and their family members, and other caregivers, with professional ethics and boundaries in mind.

STAYING FOCUSED ON PROFESSIONAL RESPONSIBILITIES

The primary responsibility of health-care professionals is to deliver and manage patients' treatment protocols and advocate for patients in terms of monitoring their ongoing well-being. When evaluating how to handle communication problems with patients and their families, it is best to consider any actions from this perspective. If the communication between patients and their family members directly impacts treatment, including caregiving responsibilities and compliance with treatment regimens, it may be necessary for health-care professionals to become involved.

KNOWING ORGANIZATIONAL GUIDELINES

Most medical offices or health-care facilities have formal or informal guidelines for addressing nonmedical issues, including psychosocial ones, which include family communication. Before intervening in patient-family communication, health-care professionals should know any guidelines. According to Health Insurance Portability and Accountability Act (HIPAA) guidelines, health-care professionals may discuss no patient's situation with anyone the patient has not specifically designated.

RECOGNIZING WHEN TO USE OUTSIDE RESOURCES

Based on both experience and training, health-care professionals are often qualified to offer assistance when communication issues arise. However, it is important for the professionals to know when the line between medical care and mental-health care is being crossed and when other resources are better equipped to step in. Large health-care institutions may have social workers or counselors on staff who can get involved when psychosocial issues arise, and medical offices often have referral resources available, which staff can pass to patients. In addition to formal and informal guidelines, conversations with supervisors can help clarify which options are appropriate.

IDENTIFYING WHEN PERSONAL BUTTONS ARE BEING PUSHED

Family relationships are always complicated. Childhood memories of family may be positive and negative, and adult relationships may have periods of disagreement.

When health-care professionals observe patient-family interactions, they are often reminded of their own family relationships. When the observations are highly similar to professionals' experiences, the professionals may experience some of the same emotions as their patients and their patients' families. At all times, health-care professionals should be aware that this could happen. Otherwise, they may lose track of professional boundaries and say things, or otherwise become involved, in inappropriate

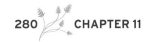

ways. Some may try to fix patients' families in subconscious attempts to fix their own. When boundaries are at risk, health-care professionals should get coworkers or supervisors involved.

STAYING NEUTRAL

It is natural for people in conflict with other people to seek allies. When, for example, family members want to persuade patients or influence their treatments, they may seek allies. Patients may also seek allies. Often, because they are uniquely positioned in the system, health-care professionals are the desired targets. Even the professionals' agreement on minor issues can cause patients or family members to feel the professionals are on their sides.

In addition to causing discomfort, this dynamic can present ethical issues. The health-care professionals' first responsibility is to ensure that patients receive the best care possible. Beyond that, clear neutrality to patients and family members is recommended.

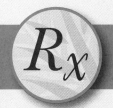

Discussing Communication between Patients and Their Loved Ones

Angela, the family member who was concerned about her husband's medical care at the beginning of the chapter, was hoping that Charlotte, the LPN with whom she had formed a relationship, would intervene with her husband and persuade him to request another oncologist. Charlotte knew that she ethically could not be involved in this conversation and was concerned as to how to help Angela without overstepping boundaries and/or making the situation worse. She asked Betty, the nursing supervisor on the floor that evening, to get involved. The three women met in the conference room.

BETTY: Hi, Angela. We haven't met before, but I'm Betty. I'm an RN, and I'm the supervisor on duty tonight. Charlotte tells me you have some concerns about your husband's treatment.

ANGELA: Hi, Betty. Yes, I have a lot of concerns, which I mentioned to Charlotte. Didn't she tell you?

BETTY: She did talk to me, but I thought you, Charlotte, and I could have a conversation together to see how we can help you. I'd really like to start by hearing directly from you what's going on.

ANGELA: Okay. I don't think my husband, Logan, is getting the best care. I don't like his doctor, for one thing. And I can't seem to persuade Logan to consider my request to bring in another one.

BETTY: How were you hoping the nurses could help you?

ANGELA: It's obvious that you are more involved with Logan's care than the doctor is because you're with him all the time. And since Logan and I both like Charlotte, all I did was ask her to have a little chat with Logan and maybe suggest another doctor on staff here that he might consider. Since Charlotte agrees that we have a problem, and Logan seems to trust her, I thought he might listen to her more than he is willing to listen to me. Was I wrong?

BETTY: I understand, Angela. You were hoping that Charlotte might talk your husband into working with another doctor?

ANGELA: That's exactly right.

BETTY: Did you want to say anything, Charlotte?

CHARLOTTE: Sure. We see a lot of family members on this floor who are worried about their family members. It's only natural that they would want the best care possible and want to do anything possible to make sure they are getting it. I want to make that clear. But as I said earlier, it wouldn't be ethical for me to get involved in trying to influence your husband's care.

BETTY: We really have strict guidelines on giving patient's advice, Angela, and Charlotte is right. This is really between you and your husband.

ANGELA: So I guess you're telling me you can't help me, even if you can see the doctor is making bad decisions. I mean, how much sense does it make to wake a patient up at night and give him a strong sleeping pill?

BETTY: Can I make a couple of suggestions, Angela?

ANGELA: I guess.

BETTY: First, let's take a look at what happened last night. I can check your husband's chart to see why he received a sedative last night. There may have been a reason we don't know about. I'll get back to you with an answer. We can also talk to the doctor about recommending a milder sedative if he thinks that would be appropriate, okay?

ANGELA: I guess that would be a start.

BETTY: I would also like to talk about the experiences we have had with other family members in your situation. Would that be okay?

ANGELA: Sure.

BETTY: A medical diagnosis places a lot of stress on everybody involved. I don't know Logan, but I know that patients often want to feel like they are in charge of their medical care. They may also want to protect their loved ones from having to make painful or scary decisions. Because of this, it may not seem like they are listening sometimes.

ANGELA: Yes, that sounds like my husband.

BETTY: And family members are often feeling pretty helpless in these situations. After all, facing a diagnosis is scary, and dealing with hospitals and medical professionals is a new experience. And so they worry about everything and, when something doesn't seem to be going right, like when you found Logan sleeping this morning, they want to jump in and make any changes they can think of to try and make everything better. Does that make sense?

ANGELA: Yes, I understand what you're saying.

BETTY: Then I have a couple of suggestions. You might have a talk with your husband about how you're feeling and see how you can work together better. Also, it's important for you to have support while you go through this. We have a counselor on staff who I could ask to get in touch with you, if you think you might want to talk to him.

ANGELA: I appreciate your concern. I'll give all of this some thought.

CHARLOTTE: Why don't I walk back to Logan's room with you? I need to give him his evening meds.

Guidelines for Conversing with Family Members

Following are guidelines to consider when having discussions with family members about how to communicate with newly diagnosed patients:

1. *Clarify roles.* Clarify the roles of the health-care professionals involved in the conversation. This is especially important when more than one health-care professional is present.

2. *Clarify the issue.* Begin the conversations with common understandings of the issues from the perspective of the family members, as well as the patients if they are involved in the conversations. This way, everyone involved in the conversation knows the purposes of the discussions and the concerns being addressed. Most likely, Charlotte had given Betty an accurate description of Angela's expectations. However, by asking Angela to repeat her request for Charlotte to talk to her husband, as well as what Angela hoped to gain from this request, Betty was able to speak directly about Angela's expectations, and Angela was better able to receive the message.

3. *Keep everyone involved.* While health-care professionals in supervisory roles, like Betty, may be called on to facilitate conversations like these, all who play roles with the family members and/or patients should contribute to the conversations. Betty asked Charlotte if she had any comments. Given that Charlotte was more involved with Angela than Betty had been, this was a sign of respect for Charlotte, as a professional, as well as an acknowledgement to Angela that Betty understood the relationship between Angela and Charlotte.

4. *Normalize the situation.* Family members, like patients, can benefit from being told that their expectations and concerns are normal. Family members may feel that health-care professionals fail to understand them or that they should be feeling or reacting differently. Reassuring family members that their reactions are normal serves both to validate their feelings—especially feelings of helplessness—as well as communicate that the health-care professionals have experience with their situations and are therefore able to offer appropriate guidance. Betty reassured Angela that she and the other professionals working on the floor were experienced with family members under stress and that she understood how Angela was feeling. Later in the conversation, Betty also acknowledged Angela's frustrations regarding Logan's sedation.

5. *Stay tentative.* Family members are feeling helpless and are fearful about the patient's well-being. Given that emotions are fragile, they may react strongly to the perception that the health-care professionals are somehow "ganging up" on them. Therefore, professionals should remain **tentative**. Betty showed sensitivity to Angela's emotional state by asking her permission to discuss other family members' experiences and to offer suggestions. Had Angela felt that Betty was attempting to dictate a solution, she most likely would have reacted defensively, and the conversation would have been unproductive.

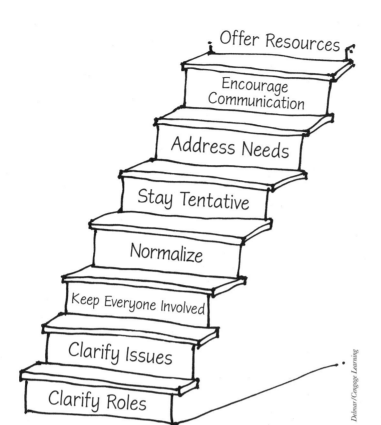

Offer Resources

Encourage Communication

Address Needs

Stay Tentative

Normalize

Keep Everyone Involved

Clarify Issues

Clarify Roles

Delmar/Cengage Learning

6. *Address the immediate need.*　One situation may cause family members to generalize negative feelings to greater issues. Recall that Angela was concerned about whether her husband was being treated by the right oncologist. As an example of what she viewed as poor care, she related that she had arrived by her husband's bedside in the morning and assumed that he had been heavily sedated. As the supervising nurse, Betty assured Angela that she would look into how her husband's nighttime sedative was being administered. This answered Angela's immediate concern and was within Betty's responsibilities to address.

7. *Encourage communication.*　Patients and family members will at some point need to communicate better. While health-care providers may be unable to facilitate that communication, they can help by offering encouragement.

8. *Offer resources.*　Whenever possible, health-care professionals should offer family members resources that might provide added relief. Betty knew of resources for family members at the hospital and opened the door for Angela to learn more about them.

SUMMARY

When a family member is ill, the whole family is affected. Emotions like fear, sadness, anger, and helplessness can greatly stress family members, and often, the communication between family members and patients suffers. When patients and family members work together, treatment decision making, compliance, mental health, and other aspects of the patient's treatment and ongoing care are enhanced. Health-care professionals can play a role in improving the communication between patients and family members.

Chapter REVIEW

Multiple-Choice Questions

1. When one family member is diagnosed with a medical condition, all family members "get sick" because:
   a. Illness conjures strong emotions for patients and their loved ones
   b. Other family members may have to assume new household responsibilities
   c. Family members must help patients make treatment decisions
   d. All of the above

2. Family members are especially likely to have to make treatment decisions for patients in _____ reaction.
   a. Flight
   b. Freeze
   c. Fight
   d. None of the above

3. A patient in _____ reaction may want no input or support from family members, which may cause conflict.
   a. Flight
   b. Freeze
   c. Fight
   d. None of the above

4. When the family members of newly diagnosed patients avoid talking about their feelings, health-care professionals can help by:
   a. Encouraging family members to focus on the patients for the short term
   b. Reminding family members that everyone is affected by a patient's illness
   c. Encouraging family members to help the patients keep a positive attitude
   d. Reminding family members that getting too emotional will prevent them from giving care effectively

5. When family members become concerned about patients to the point that they focus totally on the patients' illnesses and not the patients' ability to care for themselves, health-care professionals can enhance communication by saying:
   a. "She can't do much for herself, so just handle it for her."
   b. "Why don't we get together and talk about what everyone's role is going to be?"
   c. "Don't treat her like a sick person."
   d. "It would be easier on everyone if you didn't confuse him with more decisions to make."

Fill-in-the-Blank Questions

1. A family member's attempt to become overly involved in patient decisions or avoidance of discussing the diagnosis may both be motivated by _____.

2. Gently telling a family member that feeling sad or angry when a loved one is diagnosed with an illness may help to _____ the person's reactions.

3. Family members who were expecting worse diagnoses than patients receive may feel a sense of _____.

4. Caregivers who pay no attention to their own _____ _____ are at risk for burnout.

5. _____ and _____ are two emotions both newly diagnosed patients and their family members experience as they consider the changes they may soon be facing.

Short-Answer Questions

1. Just as a newly diagnosed patient asks "Why me?" family members may ask "Why us?" What motivates the family's question?

_____

_____

_____

2. When family members encourage patients to "think positive," how do patients tend to react?

_____

_____

_____

3. What causes a patient's family to begin viewing the patient as a "medical condition" and not as a whole person?

_____

_____

_____

4. What does it mean for patients and families to treat each other with compassion?

_____

_____

_____

5. A family member who demands that the patient "do something for himself" is most likely experiencing what emotions?

_____

_____

_____

Critical-Thinking Questions

1. Newly diagnosed patients and their families avoid discussing the "elephant in the room," which is an expression for the uncomfortable feelings they may be sharing, including helplessness and fear. How does culture impact the willingness of family members to discuss their feelings? For example, are some ethnic groups in the United States more likely to be straightforward than others? Do people in different regions of the country exhibit differences?

_____

_____

_____

_____

_____

_____

2. Witnessing patients and family members experience conflict can remind health-care professionals of their own family issues. What is the best way for health-care professionals to protect themselves from losing their objectivity and not becoming overly involved when they are having their own strong emotional reactions? Is this something professionals can avoid? What is the best way to deal with these feelings when they arise?

_____

_____

_____

_____

_____

_____

3. Health-care professionals often advise family members that if they pay no attention to their own care, they will experience burnout and become less effective caregivers. What can family members, who may have daily responsibilities for caring for their loved ones, do to care for themselves? How can health-care professionals set an example for family members?

_____

_____

_____

_____

_____

_____

Internet Exercise

Using the Internet, identify online resources that offer support for the family members and caregivers of patients facing health challenges. Consider the issues that may arise, including respite care, emotional conflicts, finances, legal problems, communication inside and outside the health-care system, and relationships with partners and children. Look for sites that might provide information and guidance, as well as community resources that might offer support to family members and caregivers.

   If you were going to provide a patient's family members or other caregivers with resources, which ones would you recommend? Why?

_____

_____

_____

_____

_____

_____

_____

_____

CHAPTER 12

Creating a Vision
for the Future

OVERVIEW

After reading this chapter, you should be able to:

- Define and use the keywords of creating a vision for the future.

- Understand how a medical diagnosis can affect a patient's vision of the future.

- Know when it is appropriate for health-care professionals to intervene with patients who have bleak future outlooks.

- Explain how to help newly diagnosed patients express feelings of fear and helplessness.

- Discuss how to identify either-or thinking for patients, and encourage them to consider alternate views.

- Describe how accurate information and emotional support provide a foundation for reassessing the future realistically and hopefully.

- Identify the outside resources that would most benefit patients and know when to recommend them.

- Understand the relationship between an optimistic vision of the future and compliance as a basis for encouraging patients to remain compliant.

- Know how to converse effectively with newly diagnosed patients who are doubting the future.

Assumptions   Either-or thinking   Uncertainty

Distraught   Role model   Vision for the future

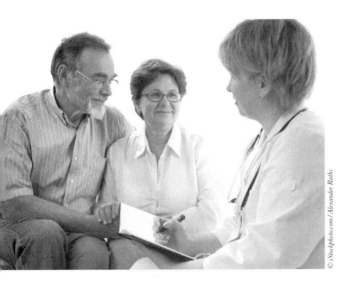

© iStockphoto.com / Alexander Raths

Case Study

Rosalie and her husband, Bob, had their dream vacation all planned. They had been saving for a cruise to Alaska, which would begin with a flight to Seattle, their cruise departure point. This was the first cruise for the couple, but they were hoping to take more and do other traveling when they retired in 10 years. Bob often joked that, when they finally retired, they would spend their time visiting their children who, by then, would be spread throughout the country.

Bob and Rosalie's vision for the future changed when Rosalie's physician informed her that, due to her pulmonary hypertension, it was not safe for her to fly for the foreseeable future, at least until her physician was certain her medication regimen was effective and her condition was stabilized. Bob was with Rosalie when her physician delivered the news. True to form, Bob tried to be as upbeat as possible, telling his wife that this would be an excuse for him to buy an SUV and a camper or for the two of them to take a train. "After all," Bob comforted, "we won't be in a hurry anyway."

> **KEEP IN MIND**
>
> Newly diagnosed patients may feel as if their plans for the future are completely out of their reach. If you were a newly diagnosed patient, how might a medical diagnosis impact your vision for the future? How does this phenomenon impact your responsibilities as a health-care professional?

For Bob, Rosalie tried to stay upbeat, but when she was alone later with Sammy, one of the medical assistants at the clinic, her attitude deteriorated.

"I feel like my future is suddenly up for grabs," Rosalie admitted resignedly. "I have no idea what to expect."

She told Sammy about how she and her husband had planned for years to take the cruise to Alaska. For years, the couple had actively explored nature, and they wanted to visit as many different parts of the world as possible. The trip to Alaska was only supposed to be the beginning.

To Sammy, Rosalie worried about how her diagnosis would affect Bob. He had been counting on Rosalie to be his partner in these adventures, and they had extensively researched places to visit and identified relatively low-cost ways to travel. The two of them had even made a list of places to visit and had started to think in terms of an overall travel schedule. They thought, for example, that they would spend their 30th wedding anniversary in the Amazon rain forest.

While Rosalie had had a long history of high blood pressure—her mother had also had it—she had not realized her condition had worsened until she began to have some of the symptoms her mother had experienced. Her recent diagnosis had confirmed her worst fears.

"This is a big disappointment to you, Rosalie," Sammy started. "And I know this is difficult. Do you want to talk about it after I finish with your lab work?"

"I'm not sure what there is to say at this point," Rosalie answered. "I think the doctor has already said it all. There's not much to look forward to at this point."

Sammy knew that Rosalie was going to need to be motivated to stay healthy if she was going to stay on top of her condition. That would mean watching her diet, maintaining a moderate activity level, and being consistently compliant with her medication regimen. A defeated attitude would render Rosalie less likely to be actively involved in her health care. The health-care team, for its part, would need to be able to depend on Rosalie to monitor herself and report any concerns that come up.

"Can I talk to you about a few things?" Sammy asked.

Introduction

"My future has been taken from me."

Previous chapters discussed the questions newly diagnosed patients have about their future. Patients worry about their treatments and how those treatments will affect them. They fear that they will have to change their daily lives in ways that will seem abnormal. They also worry about how their personal relationships will change moving forward. Chapter 10 described the spiritual crisis newly diagnosed patients may experience, prompting them to question the meaning of life and destiny.

This chapter discusses patients' visions of the future from a practical perspective. It is human nature to have a vision for the future—its successes, relationships, and activities. Unfortunately, medical diagnoses can make those visions feel uncertain or limited. Eventually, patients' **assumptions** about their futures may give way to an overwhelming sense of helplessness and loss.

When newly diagnosed patients feel they have no future, they lack the motivation to comply with treatment, which affects the ability of health-care professionals to provide them the best care. Health-care professionals can help patients by encouraging them to gather accurate information about their conditions and how those conditions may affect their future. Further, professionals should prompt patients to use the information they have gained to consider realistic alternatives.

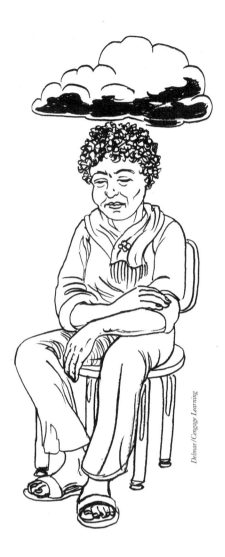

Delmar/Cengage Learning

Melding a Medical Diagnosis with a Vision for the Future

A medical diagnosis's effect on a newly diagnosed patient's **vision for the future** really begins and ends with the patient. Patients' reactions to their diagnoses are one factor shaping their forward views. Some patients are simply more able than others to handle the changes diagnoses bring. Like reactions, patients' expectations for treatment impact their projections for normalcy moving forward. Whether diagnoses are chronic, acute, or catastrophic also helps shape patients' views of their future.

WORKING WITH HOPES, DREAMS, AND ASSUMPTIONS

All people have visions for their future, even if they do not think of them as visions and even if the visions are less than positive. It is human nature, though, to envision a future of success, prosperity, and a happy home life surrounded by friends and family. To assume that this is possible simply by doing the "right things" is only natural.

Most newly diagnosed patients view their future optimistically but realistically, reflecting the belief that they will be able to continue their current activities, jobs, and relationships with family and friends. Basically, patients tend to base their visions of the future on the assumption that life will go on as it has been, that changes arising

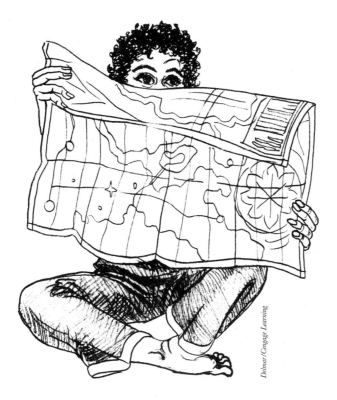

Delmar/Cengage Learning

from diagnoses will be minor, and, if changes do occur, that they will be, for the most part, controllable.

WEATHERING A CRISIS OF MEANING WITH PRACTICAL QUESTIONS

Newly diagnosed patients often describe their assumptions about the future as just that: assumptions. They realize that their future is not going to be exactly as they had planned. As discussed in Chapter 10, which focuses on meaning and spirituality, a medical diagnosis can suddenly introduce the ideas that the future may not necessarily unfold as expected and that life is uncertain. Patients may question what their future will be like, how they will change, and, in some cases, whether they will have a future at all. For most, these questions inspire spiritual crises, crises of meaning.

From a practical perspective, newly diagnosed patients must be able to reassess their visions of the future. Medication regimens, lifestyle management needs, and, possibly, the progressions of their conditions may require patients to modify their hopes and plans. Health-care professionals may find themselves helping patients address both questions about the meaning of life and questions of practical application of treatments.

FOCUSING ON THE "NUTS AND BOLTS" OF THE FUTURE

Health-care professionals can help newly diagnosed patients hone their visions of the future by focusing on the ways in which the patients' diagnoses may or may not affect short and long term daily life. Practical, medical considerations—the "nuts and bolts" of the future—will help determine which aspects of patients' visions for the future can stay and which must change. By focusing on practical issues, health-care professionals can encourage patients to view the future with informed, realistic, and optimistic attitudes.

Helping Patients Cope with Uncertainty about the Future

Newly diagnosed patients sometimes directly express that they feel they have no future or have visions of the future that are changing for the worse. More likely, however, patients express bleak attitudes toward the future through such body language as downcast eyes, slumped posture, or faces covered with the hands. Health-care professionals can help patients turn this thinking around by offering alternate viewpoints when they recognize warning signs like these.

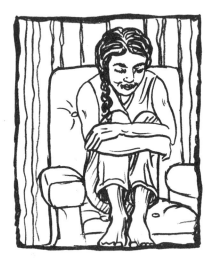 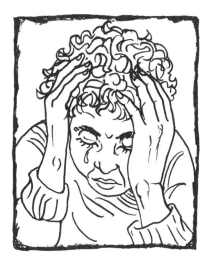 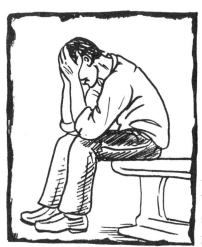

Delmar/Cengage Learning

CONFRONTING THE FEAR FACTOR: JAYDEN'S STORY

When Jayden received his diagnosis of non-Hodgkins lymphoma, he was overcome by fears about his treatment, the effects on his family, and his future. He was still in the process of establishing his small business, and he dreamt of growing it much larger to provide a secure future for his family. While Jayden's health-care team was able to help him cope with his treatment and his family showed him they could work together to keep his business going during treatment, Jayden doubted what he could expect in the future.

> *"It scared me so much to find out that I was sick. All I could think about was how afraid I was. I had so many plans for the future. But after my diagnosis, the future seemed to fade into a big patch of darkness. I was so scared I couldn't bring myself to think about what might still be possible and what might be different. It seemed like I wouldn't have anything I wanted."*

Intervening with the fear factor. Newly diagnosed patients may think they should lack fear, face their diagnoses optimistically, and take charge of their future. Alternatively, they may give into their fear to the extent that they assume that the best they can do is to admit defeat and accept their fate.

Of course, health-care professionals cannot promise newly diagnosed patients that their diagnoses will not change their future. They can, however, help patients by identifying the patients' fears about their diagnoses, normalizing their fear responses, and providing some education.

KEEP IN MIND

Health-care professionals can help newly diagnosed patients greatly by focusing on the practical considerations of diagnosis and treatment. What practical concerns might patients want answered while redefining their visions of the future?

"Jayden, I know your diagnosis is totally unexpected, something you never thought would happen. It's normal to feel scared, and it's also normal to fear that your future is not going to be anything like you planned. Patients newly diagnosed like you often have the same fears about the future. But I can tell you from experience that, as they begin to deal with their diagnoses day to day, and get informed, they better understand what their conditions will mean moving forward. The unknown can be scary. Knowledge is power, though, and can take some of that fear away."

IDENTIFYING THE EFFECTS OF HOPELESSNESS: ISABELLA'S STORY

Isabella could not explain why, or when, she had concluded that she had, in her words, "very little future." When she first received the diagnosis of a tumor in her nasal system, she was so unfamiliar with her diagnosis that she had no idea how it might affect her life. Most likely, her perception of her future changed when she learned that the extensive surgery she would need would change her appearance. Isabella had hoped for a future that would include a husband and children, but now, with facial disfiguration ahead, she felt it was useless to even try to find a life partner.

"All my plans had revolved around building a nice life for myself, including a career and family. I was dating, and, I felt, meeting guys who might be good husbands. Might in the future. Or might not, at this point. It seems like trying to find a man who would want to marry someone who doesn't look normal, and who clearly has had health problems, is an impossible dream. Who would want to take on all those problems? It all seems hopeless right now."

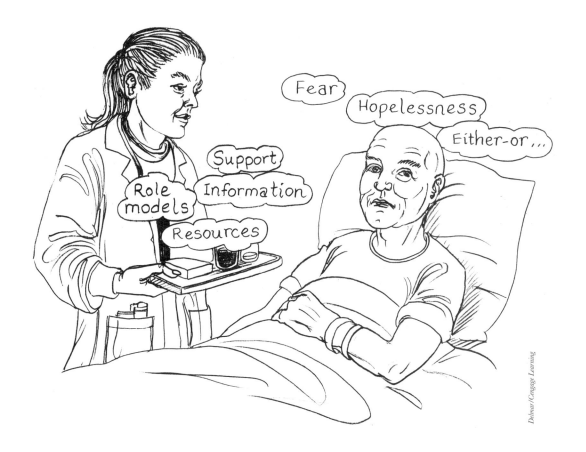

Intervening with hopelessness.   Because she anticipates being unattractive after her surgery, Isabella has decided that she will not find someone to build a home and family with. When newly diagnosed patients view their future as hopeless, as Isabella does, health-care professionals should get them to acknowledge their hopelessness, normalize the feeling, and offer suggestions and information. Reminding patients that many newly diagnosed patients feel hopeless about the future can be particularly helpful in encouraging patients to change their worldviews.

> *"Isabella, I can understand why the future may look hopeless to you right now. It's normal to wonder how people are going to react to changes in your appearance after the surgery and to think that it's going to be impossible to find a man who wants to be with you. Other patients in your situation have felt the same way. But I would encourage you to stay open-minded about the future and to not assume the worst. Let's take this one day at a time."*

EXPLAINING THE EFFECT OF EITHER-OR THINKING: BARBARA'S STORY

Barbara had intended to leave the business world in her fifties and go back to college to get a degree in social work. She wanted to do something that would give her an opportunity to contribute to her community in a new way. However, a few months before she was to begin her studies, she received an unexpected medical diagnosis of ovarian cancer. Her physician recommended that she stay in her job for the near future, because it provided excellent health benefits and would allow her to go on disability during her lengthy recovery. Her physician candidly told Barbara that she did not think she would have the energy to undertake college at this point or to start a new

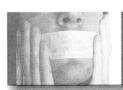

SELF • talk

Following are examples of negative self-talk about the future:

I have no future. I have nothing left to live for.

I had everything planned exactly as I wanted it to be, and now it has all blown up in my face.

If I can't give my loved ones what they need, what good will I be?

I worked so hard to build for my future, and it's been taken from me.

I have no idea what's going to happen to me.

Antidotes to negative self-talk about the future include the following:

The future is not going to be what I had envisioned, but I still have a lot to live for.

What's important is the people I love, and they are going to see this through with me, no matter what.

Life is an adventure, and I'm going to see where my path will take me.

I'm determined to make the best of my situation and create the best future possible.

No one gets to say exactly what their future will be like. All I see ahead of me is possibilities.

career in the near future. Barbara reacted with sadness and frustration and felt like her future had been taken from her.

> *"I've been ready to move on to my new career for the last few years and was waiting until I had fully vested in my pension plan and had saved enough money to go to school full time. I was preparing to close this chapter in my life and move forward into achieving what I really wanted at this point in my life. My whole future was about being a social worker and helping people. Now I feel like this has all been taken away. I can hang on to a career that I have outgrown for as long as I can physically and emotionally stand to, or I can go on disability. That is not a future."*

Intervening with either-or thinking.   As implied in the discussion of fear and helplessness, stress, like that accompanying medical diagnoses, tends to inspire **either-or thinking**, or thinking in extremes. It follows, then, that newly diagnosed patients often see their future in black-or-white or either-or terms. They focus on one extreme or the other without considering that there may be middle ground in between, with other possibilities. Instead of considering other career options, Barbara assumed that if she could not pursue a social work career she would achieve no success in the work world.

Health-care professionals can help combat either-or thinking by pointing out the thinking pattern to patients, suggesting that the patients consider other possibilities, and offering to discuss some of those possibilities with the patients. As it is with many patient reactions, normalizing patient feelings is important.

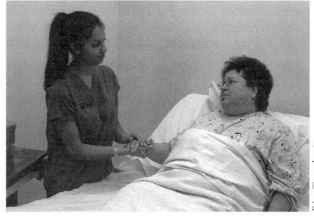

> *"Barbara, I know your diagnosis is a shock to you and that it feels like your future has now become out of reach. I've talked to other newly diagnosed patients who felt the same way. From what you told me about your plans, it sounds like you were hoping to reach out to people in need in your community. Would you like to brainstorm some other ways to do that while you see how your recovery goes? Taking some time to talk this through with someone might help you see that you have some other options."*

EMPHASIZING THE IMPORTANCE OF ACCURATE INFORMATION: ADAM'S STORY

When Adam received his diagnosis of liver disease, a nurse practitioner, Mark, talked to him about his treatment and how his life might be affected. Mark gave Adam some information to read, but Adam did not read it because thought he knew all he needed to know after recently seeing a documentary about someone with his condition. While he did not remember all the details of the program, he did remember that the man featured in it had a poor prognosis. In fact, the man's health had declined rapidly despite treatment. Adam did not tell Mark that he had seen the program, which was always on his mind in the days following his diagnosis.

> *"I knew all I needed to know. I'd watched a man about my age in this documentary who had received the same diagnosis. They showed what his life was like after his diagnosis, and I can tell you he didn't have much of a future at all. He went downhill so fast, you wouldn't believe it. I remembered his story, so I decided that maybe the best thing for me to do was to just give up so I wouldn't be disappointed."*

Intervening when information may be incomplete or inaccurate. As discussed in Chapter 7, newly diagnosed patients are often so overwhelmed by their diagnoses that they have difficulty processing information. Consequently, they may have no understanding of their diagnoses or, like Adam, they may be basing their understanding on incomplete or biased information. As discussed previously, when lacking information, it is human nature to complete the story with assumptions and worst-case scenarios. The stories that newly diagnosed patients create around their diagnoses often extend into the future, distorting the visions of what lies ahead.

Health-care professionals can be most helpful to newly diagnosed patients in this situation by helping them increase their information, beginning with understanding what patients know or think they know and how they received their information. Physicians or other members of the health-care team can offer additional perspectives. In essence, health-care professionals should "fill the gaps" for their patients.

> *"Adam, I know you saw a documentary about someone with your condition and that made you feel like your future was pretty bleak. But can I offer an additional perspective? You saw one patient's story. You were not necessarily shown what every patient experiences. A lot of factors are involved in determining how a medical condition affects one patient versus how another patient experiences it."*

RECOGNIZING THE VALUE OF SUPPORT: EDEN'S STORY

Eden's medical diagnosis completely changed her future. Plans for working overseas, and the social and career opportunities that would follow, would have to be put aside so she could be close to the medical center where she was being treated for heart disease. Eden's physician had advised her to remain in the area for at least the next year, and possibly beyond, so the health-care team could closely monitor her condition. Even if her situation improved, Eden doubted that a similar opportunity would be available again. If it did, she did not know whether she would feel strong enough to accept it. Eden felt like her future had been taken away her.

> *"I looked around my hospital room and said to myself, 'You're going to be spending a lot of time in rooms like this, trying to stay ahead of this medical condition that has already taken your future.' I felt like I was at Square 1 in my life, with no place to go but farther down. It seemed like I was left alone to face all of this."*

Intervening when patients are isolating themselves. Newly diagnosed patients like Eden benefit from knowing that they have support systems they can rely on to face the future. While Eden may be unable to pursue her plans as she had imagined them before her diagnosis, knowing that she has a caring support system behind her can help her gain some perspective of the life she has ahead.

Educational Moment

Embracing Grief and Change

A medical diagnosis is like a death in that plans and expectations cease to exist in their former states. As a result, patients may grieve the loss of their future. Health-care professionals are responsible for helping patients accept their loss and encouraging them to consider what may be possible looking ahead. The goal is to change the focus from loss to possibilities.

Health-care professionals can encourage patients like Eden to open themselves to the possibility of support by first reminding them of the value of being supported. As they adjust to their diagnoses and begin revising their visions of the future, health-care professionals can help them recognize the people in their lives who can travel with them on their journeys.

"Eden, I know this is a setback for you. The future doesn't look at all like it did before your diagnosis. But you're definitely not alone. You have people in your life who want to be there for you while you go through your treatment and who will stand by you as you face the future. Can you think of yourself as someone with a future that includes a lot of people who care about you?"

KEEP IN MIND

Patients who are in treatment or have completed it can help newly diagnosed patients struggling with what to expect in their future. What messages from experienced patients would most help newly diagnosed patients? Why? As a health-care professional, what is your role, if any, in delivering messages like these?

INTRODUCING ROLE MODELS: ENZO'S STORY

Enzo could not imagine facing the rest of his life. In addition to major changes in his daily life—limited activities, a changed diet, modified bathroom routines—his treatment for a serious bowel inflammation was going to require extensive surgery, including a colostomy. In short, the adjustments his health-care team had shared with him were overwhelming. He had never heard of anyone having to make the changes he would. If they had, he thought, they were hiding them, which is exactly what he planned to do.

" 'How was a guy supposed to live like this?' I asked myself. How would I be able to respect myself, and who else would respect me? I felt like I was going to have to go into hiding to avoid being embarrassed. If anybody found out what I was dealing with, I would feel like some kind of a freak. I wanted to go to a desert island and stay there."

Intervening with a patient in need of a role model.   Newly diagnosed patients commonly fear how their diagnoses will affect their daily lives. While health-care professionals can help allay patients' fears about their future by providing objective information and describing the experiences of other patients, patients' emotional needs may go unfulfilled. They may listen selectively, fail to comprehend fully, and fill any gaps with assumptions, good and bad.

Exposure to patients with the same conditions, who are coping with the same challenges and limitations but moving forward with the future, can be invaluable for newly diagnosed patients. Enzo had assumed the worst about his future in part because he lacked experience with other patients with his condition. As **role models** for new patients, experienced patients can answer questions about their personal experiences, talk honestly about their challenges, and provide their own perspectives on the future. The closer new and established patients are in age, diagnosis, and background, the more valuable the modeling experience. Support groups often provide speakers' bureaus or buddy systems with experienced patients who are willing to reach out to new ones.

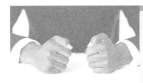

Body Language

Newly diagnosed patients may reflect their **uncertainty** or hopelessness in body language that includes the following:

- Sad facial expression or lack of expression
- Staring
- Crying
- Slumped or stiff posture

"Enzo, we have other patients in the practice who are also being treated for your condition and who might have a lot in common with you. Some of them meet each Tuesday evening in the office where I lead a support group. It might help to meet a couple of them and learn about how they are coping with their conditions. If you're interested, you're welcome to join us. Of course, we would protect your confidentiality. Think about it, and let me know."

REFERRING TO OUTSIDE RESOURCES: BREE'S STORY

Bree was initially upbeat after receiving her diagnosis. She was not looking forward to the treatment she would need, but she assumed the process would be similar to her friend's, who had been diagnosed with the same thing. Certainly, Bree did not look forward to her treatment, but she felt she could handle it.

After giving Bree some time to deal with her news, her physician sat down with her to talk specifically about what she would face going forward. As the two talked, Bree realized that her situation was much different from her friend's. Not only would her treatment be much more extensive, her future was uncertain. Initially optimistic, Bree now felt like she had received a death sentence.

"I didn't see how I was going to go on. In the blink of an eye, as they say, my future turned from hopeful to hopeless. Forget being around to see my grandchildren graduate from high school. I wasn't sure if I was going to see my daughter complete the third grade. I told myself that I needed to put one foot in front of the other and do whatever I needed to, but I wasn't sure if I could even walk to my car and drive home. My vision of the future had turned from bright to dark and foggy."

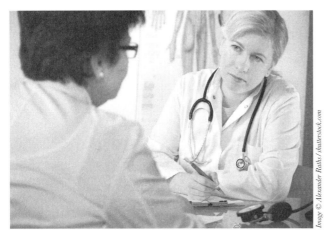

Image © Alexander Raths / shutterstock.com

Intervening when outside resources are needed. Newly diagnosed patients like Bree may need more than encouragement and suggestions to change their visions of the future. Some may need the support of mental-health professionals. Bree might have benefited from a referral to a mental-health professional or to a support center focused on her condition. Treatment centers and hospitals may offer patients additional support services.

If patients like Bree do not receive the mental-health support they need, they may feel so hopeless about their future that they either fail to follow through on treatment recommendations or do so only halfheartedly. In the worst cases, patients become self-destructive. Recall that health-care professionals can play critical roles in recognizing extreme hopelessness in patients and making appropriate referrals. To review guidelines for mental-health referrals, see Chapter 3.

> *"Bree, I can see that you're really feeling discouraged about your future right now. I would like to talk to you about some resources that we're familiar with that offer counseling services. We've referred other patients to them, and those patients have reported that they received the help they needed. I'd like to give you this information and encourage you to follow up. I'll help you make the connection if you need me to. What do you think?"*

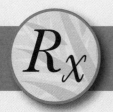

Discussing the Future with Newly Diagnosed Patients

Rosalie, the hypertension patient whose case was discussed at the beginning of the chapter, had learned from her physician that her condition would restrict her from air travel. Because she and her husband, Bob, had planned to travel extensively once they retired, Rosalie felt that her medical condition had robbed her of her future. She talked with Sammy, one of the medical assistants at her clinic.

SAMMY: Rosalie, you look really upset about this. I remember you'd been talking about your upcoming trip to Alaska.

ROSALIE: You mean my formerly upcoming trip? I don't know if I'm ever going to be able to leave town again, except to maybe drive an hour away or so, assuming that that's not going to make me feel dizzy or send my blood pressure skyrocketing. Who knew my condition was this bad?

SAMMY: What's your understanding of what the doctor told you about travel?

ROSALIE: Basically, he told me that my condition is under control but that flying was a bad idea for the time being, if not always. Right now, he wants to focus on keeping me stable. I understand that. The last thing I want is a stroke or heart attack. But I didn't know that trying to stay healthy could be so boring. And look what it's doing to my husband. He wanted this as much as I did!

SAMMY: It feels like your future is out of your control right now and that you can't do much about it.

ROSALIE: Exactly. I had all these plans. But as of today, I think maybe I don't have any control at all.

SAMMY: Well, it's always scary not to be in control. But it sounds like you realize that your doctor wants to keep you as healthy as possible, and that means managing your hypertension.

ROSALIE: Oh, yes, I know that. I watched what hypertension did to my mother's health.

SAMMY: Of course. But you know, Rosalie, I'm also hearing you say that if you aren't going to be able to travel by air, you don't have any future at all. Am I right?

ROSALIE: Exactly. That's exactly what it feels like.

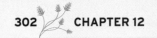

SAMMY: I don't know a lot about travel, but I'm wondering if there might be some kind of middle ground here, maybe some ways to do some trips that don't require air travel but that might still be fun. I'd be happy to brainstorm with you, just to get you started, if you think that might be helpful.

ROSALIE: If your first idea is to walk, I'm going to have to say no. I mean, it's a long walk to Alaska.

At that, Sammy and Rosalie both laughed.

SAMMY: I can't argue that. But to get the brainstorming started, I wanted to remind you that you said your husband was considering driving or taking a train.

ROSALIE: Yes, but that's not what we had planned and, to be honest, it doesn't sound like much fun.

SAMMY: I understand. Still, is it possible that you and your husband could do some investigating about car and train travel and find some opportunities that might be fun?

ROSALIE: I guess anything is possible.

SAMMY: Great. If you want to toss around other ideas sometime, let me know. You might also want to see if your husband wants to do some strategizing with you. You know that expression, "Think outside the box."

ROSALIE: Not a bad idea, Sammy.

SAMMY: And if you don't mind, I have another idea.

ROSALIE: Okay.

SAMMY: We have a lot of patients being treated at the clinic who are also dealing with lifestyle changes to accommodate their hypertension. We have an informal support group that meets on Tuesday evenings. Would you be interested in checking it out sometime? You might pick up some useful ideas. One of the staff members also attends and can answer any questions that come up. You and your husband would both be welcome.

ROSALIE: You know, it might help to talk to a few other patients. I'll ask Bob if he's interested.

SAMMY: Well, I just want to congratulate you on taking action on your hypertension by coming in to see the doctor and getting your treatment under way. Not everybody is willing to do that because they don't want to hear the bad news or find out they have to make changes in their lives. As the doctor said, if you stay with the program, you'll have a much better chance of staying healthy.

ROSALIE: Don't I know that!

Guidelines for Talking about the Future

1. *Acknowledge feelings of helplessness.* As discussed previously, helplessness is a major source of distress for newly diagnosed patients. Further, helpless feelings can distort patients' views of the future. Patients may think their future will be unrecognizable or nonexistent. Patients may be so inconsolable that their health-care professionals will be unable to comfort them. Family members are not usually good sounding boards, because they are addressing their own feelings of helplessness. The best health-care professionals can do is create environments in which patients feel safe admitting to, and talking about, their helplessness. Once they do, patients will often feel relieved and more normal. Sammy began the preceding conversation by acknowledging that Rosalie was feeling out of control.

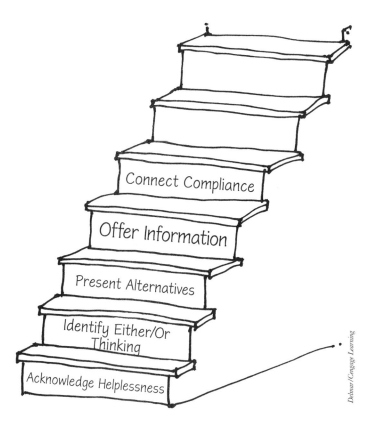

Delmar/Cengage Learning

2. ***Point out either-or thinking.*** Sammy gently pointed out to Rosalie that she was assuming that if she could not fly she could not travel with her husband. Since her vision of the future revolved around travel, she had concluded that she might have no future. As part of patients' support systems, health-care professionals may need to offer their patients balanced perspectives. While patients may not be ready to accept this feedback, recognizing self-defeating attitudes is a step toward expanding the vision of the future.

3. ***Invite patients to consider alternatives.*** Newly diagnosed patients who are overwhelmed by fear and helplessness may be closed to alternate versions of their future. They may be so invested in their views that they will reject any alternatives they sense are being forced on them. Instead of forcing issues, health-care professionals should invite patients to consider alternatives in collaborative discussions. Such an approach has two main benefits. First, it introduces the possibility of reexamining and redefining the future. Second, it can kick-start the acceptance process. In the example, Sammy did not in any way demand that Rosalie consider alternatives. Instead, she suggested that there might be a middle ground that Rosalie should consider. To solidify their partnership, she offered to help her brainstorm options. In essence, Sammy planted the seed that Rosalie could still have a future, albeit a different one than the one she had envisioned.

4. ***Emphasize the value of staying informed.*** A realistic vision of the future is based on reliable and accurate information. By being informed, newly diagnosed patients create visions that take into account the day-to-day responsibilities and challenges of their medical conditions, including any

potential complications. When patients are not completely informed, they fill the gaps with fears and assumptions. While accurate information can scare patients, it may encourage them to accurately understand their conditions and future. In the case example, Sammy encouraged Rosalie to attend a support group that would provide both accurate information and emotional support.

5. ***Connect the vision with compliance and wellness.*** The connection points between the health-care professional and the newly diagnosed patient's vision of the future are compliance and wellness. In other words, the goal is to promote the patient's realistic and optimistic attitude regarding the future. For health-care professionals, this type of attitude helps ensure that patients stay motivated to comply with their treatments and lifestyle adjustments. Professionals can nurture this connection by promoting hopeful visions. In the case example, Sammy gently reminded Rosalie of the importance of taking care of herself and reinforced her behavior by complimenting her for taking charge of her health care. In closing, she reminded her that it was important to "stay with the program."

SUMMARY

Newly diagnosed patients often react to their diagnoses by questioning their future. Many times, they see their future as differing from their visions and therefore non-existent. Health-care professionals should be particularly vigilant to these types of patients, because they may feel it is futile to comply with medication regimens and lifestyle adjustments. Professionals can help patients better understand how their diagnoses may affect their day-to-day lives and encourage them to consider alternatives. The goal is a realistic, but optimistic, view of the future.

Multiple-Choice Questions

1. Newly diagnosed patients question the future in terms of:
   a. Relationship changes
   b. Lifestyle changes
   c. Effects of treatment and medications
   d. All of the above

2. Newly diagnosed patients who feel they have no future if that future cannot be as they had envisioned it demonstrate _____ thinking.
   a. Superstitious
   b. Either-or
   c. Magical
   d. Confused

3. Newly diagnosed patients with inaccurate or incomplete information about their conditions may do which of the following?
   a. Fill information gaps on their own
   b. Process no information
   c. Both a and b
   d. None of the above

4. A patient with a bleak outlook on the future might find which of the following resources particularly helpful?
   a. Home health care
   b. Physical therapy
   c. Mental-health counseling
   d. Housekeeping services

5. The fear of being unable to live life to its fullest is often based on:
   a. Helplessness
   b. Hopefulness
   c. Anger
   d. Sadness

Fill-in-the-Blank Questions

1. By focusing on practical issues, health-care professionals can help newly diagnosed patients have _____ _____ views of the future.

2. Helping patients be more optimistic about the future may involve facing the _____ factor.

3. It is human nature to fear _____, because we want to know exactly what we can expect day to day.

4. An experienced patient who has gone through treatment and is adjusting to change can serve as a(n) _____ _____ to a newly diagnosed patient who fears the future.

5. Fear of the future is often based on _____ about what life might be like rather than rational information.

Short-Answer Questions

1. What are some of the specific concerns newly diagnosed patients tend to have in terms of how their conditions might affect their future?

_____

_____

_____

_____

2. When discussing the future, what kind of body language may indicate that a newly diagnosed patient has a bleak attitude?

_____

_____

_____

_____

3. How would you discuss the potential need for mental-health counseling when talking with patients who feel they have no future?

_____

_____

_____

_____

4. How would you describe either-or thinking about the future to a patient?

_____

_____

_____

_____

5. What is the role of support in terms of helping patients be optimistic?

_____

_____

_____

_____

Critical-Thinking Questions

1. Ideally and realistically, how should newly diagnosed patients view their future? What is the best that patients can expect? Couch your answer in terms of a range of diagnoses.

_____

_____

_____

_____

_____

_____

_____

2. What are the pros and cons of withholding condition and treatment details as a means of fostering optimism in patients? When might this be the best approach?

_____

_____

_____

_____

_____

_____

_____

3. To encourage newly diagnosed patients to have broader views of the future, and thereby boost their attitudes, what aspects would you emphasize?

_____

_____

_____

_____

_____

_____

_____

Internet Exercise

Imagine working with patients with various diagnoses, such as cancer, diabetes, HIV, or fibromyalgia. Suppose that you wanted to help each of these patients understand that they can still have a future with their condition. For each condition, find Web sites that might help the patient see possibilities for life after diagnosis. Consider Web sites that discuss staying as active as possible, coping effectively with disease progression and treatment, leveraging inspirational role models, and other future-looking strategies.

What did you learn from the information on these Web sites? What information would be most beneficial to patients? Why?

CHAPTER 13

When Diagnoses Involve the End of Life

OVERVIEW

After reading this chapter, you should be able to:

- Define and use the keywords of end-of-life issues.

- Explain how health-care professionals can prepare themselves emotionally and intellectually to interact with newly diagnosed patients facing the end of their lives.

- Identify the ways in which newly diagnosed patients react to the news that their conditions are untreatable.

- Appreciate the value of being a compassionate listener for patients.

- Describe how patients' families and other loved ones react to the knowledge that the patients will not survive.

- Name the options for referring patients for additional end-of-life support.

- Give the guidelines for conversing with patients who are newly diagnosed with terminal conditions.

KEYWORDS

Agitation

Being present

End of life

Hospice

Listening ear

Palliative care

Terminal

Urgency

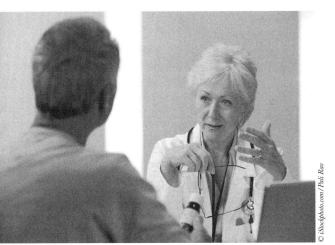

© iStockphoto.com / Pali Rao

Case Study

Marcus remembered that his oncologist, Dr. Martinez, had described his pancreatic cancer diagnosis as "one of the most lethal." After that, he remembered little, except that the physician had emphasized that she and the rest of the health-care team would do everything possible to keep him comfortable, and that he would survive at most another year.

At 42, that was one of the last things Marcus had expected to hear, especially when he was not feeling very sick. "Are you *sure* this is happening to me?" he had asked his doctor.

"I'm so sorry to have to give you this news," Dr. Martinez had answered. "But yes, I'm sure."

> ### KEEP IN MIND
>
> Being informed that they have untreatable medical conditions are likely the darkest moments patients experience. If you were one of these patients, what thoughts, images, and feelings do you think you would have? If you were a professional on one of these patients' health-care teams, how would you get started in preparing the right support?

After Dr. Martinez delivered Marcus's diagnosis, she sat with her patient to inform him of her plans for treating his cancer. She used words that were both familiar and frightening to Marcus, including "palliative care" and "hospice." Marcus tried to listen, but all he could think about was that his life was ending—much earlier than he had expected—and that he was afraid.

Before his diagnosis, Marcus was an attorney working in the public defender's office. He was active in his community. He was active in community theater and was spearheading an after-school mentoring program for inner-city children. As Dr. Martinez talked, Marcus could not help but wonder what would happen to the people who depended on him—his coworkers and his fellow community volunteers. It just did not seem fair.

"I'm prescribing some chemotherapy as part of your palliative care," Dr. Martinez said. "If you don't have any questions for me right now, I'd like to ask you to meet with our nurse who coordinates patient care, Ellen, and the IV therapist, Sarita. Would that be okay?"

"I guess," Marcus answered.

> **KEEP IN MIND**
>
> As a health-care professional, you could be called on to meet with a newly diagnosed patient whose condition is terminal. What concerns would you have as you prepared to meet with this patient? What would you want to be able to accomplish with this patient from both medical and emotional perspectives? What words would you have for your patient?

Sarita and Ellen entered the examination room where Marcus sat. They introduced themselves, and then sat across from him.

"How are you doing?" Sarita asked.

"Not so great today," Marcus responded. Instantly, he brought his hands to his face and began weeping.

"Take your time," Ellen said. "It's okay."

Ellen handed Marcus a box of tissues, and they sat quietly as Marcus cried.

Introduction

"The doctor says things don't look good."

While advances in modern medicine have resulted in breakthrough treatments for medical conditions that were once catastrophic, including cancer, heart disease, and HIV, to name a few, not all conditions can be cured by modern medicine. Inevitably, for some patients, prognoses are **terminal**. Terminal diagnoses can introduce issues on top of the traditional, further challenging patients and their loved ones and caregivers. Patients newly diagnosed with terminal diagnoses have emotions, beliefs, and experiences unique to them that influence how they react to the news that they will not survive. The initial shock of a diagnosis may be intensified when the underlying condition is terminal, and the emotions that follow

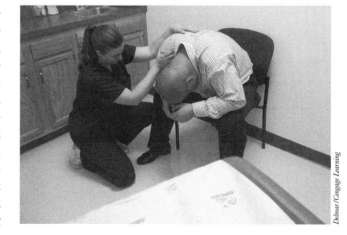

Delmar/Cengage Learning

may be more intense. Sometimes, patients' reactions coincide with those of their health-care professionals. As humans, health-care professionals have their own emotions, beliefs, and experiences about the **end of life**—fears, hopes, and spiritual beliefs—which they bring when encountering patients who are facing terminal diagnoses. Strong personal convictions regarding how one should face death, and beliefs about life after death, can impact how health-care professionals approach end-of-life discussions with their patients. Fears about death on either side of the health-care relationship can make discussing the end of life difficult.

As they approach their work with terminal patients, health-care professionals should know their beliefs about the end of life, as well as their comfort levels and limitations, so that when they are called on for support, they can provide it as effectively as possible. This chapter is not intended to discuss end-of-life issues in depth or to provide extensive guidelines for helping patients navigate this process. Instead, this chapter is meant to highlight the issues that may arise for health-care professionals and patients alike when patients receive terminal diagnoses and to make suggestions for helping patients during their initial days and weeks after diagnosis.

> **KEEP IN MIND**
>
> The medical diagnoses of terminal conditions are undeniably difficult situations for all involved. What words, if any, might be effective in this situation?

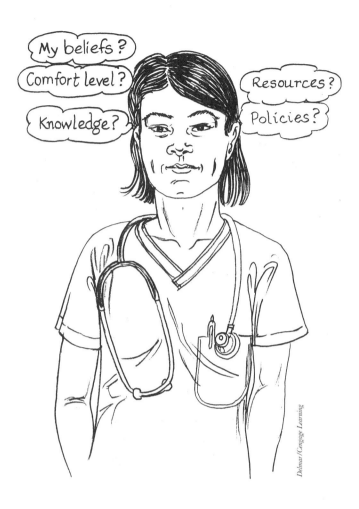

Delmar/Cengage Learning

Facing the End of Life as Health-Care Professionals

When working with newly diagnosed patients who are facing the end of life, health-care professionals must focus on medical issues. However, they must also address the range of personal emotional and spiritual issues that arise due to the terminal nature of the patients' conditions. Professionals may find, for example, that their patients' terminal diagnoses raise their own uncomfortable and confusing fears and questions about death.

Because it is normal to react to patients' terminal diagnoses, health-care professionals should complete their own "inner work" before working with terminal patients, being clear about their personal beliefs and their unique challenges so they can effectively help patients cope with their diagnoses.

The following sections outline specific suggestions for health-care professionals helping usher patients through the end of life.

DEFINING PERSONAL BELIEFS ABOUT DEATH

It is human nature to want to avoid thinking or talking about death, because it is inherently a difficult topic. For patients and health-care professionals alike, death inspires strong reactions, ones not necessarily grounded in spirituality or religion. However, health-care professionals who take time to define their own feelings about death are better able to appreciate patients' perspectives, because they have already identified their uncomfortable questions and viewpoints and are better equipped to draw parallels with patients' emotions. Interestingly, it is not necessary for health-care professionals to have religious or spiritual training in end-of-life issues or even to know all the answers. Indeed, sometimes it is enough for professionals to understand patients' difficulties and to be comfortable not knowing what the end of life might bring.

ASSESSING PERSONAL COMFORT WITH DEATH

Death is not an easy subject to discuss. Some health-care professionals are naturally comfortable talking about death and find themselves reaching out to patients newly diagnosed with terminal conditions. Patients, in turn, gravitate to these professionals to discuss their concerns as end-of-life issues arise. Health-care professionals should gauge their comfort levels with death and related topics so they can either provide support as these opportunities arise or ask their health-care team members to step in. Sometimes, added exposure and deeper personal understanding can render health-care professionals more comfortable serving in this role over time.

WORKING WITHIN APPROPRIATE BOUNDARIES

The helplessness health-care professionals may feel when working with terminally diagnosed patients can have negative consequences. For one, professionals may become emotional, thereby unintentionally interfering with the patients' emotional recovery. For another, health-care professionals may make decisions for patients and become overinvolved in family situations. Health-care professionals with strong religious beliefs may try to instill their beliefs in their patients.

While health-care professionals may have well-meaning intentions, they can emotionally damage patients and harm their therapeutic relationships. Professionals who are unclear on appropriate boundaries are more likely to approach end-of-life situations hesitantly, because they are unsure of what they can and should do for patients and what they should avoid. By staying aware of their emotional reactions to patients and understanding their professional boundaries, health-care professionals can be compassionate while staying focused on their primary therapeutic responsibilities.

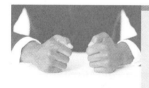

Body Language

Newly diagnosed patients who are facing terminal conditions may have body language that includes the following:

- Weeping, holding hands to the face or across the chest
- Slumped posture
- Jerky, agitated movements
- Looking down or otherwise avoiding eye contact
- Inability to sit still or relax
- Covering the face with the hands or rubbing the temples

BECOMING FAMILIAR WITH ORGANIZATIONAL POLICIES

Hospitals and clinics often have policies for communicating with terminally ill patients. For example, such policies often govern how health-care professionals should deliver terminal diagnoses and how they should involve the patients' family members in diagnosis news. Physicians and other health-care professionals in management positions may help shape their organizations' policies. All staff must observe Health Insurance Portability and Accountability Act (HIPAA) and other confidentiality guidelines in this arena, because they have legal implications.

Diligently following all guidelines, and using sensitivity and common sense, helps health-care professionals ensure that that their communications with terminally ill patients meet the highest standards of professionalism.

KEEP IN MIND

Communication with newly diagnosed patients facing the end of their lives requires preparation and skills beyond what is normally needed. As a health-care professional, what skills do you have that equip you to help support these kinds of patients? In what areas might you currently be deficient? Which skills might prove most beneficial in end-of-life situations?

Understanding How Patients Cope with Terminal Diagnoses

As mentioned earlier, newly diagnosed patients respond uniquely to their terminal diagnoses. Some use their strong beliefs about death as sources of strength. Others struggle to accept the inevitability of death.

The ways in which newly diagnosed patients react to the diagnosis play a key role. Patients in fight reaction are most likely to take the diagnosis in stride, or even to decide to fight it in any way possible. Some fighters will succeed in at least delaying the progress of the condition, and living longer than expected, by becoming actively involved in making optimal treatment decisions and lifestyle changes. A minority may find an alternate treatment that results in remission if not a cure, even if it means traveling to another state to be treated. However, patients in fight reaction nevertheless often experience shock, and extreme emotional reaction, when initially learning of the diagnosis. Patients in flight reaction will retreat into their emotions and be inconsolable, and may use their emotions as a wall to avoid discussing or otherwise considering the possibility of death. Those in flight reaction are also prone to unquestionably attach themselves to a "miracle" treatment that may or may not be recommended. Patients in freeze reaction are likely to shut down emotionally and give themselves up to fate and/or allow others to make any needed decisions for them.

Coping with a terminal medical condition is an ongoing process, and much has been written about how patients come to accept their diagnoses, both from psychosocial and spiritual or religious perspectives. In her 1969 book, *On Death and Dying*, Dr. Elizabeth Kubler-Ross wrote about the process, introducing the following five stages patients with terminal conditions complete as they address their diagnoses:

1. Denial, expressing disbelief that the terminal diagnosis is possible
2. Anger, recognizing that the diagnosis is terminal and expressing anger over the situation's unfairness

3. Bargaining, hoping that death can be postponed by making promises to a Higher Power to live in a way that is more productive or beneficial to others

4. Depression, as the patient begins to accept that death is inevitable, feeling sadness and grieving, possibly avoiding others during this time

5. Acceptance, with the realization that death is inevitable, accompanied by a sense of peace

Using case studies, the following sections give examples of each stage.

BATTLING DISBELIEF: LARA'S STORY

When Lara's physician informed her that her cancer was not treatable, her first reaction was disbelief. While her physician had said her cancer could return, she had been cancer free for a few years and had assumed that that would continue for the rest of her life.

"First, I thought that I had misunderstood him, or even that he was kidding with me. I just couldn't believe that not only had my cancer returned, but that he didn't think he would be able to treat it this time. He actually told me I should begin preparing for death and that he would break the news to my family if I didn't want to. It was like everything went into slow motion while I stood there watching. All I could manage to say was, 'This can't be happening.'"

What the patient is experiencing: Much like patients who receive any medical diagnosis, patients with terminal diagnoses often react initially with shock and disbelief. Such unexpected, final news is difficult to grasp, both intellectually and emotionally, and emotions are intensified when the outcome is end of life.

Terminal patients may need time to "sit with" their news, to sort it out in terms of what it means to them and how they feel. If they cannot come to terms with their diagnoses, they may progress into denial. Patients who continue to deny the finality of their diagnoses will suffer emotionally, fail to comply with ongoing care recommendations, and participate less than fully in decision making. The result is an increased burden on patients' family members and other loved ones, as well as on health-care teams.

FACING FEAR: FELIX'S STORY

Felix felt fear when his physician gave him his diagnosis, the worst of his life, when his physician explained that his condition was rare and that most patients with his condition did not survive beyond a year. Felix had assumed he would have a normal life. He had never thought much about the possibility of dying.

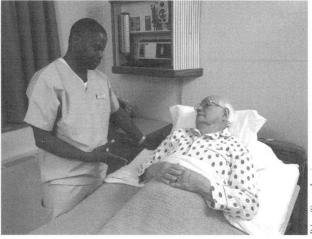

"The idea of death, when I allowed myself to think about it at all, was always terrifying to me. So when the doctor gave me the news, I felt such profound terror that I thought I might pass out. All I could think about was struggling to stay alive and feeling myself slipping away. I reached out and grabbed my wife's hand and squeezed it hard, as if I was trying to keep from being pulled into the next world, whatever that was going to be. I have never felt that afraid in my life."

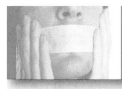

SELF • talk

Negative self-talk around terminal illness includes the following:

If I'm going to die, why bother to live?

I must have done something to deserve this.

I'm so afraid of what I'm going to have to go through before I finally die.

Nobody is going to want to have to face this with me. I'll be left alone.

I can't face this.

Antidotes to negative self-talk about terminal illness include the following:

I can face this with acceptance and dignity.

I have a lot of supportive people around me.

Death is a part of life, and I'm ready to face this.

I'll continue to do everything possible to take care of myself and to be there for the people who love me.

What the patient is experiencing: Fear is often present when patients face medical diagnoses. They fear losing what is most important to them in life, including vitality, control, financial security, and relationships. They fear the unknown: the process of decline and death and how that process will affect them and their loved ones. Terminal diagnoses confirm patients' worst fears, because they signal the end of life.

FEELING URGENCY: KATIE'S STORY

Katie, and those around her, had always considered her a "hard charger," balancing a career with being a wife and mother. She never seemed to stop running, somehow managing to excel professionally while being actively involved in her children's lives. When she was diagnosed with her terminal condition, the first thing Katie did was to list everything she wanted to accomplish before she died. Most of the items on the list focused on the needs of her family.

> *"I have all these things I want to finish, some probably kind of silly, like remodeling the living room, and others really important, like making sure my daughter finishes all her college applications. I know I'm sick and I can feel my energy declining, but I'm going to push myself as hard as I can to accomplish everything on my list. This is what I have to do for myself and for the people I love."*

What the patient is experiencing: Patients facing terminal illnesses may feel a sense of **urgency** to accomplish as much as they can before they die. They may want to make sure their loved ones are taken care of, or they may want to leave legacies behind. Staying active is a way for patients to deny their helplessness and powerlessness. Superstitious thinking may convince some patients that they can outrun death by staying active or that they can be so needed that they cannot die.

WORRYING ABOUT OTHERS: GABRIEL'S STORY

When Gabriel heard his condition was fatal, he felt extremely sad for his mother. She had been devoted to him his whole life, and he to her, and he knew that, while his siblings would watch over her, she would never get over losing him. He imagined her sitting alone in her home and missing him. He worried that she would cry often and that she would be so overcome with sadness that she would not care for herself. When he had these thoughts, Gabriel cried for himself and for her.

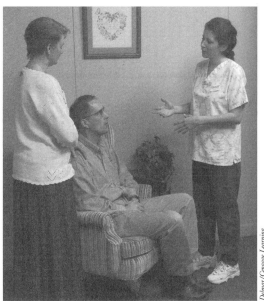

"I don't know how my mother will live without me. She's so dependent on me. I call her every day and talk about my day, and she tells me about hers. We have dinner together at least once a week, and I often bring her to my home to spend some time on the weekends. When I'm gone, all this will end. I don't know how she can possibly replace me. I'm afraid her life and health will decline."

What the patient is experiencing: Patients who know they are dying often begin grieving. They grieve for the losses of their own lives and for the losses their loved ones will soon experience. They worry that their loved ones will be unable to handle the losses, and they may spend large amounts of time imagining what life will be like for their loved ones, how their loved ones' grief will emotionally debilitate them and erode their well-being.

SENSING THE END: JANIS'S STORY

When Janis heard her physician say, "There's nothing more I can do," she burst into tears. That was the last thing she thought she would hear from her, and she felt as if she was being abandoned. Her physician continued with a description of what Janis could expect in terms of care, but Janis had stopped listening. When she left the office, she called her husband at work and said, "I've only got a week to live."

"My mind completely shut down once she said my condition was not treatable. I just saw my life crumbling before me. What would my husband do? I wasn't ready to die. I was terrified. The doctor said something about what I could expect, but I wasn't able to really listen. So I left her office with the worst possible scenario in mind: that I would be gone in a week. A couple of days later, my husband and I talked to the doctor together, and she told us I might live another year. I realized then how distraught I was."

KEEP IN MIND

You can honor another person by being a patient and nonjudgmental listener or simply by being willing to sit with the person in silence. These are among the greatest needs of patients facing death. As a health-care professional, how will you fulfill this need for your patients?

What the patient is experiencing: The shock of learning they have fatal conditions can so unsettle patients that they assume the worst. Often unable to listen any further, patients may make assumptions and further distress both themselves and their loved ones. As has been mentioned before, lacking adequate information, it is human nature to create stories to fill the gaps.

"Being Present" with Patients

Health-care professionals who have little experience working with patients newly diagnosed with terminal medical conditions often fear they will lack the words to comfort the patients, or they fear they will say something wrong. Just as patients have no words to adequately describe their diagnosis reactions, health-care professionals have no words to make things better for patients. Because health-care professionals may be feeling helpless, they may be unable to offer the support that could help patients.

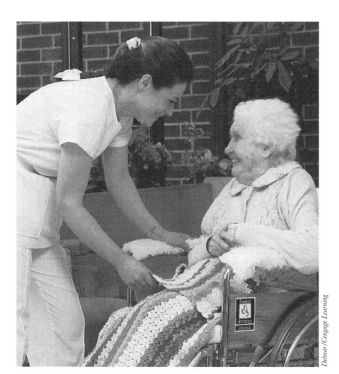

What terminal patients most need upon receiving their diagnoses are not broadscale solutions or road maps to their futures but willing, able, and skilled listeners. Often, patients' families cannot talk about death, at least not initially. Sometimes, patients delay informing their family members of their diagnoses until they have had chances to process the diagnoses themselves.

Health-care professionals can benefit terminal patients by **being present**—by being willing to sit and listen silently to patients' fear, anger, and sadness. To do this requires only patience and compassion, not spiritual insight or mental-health counseling skills. Health-care professionals can also help patients by offering objective medical information and encouraging patients to talk with their physicians. As discussed previously, because patients may shut down emotionally upon hearing that their conditions are fatal, they may miss valuable information that their physicians offer while sharing diagnoses. To help ensure patients have all the tools they need, health-care professionals can offer to discuss physician information with patients and serve as **listening ears** as the patients process it. Suggestions and outside resources are additional ways for professionals to offer patients aid. It is important that health-care professionals give patients information they can read on their own, once they feel stronger and have gathered their thoughts.

Helping Families through Patients' End of Life

The family members and other loved ones of terminally diagnosed patients experience many of the same reactions as the patients themselves. Families and friends experience fear—for the patients and their own futures. Diagnoses may be so shocking that family members initially react with disbelief and denial. They also feel sad, sad that they will lose people they love as well as their hopes and dreams for the future. Of course, family members and loved ones feel anger at the unfairness of life and helplessness at their inability to change their situations. Concerns over finances may also arise. Often, patients' loved ones simply feel powerless as they face a health-care system they feel has let them down and is failing to treat the patients sensitively. The net result is stress and interpersonal conflict.

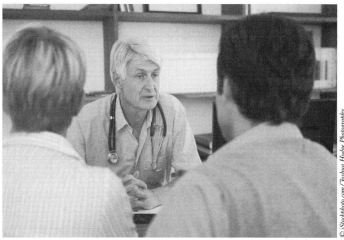

The reactions of family members and other loved ones affect patients directly. At least initially, patients' loved ones tend to rally, offering the support patients need. Unfortunately, feelings of helplessness may drive family members to become overinvolved in patients' health care and thereby inadvertently rob patients of their sense of control. Hoping to avoid further turmoil, patients may avoid expressing their feelings or asking for help.

Strained family dynamics can challenge health-care professionals. For example, professionals may receive directions from family members that conflict with patient desires. Patients may be left feeling that they have been abandoned by their families, even temporarily. When relationships are strained, the health-care team must shoulder the added responsibility of encouraging patient-family communication or making referrals to community agencies.

Much like family-patient strain can challenge health-care delivery, unresolved family issues can negatively affect patients, amplifying stress when patients really need more care and comforting. Given the stress that both patients and family members may be feeling, health-care professionals can help by being sensitive to its signs, including crying, **agitation**, arguing, or communication avoidance. When stress or conflict appears in patient-family relations, health-care professionals should notify the physicians or others leaders on the health-care team so appropriate intervention or referrals can occur.

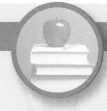

Educational Moment

Approaching the End of Life

Newly diagnosed patients experience fear, helplessness, and other emotions when first learning that their diagnoses are not treatable. With terminal illnesses, part of the acceptance process is having the opportunity to express emotions and feel listened to and supported. Health-care professionals can support this process by encouraging patients to talk, being willing listeners, and providing printed information for later reference.

Identifying Referral Options for End-of-Life Care

Numerous resources are available for patients facing the end of life, some of which appear in Appendix A. The sections that follow describe some of the resources health-care professionals should consider for patients newly diagnosed with terminal conditions, as well as their families and other loved ones.

ACCESSING MENTAL-HEALTH COUNSELING

Counselors and psychotherapy can help terminal patients who are overwhelmed with emotion or who simply need objective listening ears to gain perspective. Ideally, the counselors chosen for these tasks have experience working with patients and caregivers facing end-of-life issues.

SEEKING SPIRITUAL COUNSELING

Patients and family members can call on members of the clergy or other religious or spiritual advisors for counseling. Nondenominational spiritual counselors may be available. Ideally, the spiritual or religious backgrounds of the chosen resources closely match those of the patients or family members.

ATTENDING SELF-HELP GROUPS

A number of organizations are devoted to helping people facing specific diagnoses, such as cancer, diabetes, and HIV. Large metropolitan areas often have organizations that serve patients facing death, offering counseling, support groups, and classes in things like meditation and yoga. Religious institutions may also offer groups focused on death and grieving.

SEARCHING PUBLISHED RESOURCES

As discussed in previous chapters, hospitals and clinics often maintain lists of resources for patients' psychosocial needs. Such resources might include home health care; **palliative care**; **hospice**, spiritual, and religious services; meal services like Meals on Wheels; medical transportation; and counseling and social services. Such resources help health-care professionals as well as the patients they serve. Access to resources and potential solutions can help reduce professionals' sense of helplessness.

Health-care professionals who lack in-person access to lists of hospital or clinic resources can locate such resources on the Internet or through social service organizations. The World Wide Web has any number of sites offering end-of-life-related information and inspiration. Health organizations sponsor some sites, while religious organizations maintain others. In addition, people who have faced terminal illness personally or with others maintain blogs directed toward patients and family members. Health-care professionals should remember, however, that not all Internet information is reliable and trustworthy, and some can even be damaging. Professionals should maintain lists of the Web resources they know to be trustworthy.

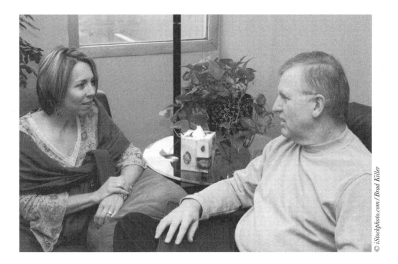

EXPLORING MEDICAL OPTIONS

After diagnosis, terminal patients may need palliative care, hospice, home health care, or other specialized services. When patients are initially diagnosed, they may not yet have been assessed for medical needs. To be prepared to make recommendations and to help answer any questions that may arise, members of the health-care team should familiarize themselves with the resources for medical options like these.

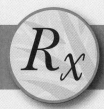 Having Conversations to Introduce End-of-Life Issues

At the cancer treatment center, Sarita and Ellen had worked with many patients newly diagnosed with terminal conditions. They were familiar with the intense emotional reactions of patients first learning of their untreatable conditions. Further, they had learned how to help such patients through these difficult times.

> ELLEN: I'm so sorry, Marcus. Please know that Sarita and I are here to help in any way we can.
>
> SARITA: Absolutely. Just let us know what we can do.

His eyes downward, Marcus nodded but did not speak. Ellen and Sarita waited patiently. Finally, Marcus raised his eyes and responded. It was clear he had been crying.

> MARCUS: I guess I can talk now, but I don't know what to say. I didn't expect to get this news today.
>
> ELLEN: Nobody expects you to say anything, Marcus. We understand how much this hurts.

Marcus cried for a few more minutes, then blew his nose.

> SARITA: You know, Marcus, we have a lot of resources here to help you. We have counselors you can speak with. We also have a social work department that can help you with anything that comes up.

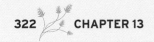

Marcus nodded.

ELLEN: What Sarita is saying is you don't have to go through this alone. You have a lot of support.

MARCUS: I don't know what I need right now.

ELLEN: That's okay. You don't need to. But I want you to know that when you're ready, we have a lot of resources to help you.

MARCUS: Okay.

SARITA: Dr. Martinez is recommending some chemotherapy, which I'll be managing. Ellen will be in charge of your treatment planning. Do you want us to go over any of this with you now?

MARCUS: I don't think I can handle that right now.

SARITA: That's alright. We don't need to. Maybe we could set up a time for you to come back in a couple of days. Would that be better?

MARCUS: Yes, I think it would.

ELLEN: I'll set up a time for you to come back, Marcus. I do want to let you know that Sarita and I are here Monday through Friday during the workday, and you can always give us a call if you have any questions or if you want any of the resources we have available. If I can't answer the phone, I'll call you back that day. We also have an emergency number during the off-hours and weekend. The staff here is never farther away than your telephone. Okay?

MARCUS: Okay.

SARITA: Now. We have to ask you, Marcus. What are you going to do for the rest of the day? It's really important that you get some support. If you don't have any available, we can set you up with some help right now.

MARCUS: I have a friend I can call. He knows I was coming in for my test results, and he offered to be available for me.

SARITA: Will you call him right away?

MARCUS: Yes. I'm going to my car, and I'll call him from there.

ELLEN: That sounds like a good idea, Marcus. If you can't reach him, please feel free to call us if you need anything today. Will you please do that?

MARCUS: Yes, I will.

ELLEN: Okay Marcus. I'll walk out with you and set up an appointment.

SARITA: We're standing by for you. I'll see you in a couple of days.

Guidelines for Having Conversations to Introduce End-of-Life Issues

The following guidelines can help health-care professionals speak with patients who have recently been diagnosed with terminal illnesses.

1. *Listen quietly.* Patients who have just learned that their conditions are untreatable do not need advice or "words of wisdom." Most likely, they would find that type of response inadequate, if not patronizing. Instead, terminal patients more likely need people who can "be present" with them, which

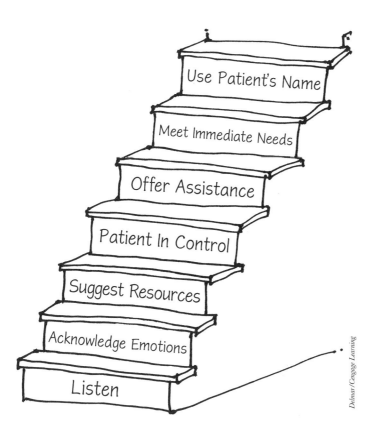

Delmar/Cengage Learning

entails simply listening quietly to their feelings and responding only when the patients are ready to talk. In the preceding example, Ellen and Sarita sat quietly as Marcus wept.

2. ***Acknowledge emotions.*** Notice that Ellen and Sarita encouraged Marcus to take his time and feel his emotions. They let him know that they understood he was hurting. In so doing, these health-care professionals helped normalize Marcus's strong feelings and conveyed that they were comfortable with his emotions. While Marcus could weep openly, other patients might need professionals' encouragement to openly express their feelings.

3. ***Suggest that resources are available.*** While newly diagnosed patients are not necessarily ready to use outside resources initially, it is important for them to know that resources are available. Ellen and Sarita informed Marcus that resources for his most immediate need, emotional support, were available, as were others.

4. ***Let the patient feel in control.*** Patients newly diagnosed with terminal conditions are most likely feeling helpless and out of control, which might cause them to resist any advice or directions they perceive as being forced on them. Health-care professionals can avoid creating resistance in patients by offering, not dictating. Notice that Sarita and Ellen remained tentative with Marcus. They made it known that resources were available if he was interested. They offered to go over information about his chemotherapy and treatment plan but allowed him to decide if he wanted to discuss it at that time. They offered to set up a return visit in a couple of days. Marcus did not control his diagnosis, but he did have a measure of control over his interactions with his treatment team.

5. ***Tell the patient how you can help.*** Patients need to know what kinds of assistance they can expect from the members of their health-care teams. They also need to know the circumstances under which they can expect this assistance. Ellen and Sarita suggested to Marcus that they could help to find resources but not that they could personally meet all his needs. They also informed him of the hours they would be available and what he could expect when they were unavailable. This helped ensure that Marcus would not have unrealistic expectations.

6. ***Ensure that immediate needs are met.*** It was clear to Ellen and Sarita that Marcus was emotionally distraught over his diagnosis and that he needed immediate emotional support. Rather than assuming that Marcus would reach out for support, they gently told him that support was important during this time and asked him what support he had available. Further, they encouraged him to reach out for support immediately. While they risked causing Marcus to become defensive if he felt they were pushing him too hard in this direction, it was their professional opinion that it was necessary for him to make an emotional connection that afternoon.

7. ***Use the patient's first name.*** Hearing one's name can be soothing during a time of stress. Notice that Sarita and Ellen repeatedly used Marcus's name when addressing him.

SUMMARY

Despite the many miracles of modern medicine, the news about a medical diagnosis is not always optimistic. Sometimes, patients' conditions are untreatable and the best they can do is accept them and prepare for the end. Each patient has a unique process of acceptance ahead, one health-care professionals can help him or her through. By understanding how patients react to the news of terminal illness, encouraging them to express themselves and ask questions, and being willing listeners, professionals can make the end of life as painless as possible.

Chapter REVIEW

Multiple-Choice Questions

1. It is important for health-care professionals to do their own inner work around end-of-life issues because patients' end-of-life issues may:
   a. Bring up memories of the professionals' experiences
   b. Raise questions the professionals have not resolved
   c. Create uncomfortable feelings for the professional
   d. All of the above

2. From a religious perspective, health-care professionals should only approach end-of-life issues with patients when they:
   a. Can provide solid spiritual guidance
   b. Are open to patients' spiritual beliefs
   c. Lack religious views or affiliations
   d. Can make referrals to clergypeople or spiritual counselors

3. When facing diagnoses of terminal medical conditions, patients in _____ reaction are most likely to seek advanced treatment, even if it requires international travel.
   a. Fight
   b. Flight
   c. Freeze
   d. None of the above

4. Patients' initial reaction to a terminal diagnosis tends to be:
   a. Acceptance
   b. Denial
   c. Shock
   d. Empowerment

5. When patients with terminal illnesses list everything they have yet to accomplish, they may:
   a. Feel a sense of urgency
   b. Try to avoid helpless feelings
   c. Stay busy to "outrun death"
   d. Any of the above

Fill-in-the-Blank Questions

1. Patients facing the end of life can benefit most from health-care professionals who are willing to _____ _____.

2. Patients may react to diagnoses with such emotions as _____, _____, and _____.

3. When terminal diagnoses cause spiritual crises, patients may request _____ to clergypeople or other spiritual resources.

4. Rather than facing their diagnoses, patients may react by _____, or not facing them.

5. Patients who feel a sense of _____ react to their terminal diagnoses by listing things to accomplish.

Short-Answer Questions

1. Briefly discuss the stages Elizabeth Kubler-Ross describes patients passing through as they come to accept their terminal illnesses.

_____

_____

_____

2. Why is it important to understand appropriate boundaries when talking to patients about terminal illness?

_____

_____

_____

3. How is a patient in flight reaction most likely to react to the diagnosis of a terminal illness?

_____

_____

_____

4. What does it mean to "be present" with a patient who is facing a crisis?

_____

_____

_____

5. What kinds of body language are common for patients diagnosed as terminal?

_____

_____

_____

Critical-Thinking Questions

1. While patients are health-care professionals' main concern, family members also go through crises when loved ones are diagnosed with terminal illnesses. From the health-care perspective, what concerns and responsibilities are reasonable for family members?

_____

_____

_____

_____

_____

2. Considering your own religious beliefs, what would you most like to say to a patient who is facing death? How does your approach relate to best practices?

_____

_____

_____

_____

_____

3. Patients who receive unexpected medical diagnoses that are terminal face two crises. What concerns should this raise with the health-care team? From an emotional support perspective, what other considerations should professionals keep in mind?

_____

_____

_____

_____

_____

Internet Exercise

Look for Internet resources related to such end-of-life care areas as spirituality, hospice and palliative care, and emotional support. Sites may be sponsored by private companies, nonprofit organizations, and religious or spiritual organizations. Choose the sites you think would be most valuable for patients facing the end of life. Why are some resources more valuable than others? Is there anything missing? If so, what would you add, and why?

_____

_____

_____

_____

_____

_____

_____

_____

_____

CHAPTER 14

Recognizing Personal Emotions as Health-Care Professionals

OVERVIEW

After reading this chapter, you should be able to:

- Define and use the keywords of health-care professionals' personal emotions.

- Understand the importance of self-care for health-care providers as a means of protection against compassion fatigue.

- Recognize the stress symptoms that may lead to compassion fatigue.

- Identify the ways of coping that help avoid compassion fatigue.

- Describe how to speak with a health-care colleague experiencing compassion-related stress.

Compassion fatigue   Objectivity   Self-care

Emotionally available   Personal qualities   Stress

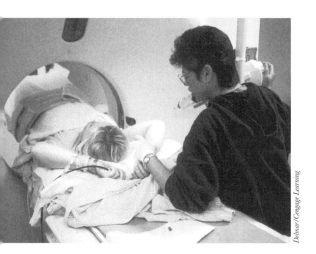

Delmar/Cengage Learning

Case Study

Monica, a radiation technician, was preparing Ryan, a young man recently diagnosed with cancer, for his first radiation treatment. Before the treatment, Monica had taken time to talk with Ryan, because he was upset. He had been shocked to discover he had cancer. Before his diagnosis, he told Monica, he had led a very active life. To help allay Ryan's concerns about his treatment, Monica had reassured him that the radiation machine was modern and well-maintained.

When she was finished with Ryan, Monica stepped into the break room and sat at the table. She rested her head on her hands and fought back tears.

> **KEEP IN MIND**
>
> Health-care professionals often listen to patients tell stories and talk about their feelings of sadness and helplessness. As a health-care professional, have you ever helped someone else address their emotions while feeling you lacked the emotional energy you needed? If so, what did you do? What should health-care professionals do in this situation?

Sean, an MRI technician, stopped in to the break room for his morning coffee break. He stood at the door and observed Monica. He knew that a lot of scared patients passed through the radiation department and that Monica always took time to be as comforting and reassuring as possible as she prepared them for their treatments. From his experience as a health-care professional, Sean knew this could be emotionally draining.

"Hey, Monica," Sean said as he entered the room and sat across from her.

"Hi, Sean," Monica answered.

"Having a rough day?" he asked.

Monica did not answer but nodded.

> **KEEP IN MIND**
>
> If you, as a health-care professional, entered the break room and saw Monica sitting at the table, would you say anything to her? Would you be concerned about getting involved? Why or why not?

Introduction

"How are you feeling?"

Previous chapters focus on understanding and supporting newly diagnosed patients, offering them emotional support, guidance, and information, and helping them comply with treatment and lifestyle management recommendations. While a deep level of patient involvement enhances the therapeutic communication between patient and health-care professional and possibly care and patient outcomes, it requires the health-care professional to have a great deal of emotional and physical energy, as well as compassion. While patient relations can be gratifying for health-care professionals, they can also be emotionally and physically draining.

Stress and compassion fatigue are common topics in the helping professions, both mental health and health care. **Stress** can result from many aspects, including emergencies and difficult patients. Ongoing stress that is not relieved can lead to **compassion fatigue** in which health-care professionals feel they have nothing to give patients emotionally. Indeed, after working with patients in extremely emotional situations, many professionals have been so exhausted that they needed to take breaks, if they were able to continue at all.

Health-care professionals assisting newly diagnosed patients are especially vulnerable in this regard, because they support patients at a time when emotions are especially raw. As discussed in previous chapters, health-care professionals have their own reactions to patients and the stories they tell. Repeatedly experiencing the trauma of newly diagnosed patients, and the helplessness this may cause, can leave health-care professionals feeling depleted and less able to be effective.

Providing Self-Care for Health-Care Professionals

Health-care professionals can prevent their own stress and compassion fatigue by being proactive in **self-care** and supportive of other health-care professionals. The following sections provide suggestions and guidelines for those endeavors.

RECOGNIZING THE SYMPTOMS OF STRESS AND COMPASSION FATIGUE

Health-care professionals are trained to look for symptoms in their patients, including stress symptoms. Ironically, they may not recognize, or acknowledge, these symptoms in themselves. The stress symptoms in health-care professionals, which are very similar to those of patients, include the following:

- Sadness, sometimes to the point of overwhelming depression

- Feeling of accomplishing nothing or adding no value

- Getting easily impatient or angry with patients, friends and family, and other professionals

- Physical symptoms that include fatigue, sleep disturbances, and appetite changes

- Changes in work habits, including sloppiness and tardiness

- Being too objective or too empathetic with patients
- Constantly feeling helpless, that nothing is in personal control

Although it is human nature to assume that stress is temporary or unacceptable and should be hidden, health-care professionals should continually monitor themselves for symptoms of stress and compassion fatigue. If they do not, they can ignore symptoms in themselves they would consider "red flags" in their patients. Being alert to concerning symptoms, in themselves and other professionals, and lending helping hands or listening ears, as described in the following sections, can be steps toward promoting the self-care of the collective health-care team.

KEEP IN MIND

Health-care professionals who know how they experience stress are better able to monitor their symptoms and reach out for help in the event they experience compassion fatigue. As a benefit to employees, organizations may offer employee assistance programs (EAPs) so employees can meet with mental-health professionals when needed. As a health-care professional, what are your personal signs of stress? What resources might you tap into upon feeling stress or compassion fatigue?

KNOWING PERSONAL STRENGTHS AND LIMITS

Professionals bring unique **personal qualities** to their careers. Some health-care professionals are comfortable interacting with patients, demonstrating good listening skills, being empathic, remaining objective, and honoring professional boundaries. While these skills can be learned to a great extent, not all professionals can execute them to the same level. Experience is a factor as well. A health-care professional who is experienced in working with patients newly diagnosed with cancer, for example, might have more to offer to another cancer patient than a professional who has never worked with the condition before.

Professionals' effectiveness may vary from day to day. All health-care professionals have days when they are feeling less able to be **emotionally available** to patients and consequently need other professionals to act as backups. Further, patients may feel more comfortable talking about emotional topics with those members of the health-care team they feel resemble them in some way, whether it is in gender, age, or background.

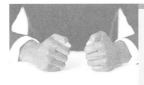

Body Language

Much like in patients, body language in health-care professionals transmits feelings. As members of their health-care teams, professionals should monitor themselves and their coworkers for signs of stress and compassion fatigue, which appear as the following postures:

- Avoidance—Arms folded, disinterested expression
- Fatigue—Leaning against a wall, tired expression
- Tension—Feet apart, broad gestures, angry expression

MAINTAINING OBJECTIVITY

People often describe being upset by books or movies that remind them of their own lives or hearing of friends' problems and remembering how they felt in similar experiences. In health care, patients' situations may bring up personal feelings in members of the health-care team. If the feelings are too painful, professionals may avoid them. If they inspire strong convictions, professionals may want to solve the patients' problems for them. Either way, the health-care professionals have lost **objectivity**, the ability to stay neutral about topics and experiences.

Objectivity means being able to view situations without personal prejudices, without judgment, and to focus instead on factual information. Being objective does not imply that essential elements in communicating with newly diagnosed patients, including empathy and compassion, are missing. To realistically assess medical situations and make appropriate recommendations, health-care professionals must be able to balance their rational and emotional sides.

SETTING BOUNDARIES WITH PATIENTS

As discussed in previous chapters, particularly Chapter 8, as much as health-care professionals may want to be emotionally available to patients and to help them as much as possible, crossing professional boundaries benefits neither the professionals nor their patients. Health-care professionals who lose their objectivity run this risk.

Generally, health-care professionals choose the profession because they are motivated to help people. Newly diagnosed patients tend to have so many needs that their health-care professionals want to "go the extra mile" with them—be available after work hours, assist with tasks outside the traditional job responsibilities, or give advice. In newly diagnosed patients health-care professionals see people who are in emotional pain, most likely uninformed about their medical conditions, and possibly lacking adequate support from families or friends. Unfortunately, health-care professionals who are too available to patients cross professional boundaries.

Of course, helping newly diagnosed patients can be emotionally draining. Assisting multiple patients on an ongoing basis can cause stress and compassion fatigue. To help combat staff fatigue, hospitals, clinics, and practice settings generally have guidelines for professional-patient interactions, ones based on best practices, ethics, and common sense. For example, professionals should give advice only within the scope of professional responsibility, because to do otherwise can have ethical and legal implications. Similarly, patients should not be allowed to become too dependent on single staff members; instead they should be encouraged to become more empowered. One aspect of professional boundary setting in health care is letting patients know that other members of the team are available to support them.

FOLLOWING THE GUIDELINES FOR A HEALTHY LIFE

Health-care professionals advise their patients to maintain healthy lifestyles of adequate rest, healthy diets, and regular exercise, but they do not always follow their own advice. Human beings who are not at their best physically are less likely to function well mentally or emotionally, and health-care professionals are no different. Health-care professionals who take care of themselves physically and do things like take regular breaks are better able to meet the demands of patient care and set examples for their patients to follow.

RECOGNIZING PERSONAL CONTRIBUTIONS

Newly diagnosed patients can be challenging for health-care professionals, because they tend to require emotional support, information, and guidance beyond the norm. When patients fail to show their appreciation, family members make unfair demands, or stressed and fatigued coworkers lash out, the health-care profession can feel thankless.

It is natural for health-care professionals to want to feel acknowledged by the recipients of their attention: patients, coworkers, and managers. Given that the focus in health care is often elsewhere, people like patients and coworkers do not always freely offer acknowledgement. Fortunately, health-care professionals can, through self-talk and self-care, learn to acknowledge and reward themselves. The knowledge that they are supporting patients through crises can be powerful, for example, as can be breaks to rest outside work and enjoy life. Sitting with good listeners can also help.

FINDING A SAFE PLACE TO EXPRESS FEELINGS

To ensure their feelings are heard, health-care professionals should take the advice they often give their newly diagnosed patients: Sit with people who are willing and able listeners, people who do not need to dictate the professionals' actions and who can hear such difficult feelings as anger and frustration. For health-care professionals, these people can be coworkers, family members, friends, clergypeople, or mental-health professionals. Safe places to express feelings, and even to ventilate, help prevent stress buildup and thereby emotional overreaction or unavailability. Should they choose to speak with anyone outside the health-care team, however, health-care professionals must remember that Health Insurance Portability and Accountability Act (HIPAA) guidelines restrict them from using patients' names.

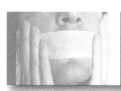

SELF • talk

The negative self-talk of health-care professionals may include:

Doesn't anybody know how hard I'm working?

There's no way I can give these patients the emotional support they really need.

I have to be a rock here, or the patient is going to have nobody.

I know I'm a terrible person, but I can't listen to another sad story today.

I don't think I can go on any longer before I'm completely emotionally drained.

Antidotes to the negative self-talk of health-care professionals include:

I know I'm going above and beyond the call of duty today. I don't have to always be told by others what a good job I'm doing.

I'm only human, too, and I don't have to always know the right thing to say or do.

I can be here for patients but also pay attention to my own need to pace myself.

Patients have me to rely on, but they also have my coworkers and other resources.

Educational Moment

Self-Care for Health-Care Professionals

Health-care professionals may try to hide how they are really feeling because they feel they cannot be themselves in their roles. Therefore, it is even more important for all members of the health-care team to look for signs of stress and compassion fatigue in themselves and their coworkers. When they see them, they should offer reminders that people are doing the best they can.

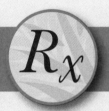

Having a Conversation about Compassion Fatigue

When Sean had experienced stress and compassion fatigue at various times during his career, other health-care professionals had reached out to offer him support. To return the favor, he reached out to Monica.

SEAN: Is there anything I can help you with?

Monica sat up and looked at Sean.

MONICA: I'm just having a bad day, you know.

SEAN: We all have them. I'm here to listen.

MONICA: My patients are facing one of the most difficult times in their lives, if not the most difficult. They're living their lives and then all of a sudden they're going through our clinic, telling me what happened and, sometimes I think, hoping I can tell them they're going to be okay.

SEAN: I know what you mean, Monica. You hear a lot of sad stories.

MONICA: Yes. And sometimes you wonder if you won't be able to listen to any more at some point. I mean, you want to help patients any way you can, but you also wonder if you can give them the help they need.

SEAN: It can be overwhelming, right?

MONICA: Absolutely. At least it feels overwhelming today.

SEAN: Can I give you some feedback?

MONICA: Sure.

SEAN: We're only human, Monica. After hearing how helpless our patients feel, and how scared they are, it's only natural that we would feel helpless after a while too. It takes a lot of emotional energy to be with so many sad and scared people, to listen to them, and to show them that we care. Sometimes, we just get tired out.

MONICA: Exactly.

SEAN: What I do is remind myself of what I just told you. I tell myself that I'm human and that I'm doing the best I can. But I also make sure I take care of myself. After a hard day, I make sure I do something I enjoy in the evening, even if it's only listening to some music I enjoy while I make dinner. Maybe I'll call a friend and talk about my day, you know, blow off some steam. And make sure I get a good night's sleep. Are you taking care of yourself?

MONICA: Kind of . . . but maybe not enough.

SEAN: And another thing. I don't take on all the responsibility for helping patients with their emotions. We're not counselors, after all. I listen. That's the best thing I can do for them at that time. And I answer their questions. But I also remind them that the clinic nurses can refer them to a counselor, and I tell them how valuable it might be for them to get some additional emotional support during this time.

MONICA: That's a good idea. I have to admit that, with some patients, I wonder if anyone other than me is taking the time to really listen to them. It's like they've never talked to anyone else about how they feel. That's a big job for me.

SEAN: And they probably *haven't* talked to anyone. It's a gift to be a good listener and to show someone you care. I don't want to not do that for patients. But I also want to make sure they get the professional support that they need, and that's where our resource file comes in handy.

MONICA: That's a great idea.

Guidelines for Having a Conversation about Compassion Fatigue

Following are guidelines for speaking with other health-care professionals about compassion fatigue:

1. *Offer to listen.* Like patients, health-care professionals experiencing compassion fatigue first need to be able to express how they feel. What they need most is someone who is ready to listen. Sean began the conversation by offering to listen to Monica. Notice that he used a tentative approach and gave her the option to open up if she chose to.

2. *Normalize feelings.* Monica initially expressed some guilt about feeling compassion fatigue and wondered if she was up to the challenge of being emotionally available to patients. As Sean reminded Monica, it is normal to feel emotionally drained when working with patients who are struggling with new diagnoses. He offered additional reassurance by telling her that he had had similar experiences.

3. *Encourage self-care.* Health-care professionals who are not taking care of themselves cannot be present for patients. Sean recommended that Monica build some relaxation into her day, do things that she enjoys, and call on friends who can offer emotional support. Again, he used his own experience as an example.

4. *Encourage the use of referrals.* Health-care professionals are part of a team that includes mental-health professionals who can be called on to help the professionals emotionally. Sean reminded Monica that their clinic has mental-health resources that patients can be referred to.

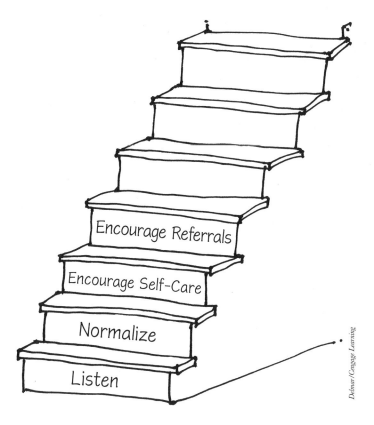

Delmar/Cengage Learning

SUMMARY

Health-care professionals are asked to be present with patients during very emotional times in the patients' lives, and the level of empathic listening and emotional support they offer to patients can be physically and emotionally draining. Caring for the caregiver is something that health-care professionals can do for themselves and for others.

Chapter REVIEW

Multiple-Choice Questions

1. Working with patients who are experiencing an emotional crisis requires:
   a. Physical energy
   b. Emotional energy
   c. Compassion
   d. All of the above

2. Experiencing stress with no relief can cause which of the following?
   a. Enhanced energy
   b. Compassion fatigue
   c. Sense of empowerment
   d. Increased stamina

3. Health-care professionals can help each other cope with their own emotional stress through:
   a. Being a listener and offering support
   b. Offering to complain to management
   c. Chastising the patient for being overly demanding
   d. Alerting management to the situation

4. Positive self-talk for a health-care professional experiencing stress would include:
   a. "I have already given more than I should."
   b. "I am the one who needs to be strong."
   c. "I can be effective and take care of myself."
   d. "I don't think I can go on any longer."

5. Helping other health-care professionals normalize their compassion fatigue includes which of the following?
   a. Acting like fatigue is a nonissue
   b. Delaying rest periods
   c. Offering better stress-management strategies
   d. Acknowledging the feeling in other professionals

Fill-in-the-Blank Questions

1. Health-care professionals who are experiencing stress may have difficulty being emotionally _____ with patients.

2. While health-care professionals are focused on patient care, it is also important for them to attend to their own _____ _____.

3. Health-care professionals with an attitude of _____ can be with patients emotionally without becoming overly involved.

4. Setting _____ is a way for health-care professionals to be conscious of where they can help patients appropriately and where they risk becoming too involved.

5. Health-care professionals feeling emotional stress may benefit most from being with colleagues who are willing to _____ to them.

Short-Answer Questions

1. What are the key symptoms of compassion fatigue?

_____

_____

_____

_____

2. What can health-care professionals do for themselves on an ongoing basis to cope with stress?

_____

_____

_____

_____

3. Why is it important for health-care professionals to recognize their own contributions to patients' well-being?

_____

_____

_____

_____

4. What does it mean to remain objective in patient interactions?

_____

_____

_____

_____

5. What can a health-care professional do to help a colleague who is experiencing stress and compassion fatigue?

_____

_____

_____

_____

Critical-Thinking Questions

1. Health-care professionals working with newly diagnosed patients may be especially vulnerable to compassion fatigue. Why might newly diagnosed patients present greater emotional challenges?

_____

_____

_____

_____

_____

_____

2. How can health-care professionals best assess their abilities to be objective, empathetic, and good listeners? How can they best avoid situations in which they might be less effective?

_____

_____

_____

_____

_____

_____

3. How can health-care professionals recognize stress and compassion fatigue in colleagues in ways that avoid offending those colleagues and honor boundaries? In what situations might it be necessary for health-care professionals to alert management to these symptoms and behaviors in colleagues?

_____

_____

_____

_____

_____

_____

Internet Exercise

Explore the Internet for resources that address the issue of stress and compassion fatigue both in health-care professionals and other helping professionals, such as counselors and social workers. Look for examples and case studies about compassion fatigue, as well as examples of any programs or techniques to address these issues. Choose a few Web sites that have the most useful content. What did you learn from them? How will this information help you? Your patients?

_____

_____

_____

_____

_____

_____

_____

_____

_____

Accepting attitude—Ability and desire to accommodate events and realities.

Activities of daily living—Set of daily, self-care activities (e.g., bathing, eating).

Agenda—List of topics to be covered during a meeting.

Aggressive manner—Strong emotional posture.

Agitation—Unsettledness, driven usually by negative energy.

Alienation—To make indifferent or hostile.

Anger—Strong negative feeling.

Anticipatory anxiety—Anxiety or concern based on the assumption that an event might occur, most likely based on a lack of information.

Antidote—Cure or remedy.

Anxiety—Concern or fear.

Appearance—Outward presentation; aesthetics.

Assertiveness—Ability to back a cause or viewpoint.

Assessment—Characterization of an entity's qualities, positive and negative.

Assumptions—Statements or facts taken to be true without validation.

Attributes—Qualities or characteristics.

Avoidance—Act of departing from or failing to engage with.

Baggage—Remnants of past events, usually emotional.

Barrier—Obstacle or challenge.

Being present—State of being open and receptive to incoming stimuli.

Beliefs—Set of thoughts or feelings.

Bias—Leaning toward a particular viewpoint.

Bibliotherapy—Therapeutic value of information.

Body image—Individual's personal notion of body's *appearance*.

Body language—Set of facial expressions, movements, and postures that together serve as nonverbal expressions of emotion.

Bond—Relationship.

Boundaries—Figurative limits to acceptable behaviors or treatments; similar to *parameters*.

Brainstorming—Gathering ideas and concepts about a set topic, free of restraints.

Burden—Load, duty, or responsibility.

Case manager—Health-care professional responsible for coordinating a patient's medical services.

Change—Render different.

Check-in—Act of ensuring an individual and/or event is satisfactory.

Clergypeople—Representatives of religious organizations.

Cognitive—Knowing; conscious intellectual activity.

Cognitive exhaustion—Fatigue from conscious intellectual activity.

Cognitive skills—Ability to knowingly process information.

Collaborate—Work cooperatively, as a team.

Comfort level—Level at which one functions easily.

Communication—Information exchange between two parties.

Compassion—Sympathy or goodwill toward another.

Compassion fatigue—Inability to perform with care and concern arising from overstimulation of negative events and overperformance of care duties.

Compliance—Act or process of fulfilling requirements.

Comprehension—Understanding.

Consciously suppressing—Actively denying expression of thoughts, feelings, or actions.

Counterargument—Standpoint from opposing view; argument against.

Counterevidence—Information from opposing view; information against.

Denial—Failure to admit reality or truth; refusal to believe or accept reality.

Depression—Profound sadness.

Despair—Sadness.

Diagnose—Evaluate; recognize a medical condition.

Disappointment—Failure in expectation.

Disempowered—Lacking strength, ability, or desire.

Distraught—Upset.

Educational moment—Opportunity for teaching or illustration.

Either-or thinking—Manner of cognition that leaves only two options.

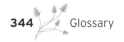

Elephant in the room—Unspoken though recognized issue.

Embrace—Hug, accept, or encircle.

Emotion—Feeling or mental reaction.

Emotional reaction—Feeling-driven response.

Emotionally available—Able to receive and provide the feedback needed for meaningful relationship exchanges.

Empowered— State of feeling able to act from a position of strength or power.

End of life—Death or expiration.

Equilibrium—Balanced state.

Ethical—Conformed to accepted standards of behavior.

Face time—In-person interaction.

Faith—Belief in; loyalty or allegiance.

False promise—Declaration made with no intention of fulfillment.

Fear—Extreme concern.

Fear factor—Strong, negative component to medical diagnosis reaction that tends to impede forward progression by preventing rational thought.

Fight—Reaction to medical diagnosis in which responder can harness both emotional and rational resources to combat a situation; ideal reaction for newly diagnosed patient.

Flight—Primarily emotional reaction following a medical diagnosis characterized by responder being unable to make objective decisions.

Freeze—Largely unemotional reaction to a medical diagnosis that prompts patient to deny emotions or adopt fatalistic views.

Frustration—Lack of fulfillment driven by defeat.

Generalize—Make sweeping statements.

Goal—Objective to achieve.

Grief—Mourning a loss.

Healthy grief—Acceptance of basic life beliefs, including death.

Hear—Sense through auditory means; perceive via the ears.

Helplessness—State of feeling unable to act.

High maintenance—Requiring a great deal of attention and/or support.

Higher Power—Entity perceived as greater than individuals.

Hope—Anticipate or expect with desire.

Hopelessness—State of feeling devoid of a future; inability to see a future.

Hospice—Care for terminally ill patients.

Hot buttons—Issues or events that inspire strong reactions, usually negative ones.

Information-gathering—Process of obtaining facts or data.

Intellectualize—Process information from purely rational view.

Interaction—Shared activity.

Judge—Critique or assess.

Judgmental—Characterized by harsh assessment.

Lifestyle—Way in which an individual, group, or organization navigates life.

Lifestyle management—Structured program aimed at promoting health and related, desirable behaviors.

Listen—Actively hear or perceive through auditory means.

Listening ear—Audience for communication, particularly negative or difficult communication.

Low self-image—Negative personal perception; see *self-image*.

Meaning—That which is conveyed via words and/or actions.

Mediation—Process of bringing about compromise or resolution.

Medical regimen—Plan or regulated course of medical treatments and activities.

Negative self-talk—Phrases that outline all nonpositive outcomes (e.g., "You'll end up an invalid").

Normalcy—State of conforming to a regular or accepted type or presentation.

Normalize—Set as expected and reasonable; characterize as normal.

Normalizing—Characterizing as reasonable and natural.

Nuance—Subtlety.

Numbness—State of nonfeeling.

Objective—Devoid of emotion; based on fact; unswayed by *bias*.

Objectivity—Reasonable approach based on fact, not emotion.

Open dialogue—Communication free of filters and/or restrictions.

Open posture—Stance indicating openness to communication and feedback; typified by things like leaning forward.

Openness—State of receptivity to outside stimuli; accessibility.

Optimism—Hope.

Organized religion—Any recognized religious group with prescribed guidelines and requirements (e.g., Catholic Church).

Overwhelmed—State of excess stimuli to the point of stress or inaction; overcome or overpowered.

Palliative care—Treatment dedicated to reducing the severity of disease symptoms, rather than halting or reversing the same.

Panic—Extreme anxiety or fright.

Parameters—Guidelines for behaviors or actions; similar to *boundaries*.

Paraphrase—Reword to achieve same meaning.

Passive-aggressively—Negative feelings expressed unassertively.

Patient empowerment—Movement to inspire patients to be accountable for their medical treatments and outcomes.

Peacefulness—State devoid of stress or *anxiety*; untroubled state.

Perceptions—Viewpoints.

Personal qualities—Set of characteristics that make an individual unique; see *personality*.

Personality—Set of uniquely individual qualities and characteristics.

Personality conflict—Discord arising from differences in personal approaches or makeups.

Prebargaining—Promising to do or be something in return for a positive medical outcome; negotiating or bartering using medical state or health; form of *superstitious thinking*.

Prejudice—Irrational leaning toward a particular viewpoint.

Process—Comprehend or understand (v); step-wise cycle with a defined beginning and end (n).

Psychosocial—Psychological and social aspects; social conditions related to mental health.

Rapport—Harmony.

Referral—Medical-process tool designed to transfer patients between providers.

Reflective listening—Receiving and comprehending information communicated by another by repeating information that is heard.

Relief—State following removal of a negative entity.

Religion—Belief in, and worship of, a god or gods.

Resistance—Opposition; motivation against.

Resources—Entities that provide support or information.

Role—Set of prescribed actions, behaviors, and responsibilities (e.g., parent or teacher).

Role model—Person viewed as a standard to which to aspire.

Sadness—*Depression* or *despair*; unhappiness.

Selective listening—Choosing to hear only that which is desired or preferable.

Self-care—Set of routine, daily activities (see *activities of daily living*).

Self-destructive behavior—Action harmful to oneself.

Self-efficacy—Ability to treat or support oneself.

Self-esteem—Respect for and/or confidence in oneself.

Self-image—Personal concept of oneself.

Self-talk—Inner thoughts or perceptions that positively or negatively impact events, actions, and attitudes.

Shame—Knowing state of guilt or responsibility.

Shock—State of disbelief.

Shorthand—Abbreviated version of written messages.

Social work department—Group in health-care organization dedicated to social welfare and societal change.

Socioeconomic status—Combination of social and economic factors that determines level at which one functions in society.

Spiritual community—Formal or informal organization of individuals with like viewpoints of *religion* or a *Higher Power*.

Spiritual connection—Bond predicated on shared views of *religion* or a *Higher Power*.

Spiritual counselor—Individual responsible for directing and coaching pursuits related to *religion* or a *Higher Power*.

Spiritual direction—Path (see *spiritual path*) or goals related to *religion* or a *Higher Power*.

Spiritual issues—Topics related to *religion* or a *Higher Power*.

Spiritual path—Direction (see *spiritual direction*) or goals related to *religion* or a *Higher Power*.

Spiritual practices—Activities and behaviors related to *religion* or a *Higher Power*.

Spirituality—Set of beliefs related to *religion* or a *Higher Power*.

Stress—Influence or force with negative or deleterious effects.

Subconscious—In an unaware state; below a knowing or conscious level.

Superstitious thinking—Believing that kindness or goodness will prevent negative events and ensure positive ones.

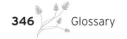

Support—Assistance or aid.

Suppress—Hide or withhold.

Suppressed feelings—Emotions denied expression.

Teamwork—Collaboration of multiple people toward a shared goal.

Tentative—Uncertain.

Terminal—Related to an ending point or a boundary; see *end of life*.

Trust—Faith in another.

Uncertainty—Indefinite or unreliable.

Unconscious—Unable to process information; state of unawareness.

Unemotional—Lacking feeling.

Urgency—Pressing or insistent quality.

Ventilate—Express or communicate animatedly.

Ventilation—Enthusiastically express feelings and emotions.

Vision for the future—Picture of what is to come.

Wishful thinking—Thought pattern characterized by desired outcomes that are not necessarily possible.

Withdraw—Pull back from.

Worship—Perform or take part in activities related to *religion* or a *Higher Power*.

Yoga—Bodily or mental exercises designed to achieve control and/or a state of well-being.

Emotions

www.nimh.nih.gov

www.helpguide.org

www.coping.org

www.mentalhealth.com

www.JustGotDiagnosed.com

Information-Gathering/Decision Making

www.WebMD.com

www.healthline.com

www.MayoClinic.com

www.medlineplus.gov

www.healthwise.com

www.familydoctor.org

www.medline.com

www.myphr.com (creating an online personal health record)

Support

www.alliancehealth.com (social networking for patients)

www.dailystrength.org

www.nurse.com/resources

www.cmrg.com (comprehensive list of resources)

www.longtermcarelink.net

Caregiving

www.caregiversupportnetwork.org

www.usa.gov/Citizen/Topics/Health/caregivers.shtml

www.caregiverresource.net

www.caregiverslibrary.org

www.thefamilycaregiver.org

Spirituality

www.spiritualityandhealth.com

www.spiritualityandpractice.com

End of Life

www.widownet.org

www.hospicenet.org

www.noahschildren.org

www.growthhouse.org

Self-Care for Health-Care Professionals

www.nursesselfcare.com

www.nursingadvocacy.org

http://topics.nurse.com/well+nurse

Chapter 3

Gary, R.; Dunbar, S.; Higgins, M.; Musselman, D.; Smith, A. Combined exercise and cognitive behavioral therapy improves outcomes in patients with heart failure. *Journal of Psychosomatic Research*, 2010, 69(2), 119–31.

Van Bastelaar, K.; Pouser, F.; Geelhoed-Duijvestijin, P.; Tack, C.; Bazelmans, E.; Beekman, A.; Heine, R.; Snoek, F. *Diabetic Medicine*, 2010, 27(7), 798–803.

Vannoy, S.; Fancher, T.; Malvedt, C.; Unutzer, J.; Duberstein, P.; Kravitz, R. Suicide inquiry in primary care: Creating context, inquiring, and following up. *Annals of Family Medicine*, 2010, 8(1), 33–39.

Chapter 4

Dalgas, U.; Stenager, E.; Jakobsen, J.; Petersen, T.; Hansen, H.; Knudsen, C.; Overgaard, K.; Ingemann-Hansen, T. Fatigue, mood, and quality of life improve in MS patients after progressive resistance training. *Multiple Sclerosis*, 2010, 16(4), 480–90.

Dane, B. Thai women: Meditation as a way to cope with AIDS. *Journal of Religion & Health*, 2000, 39(1), 5–21.

Derelli, E., and Yaliman, A. Comparison of the effects of a physiotherapist-supervised exercise programme and a self-supervised exercise programme on quality of life in patients with Parkinson's disease. *Clinical Rehabilitation*, 2010, 24(1), 352–62.

Editorial Board. Pain, anxiety, and depression: Why these conditions often occur together and how to treat them when they do. Editorial board of *Harvard Mental Health Letter*, 2010, May 26(11), 1–3.

Johnson, M.; Dose, A.; Pipe, T.; Petersen, W.; Huschka, M.; Gallenberg, M.; Peethambaram, P.; Sloan, J.; Frost, M. Centering prayer for women receiving chemotherapy for recurrent ovarian cancer: A pilot study. *Oncology Nursing Forum*, 2009, 36(4), 421–28.

Kabat-Zinn, J. *Coming to Our Senses: Healing Ourselves and the World through Mindfulness.* Hyperion, 2006.

Kabat-Zinn, J. *Full Catastrophe Living: Using the Wisdom of Your Body and Mind to Face Stress, Pain, and Illness.* Delta, 1990.

Lykins, E., and Baer, R. Psychological functioning in a sample of long-term practitioners of mindfulness meditation. *Journal of Cognitive Psychotherapy*, 2009, 23(3), 226–41.

Chapter 5

Holme, A. Exploring the role of patients in promoting safety: Policy to practice. *British Journal of Nursing*, 2009, 18(22), 1392–95.

Lantz, P.; Janz, N.; Fagerlin, A.; Schwartz, K.; Ligua, L.; Lakhani, I.; Salem, B.; Katz, S. Satisfaction with surgery outcomes and the decision process in a population-based sample of women with breast cancer. *Health Services Research*, 2005, 40(3), 745–68.

Pellat, G. Patient-professional partnership in spinal cord injury rehabilitation. *British Journal of Nursing*, 2004, 13(6), 948–53.

Chapter 6

Borg, J. *Body Language: 7 Easy Lessons to Master the Silent Language.* Prentice Hall, 2008.

Engleberg, I. *Working in Groups: Communication Principles and Strategies.* My Communication Kit Series, 2006.

Chapter 7

O'Connor, A.; Drake, E.; Wells, G.; Tugwell, P.; Laupacis, A.; Elmslie, T. A survey of the decision-making needs of Canadians faced with complex health decisions. *Health Expectations*, 2003, 6(2), 97–109.

Pew Internet and American Life Project. Health Information Online, 2005, www.pewinternet.org.

Chapter 9

Coskun, A. An investigation of anger and anger expression in terms of coping with stress and interpersonal problem solving. *Educational Sciences: Theory and Practice*, 2010, 10(1), 25–43.

McKay, M., and Fanning, P. *Self-Esteem: A Proven Program of Cognitive Techniques for Accessing, Improving, and Maintaining Your Self-Esteem.* New Harbinger, 2000.

Chapter 10

Bundy, C. When communication has gone wrong between a doctor and a patient. *Diabetic Medicine*, 2001, 18, 6–7.

Coppola, F., and Spector, D. Natural stress relief meditation as a tool for reducing anxiety and increasing self-actualization. *Social Behavior & Personality: An International Journal*, 2009, 37(3), 307–311.

Foley, E.; Baillie, A.; Huxter, M.; Price, M.; Sinclair, E. Mindfulness-based cognitive therapy for individuals whose lives have been affected by cancer: A randomized controlled trial. *Journal of Consulting and Clinical Psychology*, 2010, 78(1), 72–79.

Hack, T.; Degner, L.; Parker, P. The communication goals and needs of cancer patients: A review. *Psycho-Oncology*, 2005, 14(10), 831–45.

Kabat-Zinn, J. *Coming to Our Senses: Healing Ourselves and the World through Mindfulness.* Hyperion, 2006.

Kabat-Zinn, J. *Full Catastrophe Living: Using the Wisdom of Your Body and Mind to Face Stress, Pain, and Illness.* Delta, 1990.

Kennedy, L. Communication in oncology care: The effectiveness of skills training workshops for healthcare providers. *Clinical Journal of Oncology Nursing*, 2005, 9(3), 305–12.

Richards, H.; Fortune, D.; Griffiths, C. Adherence to treatment in patients with psoriasis. *Journal of the European Academy of Dermatology & Venereology*, 2008, 20(4), 370–79.

Sears, S., and Kraus, S. I think therefore I om: Cognitive distortions and coping style as mediators for the effects of mindfulness meditation on anxiety, positive and negative affect, and hope. *Journal of Clinical Psychology*, 2009, 65(6), 561–73.

Sherr, L.; Lampe, F.; Norwood, S.; Date, H.; Harding, R.; Johnson, M.; Edwards, S.; Fisher, M.; Arthur, G.; Zetler, S.; Anderson, J. Adherence to antiretroviral treatment in patients with HIV in the UK: A study of complexity. *AIDS Care*, 2008, 20(4), 442–48.

Chapter 13

Kubler-Ross, E. *On Death and Dying.* Scribner, 1997.

thinking, superstitious, 89
upsides to, 80
"What if . . . ?" questions, 70, 86–87
feelings. *See also* anger; fight reaction; flight reaction;
 freeze reaction; sadness
 normalizing, 59
 paraphrasing patient's statements, 59
 sadness, 59
 shock, initial, of hearing diagnosis, 11, 21–23, 25
 suppression of feelings, 52–53, 62
 venting, 58
fight reaction
 cognition of patient, 98, 102
 defined, 22
 described, 25–26, 53
 empowerment, 22
 family members, 264
 information-gathering, 157, 162, 163
 misuses of empowerment, 272
 motivated by fear, 80
 patients, communicating with, 34–37
 shock, initial, of diagnosis, 23–24
finances, 72–73, 189–90
flight reaction
 abandonment issues, 272
 cognition of patient, 98
 family members, 264
 fear, 52
 overcoming barriers to information, 163–64
 patients, communicating with, 27–29
 sadness, 48
 selective information-gathering, 157
 shock, initial, of diagnosis, 23, 25–26
 working with patient in, 27–28
freeze reaction
 caregivers' interventions, 174
 cognition of patient, 98
 coping styles, 25
 defined, 22
 described, 24–25, 58–59
 family members, 264
 hopelessness/helplessness, 25, 30
 initial reaction, 23–24
 need for family support, 272–73
 panic, 24
 paraphrasing patient's statements, 27–28, 31
 patients, communicating with, 29–33
 reflecting feelings, 24, 28, 59
 selective information-gathering, 157
 self-protection, 52

shock, initial, of diagnosis, 30
suppression of feelings, 52–53, 62
working with patient in, 29, 30–31
Freud, Sigmund, 5
frustration, 51
future
 concerns about, 6–7
 diagnosis and thoughts of, 7
 hopes, dreams, and assumptions, 292–93
 practical questions, 293–94
 vision for, 292–93, 298, 303, 304

G
gender issues, 162, 169
goals of treatment, 116–17
grieving
 healthy process, 55–57
 On Death and Dying (Kübler-Ross), 314–15
 patient facing terminal diagnosis, 317
 sadness, 56
 self-help groups, 320
guidelines for health-care professionals
 communication, enhancing, 148–50
 compassion fatigue, 336
 diagnosis, discussing, 14–15
 end-of-life issues, 322–24
 ethical, 236
 future, discussing, 302–4
 information-gathering, 174, 176
 self-image, good, encouraging, 226–28
 support discussions, 204–5
 treatment decision, 116–18

H
health and wellness, promoting, 168
Health Insurance Portability and Accountability Act
 (HIPAA), 132, 279, 314, 334
health-care professionals. *See also* boundaries,
 professional
 body language, 135–36
 boundaries and compassionate care, 313
 clerypeople, as advisors, 334
 end-of-life beliefs, 313
 hopelessness/helplessness, 69, 113
 professional-patient interactions, 323, 333
 relationship parameters, 127
 responsibility to patient, 279
 self-care, 331–34, 335, 336
 self-talk, 334
 terminal diagnosis, concerns about, 313, 314